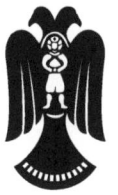

PUBLIC HEALTH
IN QAJAR IRAN

Willem Floor

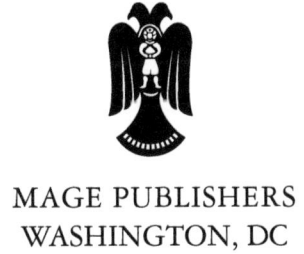

MAGE PUBLISHERS
WASHINGTON, DC

COPYRIGHT ©2004 WILLEM FLOOR

ALL RIGHTS RESERVED. NO PART OF THIS BOOK MAY BE REPRODUCED
OR RETRANSMITTED, EXCEPT IN THE FORM OF A REVIEW,
WITHOUT WRITTEN PERMISSION FROM THE PUBLISHER.

IMAGE OF ENVELOPE ON BACK COVER COURTESY OF HEINZ-JOSEPH VERGOSSEN

LIBRARY OF CONGRESS CATALOGING-IN-PUBLICATION DATA

FLOOR, WILLEM M.
PUBLIC HEALTH IN QAJAR IRAN / WILLEM FLOOR.
P. ; CM.
INCLUDES BIBLIOGRAPHICAL REFERENCES AND INDEX.
ISBN 0-934211-08-6 (PBK. : ALK. PAPER)
1. PUBLIC HEALTH--IRAN--HISTORY--19TH CENTURY.
2. PUBLIC HEALTH--IRAN--HISTORY--20TH CENTURY.
3. MEDICINE--IRAN--HISTORY--19TH CENTURY.
4. MEDICINE--IRAN--HISTORY--20TH CENTURY.
[DNLM: 1. PUBLIC HEALTH--HISTORY--IRAN.
2. HISTORY OF MEDICINE, 19TH CENT.--IRAN.
3. HISTORY OF MEDICINE, 20TH CENT.--IRAN.
WA 11 J17 P631 2004] I. TITLE.
RA533.F565 2004
362.1'0955'09034--DC22
2004008515

ISBN 0-934211-08-6

MAGE BOOKS ARE AVAILABLE AT BOOKSTORES
AND DIRECTLY FROM THE PUBLISHER.
VISIT MAGE ON THE WEB AT
WWW.MAGE.COM
OR CALL 800 962 0922 OR 202 342 1642
TO ORDER BOOKS OR TO RECEIVE OUR CURRENT CATALOG

CONTENTS

PREFACE: 7

CHAPTER ONE
Introduction: 11

CHAPTER TWO
Main Diseases: 13

CHAPTER THREE
Public Hygiene: 59

CHAPTER FOUR
Medical Knowledge: 68

CHAPTER FIVE
Medical Institutional Infrastructure: 77
Spiritual Healers: 80
Islamic-Galenic Physicians: 100
Traditional Healers: 141

CHAPTER SIX
The Progress of Modern Medicine: 168

CONCLUSION: 232

APPENDIX ONE
Mansur Sheybani's Eyes—A Case Study of Sorts: 236

APPENDIX TWO
Published and Manuscript Medical Works: 240

APPENDIX THREE
Decisions of the Sanitary Council of Khorasan: 244

BIBLIOGRAPHY: 246

INDEX: 264

PREFACE

While there are quite a few books published in Persian dealing with traditional medicine, herbs and drugs, there are as yet no books and only a few articles that deal with the actual practice of medicine in Qajar Persia. Even Elgood's *Medical History of Persia*, which describes the history of the Persian medical system, does not discuss the situation in the Qajar period in great detail. Most available modern studies usually deal with one medical aspect only (*e.g.*, drugs, a particular disease or class of diseases, medicinal plants). No study as yet has analyzed the available material to create a more or less comprehensive overview of the state of public health, medical practice and its practitioners not from a theoretical and normative point of view, but from a real and actual one.

This study provides the reader with an overview of what major diseases the population suffered from and how these were treated. Also, it provides an assessment of the extent to which the nature of public hygiene in Persia contributed or not to the public health of the nation. Moreover, I discuss what medical theories prevailed as to the understanding of the cause as well as the cure of diseases and disorders. This I further highlight by a discussion of the various medical practitioners and the variety and range of their actual interventions. Finally, I detail the impact that Western medicine made on traditional medical practice and institutions of Qajar Persia. In short, this study focuses on public health rather than on technical medical issues.

The data are mainly drawn from European observers who have reported on actual medical practice, prevalence and treatment of disease in Qajar Persia. Most of these observers had practiced medicine in Persia, often for as many as 20 years, and quite a few of them took the trouble to learn what Persian healers had to offer. These medical observers ranged from doctors in the service of the Indo-European Telegraph Department (Wills), in government service (Feuvrier, Häntzsche, Polak, Saad, Schlimmer, Tholozan), in diplomatic service (Baker, Bélanger, Clarke, Coville, Jukes, Neligan, Gilmour), in private practice (Collins) to those working as missionary doctors (Carr, Cochran, Dodson, Hume-Griffith, Lichtwardt, Sargis, Wishard). Among the latter group there also was a small number of female physicians such as Uriana Latham-Malcolm, Rosalie Morton, Elizabeth Ross, and Emmeline Stuart. Finally, there were keen, non-medical European observers (*e.g.*, John Malcolm, Fowler, Höltzer, Landor, Rice and the Sykes siblings), who were interested in the subject matter and made many useful observations or recorded those made by physicians who did not write books and articles, or were 'forced' by circumstances to operate as a rural doctor, such as Forbes-Leith and Mary Bird. To counter-balance the accusation that I am pursuing a possibly Euro-centric approach to the analysis of the medical sector in Qajar Persia, I have also used the observations made by Persian patients in their Memoirs or Travelogues on their own or other people's diseases and treatment (Basir al-Molk, E'temad al-Saltaneh, E'tesam al-Molk, `Eyn al-Saltaneh, Pirzadeh) as well as other contemporary Persian texts that comment on the public health situation of Persia rather than normative theoretical Persian medical texts.

The reason for this choice is that studies on medieval Islamic medicine have shown that "the medical knowledge and the therapeutic advice so meticulously described in theoretical works were not paralleled in the physician's medical performance. On the contrary, it appears that learned tradition served other purposes than determining medical practice."[1] It is my suspicion that the same holds for the texts written by physicians in Qajar Persia. For example, one of the Persian medical treatises written in the mid-nineteenth century states that sulfurous springs are directly communicating with hell and therefore should be avoided, "for not only did they have no healing effect, but they were positively harmful to the body."[2] In actual practice, these springs, as is shown in what follows, were much frequented by multitudes of Persians who suffered from a range of diseases. In fact, Reitlinger's Persian driver was appalled that he bathed in such a sulfurous spring, "where all the diseased people in Gilan went to be cured."[3] Relying on Persian medical texts like these for reliable information on actual medical practice in Qajar Persia would therefore be a hazardous undertaking. For, like their medieval forerunners, these authors also had a particular ideological agenda for writing their treatises.

Finally, the study makes the point that Islamic-Galenic medicine only played a marginal role in Qajar Persia as far as medical service was concerned. Although it had greatly influenced how Persians perceived illness, the number of its practitioners, however, was limited and their services were neither affordable by nor accessible to the majority of the population. Therefore, pre-Islamic theurgic folk medicine, based on traditional herb lore and trial-and-error practice, imbued with the Galenic hot-cold dichotomy, was the mainstay of the medical service provided to the majority of the population. Once it had been introduced, Western medicine became even more important than Islamic-Galenic medicine, overtaking it altogether after 1940. Despite weak opposition from some traditional Islamic-Galenic medical practitioners, Western medicine was persistently pursued by the reforming political elite and actively adopted by the new generation of formally trained physicians. It probably provided effective treatment to a larger number of people than practitioners of Islamic medicine reached by the end of the Qajar period, and, more importantly, through its advocacy for public health measures (vaccination, quarantine, public and personal hygiene) Western medicine had a significant impact in bringing about a reduction of outbreaks of deadly epidemics as well as in controlling their impact.

The reason for writing this book was to reduce my ignorance about the practice of medicine in Persia about which I did not know anything. The available literature left me

---

[1] Álvarez-Millàn, Christina. "Practice versus Theory: Tenth-century Case Histories from the Islamic Middle East," *Social History of Medicine* 13/2 (2000), p. 293; see for similar remarks with regards to the practice, or rather the absence, of surgery Savage-Smith, Emilie. "The Practice of Surgery in Islamic Lands: Myth and Reality," *Social History of Medicine* 13/2 (2000), pp. 307-21.
[2] Ebrahimnejad, Hormoz. "Religion and Medicine in Iran: from Relationship to Dissocation," *History of Science* 40 (2002), p. 94 (quoting from the *Resaleh-ye Dallakiyeh*, a manuscript extant in St. Petersburg). Although this text reflects folk medicine rather than Galenic medicine it reinforces my argument, *i.e.*, that there is a divorce between what people should do, according to theoretical lore, and what they actually do. Nevertheless, these texts offer an insight into the Persian doctors' attitude towards medicial theory, practice, and change.
[3] Reitlinger, Gerald. *A Tower of Skulls, a journey through Persian and Turkish Armenia* (London: Duckworth, 1932), p. 168.

with more questions than answers, and as a result I found myself hitting the books in search of the missing information. Because the subject of public health was unknown territory to me I have asked some knowledgeable people for comments on the final draft of this study. Jan Meulenbeld, Hormuz Ebrahim-Nejad, and Andrew Newmann have been so generous to read the entire text. Marianne Floor was so kind to read the text so as to spot any errors that I might have made in the field of medical science. Although I have benefited from their comments, I have not always entirely adopted them. Herewith, I want to thank them for having taken the time to engage me in a discussion that has improved my understanding, if not my analysis, of the development and dynamics of public health in Qajar Persia, which I submit here to the interested reader.

Finally I want to thank John Emerson (Widener Library, Harvard University) for his enormous help in getting hold of rare books and articles. Likewise I want to thank Irene Schneider and Doris Mir-Ghaffari (Halle University, Germany) for finding a few rare German publications as well as for the help in finding the meaning of some "schwere Wörter."

INTRODUCTION

POPULATION SIZE

Qajar Persia was an agrarian subsistence economy with a total population of about 5 million in 1800 and of about 9 million in 1900. The majority of the population was rural and engaged in agriculture. The urban population had been reduced to about 7 percent at the beginning of the nineteenth century due to anarchy and warfare during most of the eighteenth century. By 1900, the urban population had more than doubled and represented some 18 percent with three towns having more than 100,000 inhabitants: Tehran with about 280,000, Tabriz with 200,000 and Isfahan with 100,000. Four other towns had each 50,000 inhabitants or more.[1] More than one-third of the population was nomadic around 1860, according to Polak. However, he seems to have included seasonal migrants among his definition of nomads.[2] The percentage of people being engaged in a nomadic lifestyle dropped during the nineteenth century to 20-25 percent. In the beginning of that century, the nomads indeed may have constituted one-third of the population. In 1900, the rural sedentary population of some 5 million lived in more than 30,000 large and small villages, most of which were only accessible via dirt tracks.

THE STATE OF PUBLIC HEALTH

Mortality and morbidity rates for Qajar Persia are not known, due to a lack of any relevant statistics, which were only available for Tehran after 1922, and which are incomplete. Gilbar has estimated a mortality rate at >30 per thousand and a birth rate of 40-50 per thousand, resulting in an average annual population net growth rate of 1% in the second half of the nineteenth century.[3] These figures imply that the rate of infant deaths was higher than 50%, which seems to be borne out by impressionistic data. Merritt-Hawkes, for example, observed: "There is a great deal of illness, most children are born only to die."[4] According to Binder, infant mortality was higher than 50 percent in the village in Kurdistan that he surveyed.[5] According to one physician, who worked in Persia in the 1930s, the mortality rate was even higher, viz. "at the appalling figure of 80 percent."[6]

Data on mortality rates for individual diseases were, of course, not available either. In fact, the prevalence and incidence of what kind of diseases in Qajar Persia was not even precisely known. There was no compulsory notification of cases of infectious diseases,

---

[1] Gilbar, Gad G. "Demographic Developments in Late Qajar Persia 1870-1906," *Asian and African Studies* 11 (1976), pp. 147-49.
[2] Polak, J.E. *Persien, das Land und seine Bewohner*, 2 vols. (Leipzig, 1865), vol. 2, pp. 90, 93.
[3] Gilbar, "Demographic Development," p. 133.
[4] Merritt-Hawkes, O. A. *Persia – Romance & Reality* (London: Nicholson & Watson, 1935), p. 104.
[5] Binder, Henry. *Au Kurdistan* (Paris: Quantin, 1887), pp. 352-53.
[6] Morton, *A Doctor's Holiday*, p. 214; Jackson, Kate. *Around the World to Persia* (New York: printed only for private circulation among friends, 1920), p. 69 (70% infant mortality rate); Rice, Clara. *Persian Women and Their Ways* (London: Seeley, Service & Co, 1923), p. 123 (30-50% infant mortality rate, although she also quotes higher figures); Ibid, *Mary Bird in Persia* (London: CMS, 1916), p. 110 (over 80%).

and there was no qualified personnel to rely upon to do this correctly. Morbidity data might in theory be inferred from the limited data available from Tehran. However, even these data are not reliable either, because the cause of death is often uncertain.

> Death certificates were introduced by the municipality in 1922. Nearly all corpses are taken to the public washers of the death, who are forbidden to deal with bodies unless accompanied by death certificates. These are collected by the washers, but all do not indicate the cause of death. The poor do not seek medical advice when it is clear that there is no hope of recovery. In such cases the medical officer of the district will give a certificate when there is no suspicion of crime, but he may be quite unable to state accurately the cause of death, since the religious law forbids post-mortem examinations. The certificate is therefore in many cases nothing more than a permit to carry out the last rites.[7]

But even when the medical officer assigned a cause of death it might not be accurate and thus still difficult to interpret mortality statistics. According to Neligan, "Persian doctors used the same word *haspeh* (spotted) to signify both typhus fever and typhoid fever. In 1918 the Sanitary Council recommended that two different words should be used: the Arabic words are mothbegeh, typhoid, and mohregheh, typhus."[8]

---

[7] Government of Great Britain, *Geographical Handbook Series - Persia* (n.p., September, 1945), p. 408.
[8] Government of Great Britain, *Geographical Handbook*, pp. 415-16; Neligan, A.R. "Public Health in Persia. 1914-24, Part II" *The Lancet* March 27, 1926, pp. 692-93.

MAIN DISEASES

All the main diseases that occurred in Europe also were met with in Persia. However, according to Baker, "Phthisis, pneumonia, pleurisy and rheumatic affections are rare."[1] This may have been true when Baker wrote these words in 1885, although I doubt it, because his experience was limited to only a part of Persia, and later in the Qajar period these diseases were also found to be rampant.[2] There were nevertheless different patterns of illness among the various groups and/or regions. These different patterns were not only determined by climate, but also by lifestyle, accessibility, and elevation. Landor observed, for example, that the climate of Seistan was very healthy. Therefore, the incidence of certain maladies was much lower or more rare than elsewhere in Persia.[3] The same held, for example, for the nomadic Bakhtiyari tribe. They moved generally at an elevation of 2,000 meters and, therefore, "Ophthalmia, glaucoma, bulging eyeballs, inflamed eyes and eyelids, eczema, rheumatism, dyspepsia, and coughs are the prevailing maladies, and among men, bad headaches, which they describe as periodical and incapacitating, are common."[4] Scrofula (adenitis) or *varam-e ghoded-e lemfatiqiyeh* was a disease widespread in Gilan and Mazandaran, but rare in Tehran, Kerman and Isfahan.[5] Ivanov observed as to the Khorasan peasant population that, "it is remarkable that very few traces of small-pox are seen or cases of sore eyes and signs of venereal disease."[6] Among Armenians, who ate pork, tapeworm occurred, whereas among the Moslem population it did not. These examples demonstrate that it mattered where and how you lived. It would seem, generally speaking, that wealth was not a major factor in the incidence of the major diseases. It must be assumed, however, that because of their better diet the resistance of the moneyed class was better, while they also could afford to flee cholera and plague epidemics because of their wealth. Nevertheless, it was no guarantee and even royalty died of cholera, such as in 1822, when Mohammad `Ali Mirza, governor of Kermanshah and oldest son of Fath `Ali Shah, succumbed to cholera.

For the majority of the population, the same menu of diseases occurred. Forbes-Leith, who had medical training and spent a few years in Latgah (Hamadan district) as estate manager and as a doctor-by-necessity around 1920, observed that, in the rural districts, "disease of all kinds was rife." ... "Typhoid fever, typhus, malaria, and smallpox were

---

[1] Baker, James E. "A few remarks on the most prevalent Diseases and the Climate of the North of Persia," appendix to Herbert, "Report on the present State of Persia and her Mineral Resources," in Government of Great Britain, *Accounts & Papers* 67 (1886), p. 323. Tuberculosis (*sel-e riyeh*) was rare Polak, *Persien*, vol. 2, pp. 291, 325; Schlimmer, Joh. L. *Terminologie Médico-Pharmaceutique: Française - Persane* (Tehran, 1874 [Tehran: Daneshgah, 1970]), pp. 458 (q.v. phthisie pulmonaire), 464 (q.v. pneumonie or *dhat al-rīyeh*), 463 (q.v. pleurésie or *dhat al-janab, sineh-ye pahlu*), 489 (q.v. rhumatisme or *bad-e mofasel, riyeh-e tayyari*).
[2] Morton, *A Doctor's Holiday*, p. 215; Rice, *Persian Women*, pp. 255-56.
[3] Landor, E. Henry. *Across Coveted Lands* 2 vols. (New York: Scribners, 1903), vol. 2, p. 180.
[4] Bird, Isabella (Mrs. Bishop). *Journeys in Persia and Kurdistan*, 2 vols. (London, 1891 [London: Virago Travellers, 1988]), vol. 2, p. 75.
[5] Schlimmer, *Terminologie*, p. 16.
[6] Ivanov, W. "Notes on the Ethnology of Khurasan," *Geographic Journal* (1926), p. 148, note *

amongst the worst evils to be contended with; scabies was an almost general complaint; cases of venereal disease existed in huge numbers, and about eighty percent of the people were suffering from some form of trachoma, a painful affliction of the eyes."[7] This characterization is indeed borne out by the facts, as we know them.

In the first part of this study, I briefly discuss the prevalence and treatment of the following main diseases starting with:

MALARIA
Malaria (*nowbeh, homay-e varami, tebb-e larz*) was the most important endemic disease in Qajar Persia.[8] This debilitating and in many cases mortal disease was present all over the country, and in particular in the subtropical Caspian littoral (Gilan, Mazandaran, Astarabad). In the latter region with its rainy, subtropical climate and vast irrigated rice fields everybody was infected. The prevalence of the disease affected productivity, because people often were unable to work. At times, it even had a negative effect on crop output due to lack of sufficient labor at the critical moments of the agricultural cycle. Although the central plateau was a dry and arid place, malaria also prevailed there. This was due to irrigation practices and water storage methods as well as the fact that swamps were associated with rivers. As a result, there were areas where the incidence of malaria was almost as bad as in the Caspian littoral. Neligan mentioned in particular the fertile districts of Shariyar and Khar near Tehran, where the situation was so bad that the people around 1920 asked the government to do something, because so many people died each year. The result was a lot of advice, not enough quinine, and little result.[9]

Other affected provinces included: Khorasan, Azerbaijan, Kurdistan, Kermanshah, Hamadan, and Khuzistan. In the latter province only the area on both sides of the Karun River was infected, for in the towns of Shushtar, Dezful and Mohammerah (Ahvaz) malaria did not occur much. The Persian Gulf littoral was also heavily infected. There also was some malaria in Isfahan, Yazd, and Kerman, but Seistan and Baluchistan were free from the disease. Malaria was also present in urban areas due to the lack of urban hygiene with the occurrence of open cesspools and cisterns for drinking water. As such, malaria has been called a man-made disease, because human beings created and maintained the conditions for its distribution. In some areas of Persia, the number of

---

[7] Forbes-Leith, A.C. *Checkmate and Fighting* (London, 1927 [New York: Arno, 1973]), p. 88; Rice, *Mary Bird*, p. 110. For a list of the range of diseases seen in 1904 in the American missionary hospital in Urumiyeh see Speer, Robert E. *Hakim Sahib, the foreign doctor; a biography of Joseph Plumb Cochran* (New York: Revell, 1911), p. 328. For those occurring in Shiraz see Sirjani, Sa`idi. *Vaqaye`-ye Ettefaqiyeh. Gozareshha-ye khofyeh-nevisan-e englis* (Tehran: Now, 1361/1982), Index q.v *bimariha*; for those occurring in Ardabil see Safari, *Ardabil*, vol. 3, p. 481-83.
[8] In the seventh century, the Italians named the disease *mal aria*, meaning bad air, because of its association with ill smelling vapors from the swamps near Rome. It was also around this time that the bark from the cinchona tree was used to treat the intermittent fevers associated with this illness. However, it was not until the mid-nineteenth century that quinine was identified as the active alkaloid.
[9] Neligan, "Public Health," part II, pp. 692-93; Häntzsche, J.C., "Physikalisch-medicinische Skizze von Rescht in Persien," *Virchows Archiv* 15 (1862), p. 567.

mosquitoes was so large that they became depopulated. Those visiting the British Residency's dispensary in Bushire for treatment of malaria numbered 5,720 (1918), 4,940 (1919) and 4,892 (1920) or about 25% of the population.[10] Gilmour also confirmed Neligan's findings about the severe nature of the prevalence of malaria around Tehran. In the Karaj area (near Tehran), where Gilmour examined the population in one malaria affected village, he found that women on average had only one living child, the oldest man in the village was 45, and 85% of the children examined had hypertrophy of the spleen. Data collected among the garrison of Tehran in 1923-24, showed that malaria indeed was the disease with the highest incidence and that there was seasonal variation.[11] Among the indigenous population of Tehran itself, malaria seems to have been of a low incidence of not more than 4% in 1929, which seems to be at odds with the earlier data.[12]

Table 1: Total number of sick soldiers in Tehran and those infected with malaria (1923-24)

Month	Total # sick	Malaria cases	Malaria in %% of total
April 1923	885	171	19
May	917	188	20
June	1,037	225	21
July	1,016	295	28
August	1,091	415	37
September	1,272	521	40
October	1,153	409	35
November	890	332	38
December	847	248	28
January 1924	1,072	255	23
February	1,016	209	30
March	855	178	20
April	698	141	20
May	762	182	23
June	1,000	286	28
July	1,014	303	29

Source: Gilmour, *Rapport*, p. 49.

---

[10] Government of Great Britain *Report on the trade of the consular district of Bushire 1920-21*, pp. 1-2; Neligan, "Public Health," part II, pp. 692-93; Polak, *Persien*, vol. 2, pp. 330-343; Stark, Freya. *The Valley of the Assassins* (London, 1934 [New York, 2001]), pp. 183, (Garmrud area), 208 (Shah Rud valley), 213-18 (she suffered from malaria herself and described her treatment). Government of Iran, *Ruznameh-ye Ettefaqiyeh-ye Vaqaye`* 4 vols. (Tehran: Ketabkhaneh- Melli, 1373-74/1994-95), pp. 567, 945, 1275, 1925, 2186.

[11] Gilmour, John. *Rapport sur la situation sanitaire de la Perse* (Geneva, Société des Nations, 1924), pp. 46-49; Schlimmer, *Terminologie*, p. 281 (q.v. fièvre anticipante), 283 (q.v. fièvre intermittante); Southgate, H. *A Tour Through Armenia and Mesopotamia*, 2 vols. (New York: D. Appleton & Co, 1840), vol. 2, p. 66 ("Intermittent fever is very prevalent in Persia"); Baker, James E. "A few remarks," p. 323.

[12] Baladiyeh-ye Tehran. *Dovvomin Salnameh-ye Ehsa'iyeh-ye Shahr-e Tehran* (Tehran, 1310/1931), p. 96. Gilmour, *Rapport*, p. 48 reported a much higher rate of 20%, among those treated at the Tehran dispensary.

All three forms of malaria occurred, but quartan infection was not common. Treatment of the disease was inadequate and ineffective.

> Persian doctors use inadequate doses of quinine, and a patient is rarely treated after the temperature has fallen. The custom of waiting until the temperature drops to normal before giving quinine is widespread, and is disastrous in the case of continuous pernicious forms. Another class of patient from which quinine is withheld is pregnant women. The most and rapidly fatal cases of aneaemia are seen among them. Administration of quinine by injection is far too common, and, unfortunately, the injection is frequently badly made. Patients, however, think that there is a special virtue in the syringe, and *injection* has become a Persian word.[13]

The more traditional methods of treating malaria or the ague, as it was also referred to, were even more inadequate. The first traditional reaction to fever was bleeding, and thus "Bleeding is large resorted to for all complaints, even malaria."[14] John Malcolm, the first British ambassador to the Qajar court, related that the chiefs of a Kurdish tribe, on the border between Persia and Iraq, claimed the power to be able to cure the ague, "descended through many generations, of curing the ague, which is a common complaint in that country, by beating the patient in a very unmerciful manner. Their success in this practice is said to be great."[15] This method was also applied elsewhere in Persia.[16] According to Dr. Lichtwardt,

> a person suffering from malaria will carefully shell eleven almonds and remove the inner skin; these nuts he will take to the mullah who will duly bless them, inscribe a few holy marks on their surface, and the patient faithfully takes three almonds the first day, four on the second and the remaining four on the third, after which (he hopes) his malaria disappears. Should this treatment not be efficacious, this man, with his chills and fever, goes out into the desert at night, and listens to the howling of the jackals which will come quite near to the village in the darkness. The man pulls of his rope-like belt, and at each bark of a jackal he ties one knot in the belt; after seven barks and seven knots, he returns home with a shorter belt, but the assurance that his malaria will have disappeared.[17]

Prayer and magical formulas were, of course, also tried.[18]

---

[13] Neligan, "Public Health," part II, p. 693.
[14] Collins, Edward Treacher. *In the Kingdom of the Shah* (London: T.F.Unwin, 1896), p. 168.
[15] Malcolm, *The History*, vol. 2, p. 536 (in a note, Malcolm recounted his meeting with the chief's son in 1810. The latter had succeeded his deceased father and also had inherited his father's skill. He tied the patient up "by the heels, when the cold fit is on, and bastinado them most severely, scolding them at the same time, so asto produce heat and terror, instead of a cold fit." He always had success with the treatment, he claimed.)
[16] Fowler, *Three Years*, vol. 1, p. 60, reported for other parts of Persia that to cure the ague "they beat the patient most unmercifully, in which treatment they say they generally succeed. I did not submit to this process during the many months of my intermitting visitor."
[17] Lichtwardt, H.A. "Ancient Medicine in Modern Persia," *Annals of the History of Medicine* 7 (1935), pp. 81-81.
[18] Saad, *Sechzehn Jahre*, p. 185 ("Bism allah, al-rahman al-rahim, wa rafa`nahu makana `alay

Ignorance made that individuals did nothing to deny anopheline mosquitoes breeding places in and around their home. The government had neither the means (quinine, medical infrastructure) nor the will to undertake large-scale preventive or curative measures. In fact, the Tehran municipality as part of its own timid effort to improve the public health situation made things even worse, "by constructing a series of small tanks from which the streets are watered, and which serve as additional breeding-places." Neligan introduced the use of goldfish as larvicides, shortly after his arrival in 1906. The practice was adopted by many households in Tehran, but not by all. The measure also had its drawback, because cats liked the fish as much as the fish liked mosquito larvae. Also, when changing the water in the small garden tanks, the fish would often escape. Only the rich used mosquito nets and took quinine whenever they felt they needed it, and not necessarily against malaria. Neligan argued for a strong sanitary organization with police powers to stamp out all breeding places.[19] Oil production had a positive influence on the prevention of malaria. Dr. Ross reported "an interesting medical fact is that the oil which flows into the waters of this region [near Shushtar] prevents malaria by destroying the breeding places of the anopheles."[20]

CHOLERA

Cholera (*vaba*; also *marg-e mowt* and *margamargi*) was not endemic in Persia (it was imported from India and Russia), although it regularly decimated its population, in particular children in their second or the beginning of the third year of their life. Contemporary European authorities distinguished several kinds of cholera, which reflects the imperfect state of knowledge among physicians, whether Western or Galenic, about the cause, spread and treatment of the disease at that time.[21] Apart from the epidemic

---

Sayyid Sultan Hasan, Sayyid Sultan 'Ali ibn Sultan Muhammad. 1128 [year] or In the Name of God the merciful and compassionate, we beseech the lofty assistance of Sayyid Sultan Hasan etc.).

[19] Neligan, "Public Health," part II, pp. 693; Government of Iran, *Ettefaqiyeh-ye Vaqaye`*, vol. 1, pp. 443-54 (cause), 710, 874 (treatment). In 1880, the epidemiologic breakthrough came when Charles Lavern, a French army surgeon, observed and described the exflagellated gametes of malaria parasites in the red blood cells of man. About ten years after this, it was thought that malaria was transmitted by mosquitoes. Sir Ronald Ross then supported this theory when he observed developing plasmodia in the intestine of mosquitoes. By July 1898, malaria transmission through the mosquito was established. At that time, the Italian scientist Giovanni Batista Grassi traced the course of the parasite through the mosquito, and proved that human malarias were transmitted by species of *Anopheles*.

[20] Ross, Elizabeth N. MacBean. *A Lady Doctor in Bakhtiyari Land* (London: Parsons, 1921), pp. 57, 59 (extension of the area under rice cultivation in the Bakhtiyari lands had the opposite effect, of course).

[21] John Snow was the first (1854) to establish the link between germs and the occurrence of cholera. Nevertheless, most Western doctors continued to believe that cholera was caused by bad air or *miasmata* while others favored John Snow's germ theory. Robert Koch is often identified as the first person to identify *Vibrio cholerae* as the causative agent of cholera (1884), however, the honor rightfully goes to Filippo Pacini who first identified the organism in 1854. Dr. Cloquet, the shah's personal physician (1846-55), was a believer in the miasma cause of cholera and even sent some odd products to France of which he believed that these might cure cholera. One was a rubber-like substance called "Ganderoum," and the other a root from Central Asia called "Sambouldebali," that allegedly was used in Russia as a medicine against cholera, see Larbey, H.

deadliest form (cholera morbus or *vaba*), they also distinguished sporadic or autumn cholera (*vaba-ye pa'izi, theql-e sard*), and cholera of nurslings (in Tehran: *tabi`at kardan*; in Hamadan: *kholgh shodan*). Polak even distinguished a cholera ablactatorum, either as a kind of cholera of weaned children or as a sporadic cholera, which he referred to as *heyzeh*. However, as Schlimmer has pointed out, Persian physicians used the term *heyzeh* to refer to diarrhea of surfeit or diarrheic indigestion.[22]

Between 1820 and 1903, seven major cholera epidemics have been identified.

(1) In 1821, the epidemic started in the Persian Gulf, moved to Shiraz and Isfahan, stayed for two years in the center of the country, and then moved northwards via the Caspian littoral to Russia.
(2) In 1829, the second epidemic struck, originating in India it entered Persia via Afghanistan and via the Caspian littoral reached Tiflis in 1830, and via Russia reached Germany, Great Britain, and finally France in 1832.
(3) In 1845-47, the third epidemic occurred. The disease came from India via Afghanistan, reached Mashad and Isfahan and moved to Baghdad, Istanbul, Russia, and Europe. According to Dr. Cloquet, 10% of the population of Tehran, or 12,000 people, died in 1846. In Tabriz, some 120 persons died per day, although he did not state the timeframe for this mortality rate.
(4) In 1851-53, the fourth epidemic occurred and remained active for a number of years; it also broke out in Iraq and Russia. During this epidemic Tehran, according to Dr. Cloquet, lost 15,000 to 16,000 people to the cholera.
(5) In 1868-69, Indian pilgrims took cholera to Mecca, whence it raged from Egypt, Iraq to Persia. The cholera that had ravaged Tabriz in 1866 and since then had been dormant broke out again and swept over northern Persia. It was said to have caused 50 deaths a day in Tehran in June 1869, and in Shiraz a total death toll of 5,000 in July 1869.
(6) In 1889-90, the sixth epidemic happened. Via the Persian Gulf it spread over the entire country and reached Europe in 1892. There were 2,000 deaths at Shushtar alone.
(7) The seventh epidemic struck in 1903, when it was introduced by way of Mecca and Iraq through both the Persian Gulf and western Persia. It then continued onwards towards the east (Khorasan) and the north (Azerbaijan) and thus reached Russia, Austria and Germany in 1905. There are no data available on the total number of people who succumbed to the cholera, but it raged for three months in Tehran, where no less than 70,000 allegedly died. This figure is unlikely, because it would mean that about one-third of the population of Tehran had died. Hajj Sayyah wrote that the figure was 20,000 dead, mostly among the poor and the weak, which seems more likely.

In between and after the occurrence of these major epidemics there frequently occurred localized outbreaks. Usually, cholera was introduced from India via Basra or Baghdad.

"Notice sur le docteur Ernest Cloquet," and Dequevaullier, Dr. "Notice sur le docteur Ernest Cloquet," both in *Notices sur le docteur Ernest Cloquet* (Paris, 1856), pp. 6, 20.
[22] On this issue see the detailed discussion by Ebrahimnejad, Hormoz. "La médecine d'observation en Iran du XIX siècle," *Generus* 55 (1998), pp. 33-57, and Ibid., "Un traité d'épidémologie de la médecine traditionelle persane: *Mofarraq ol-Heyze va'l-Vaba* de Mirza Mohammad-Taqi Shirazi (ca. 1800-1873), *Studia Iranica* 27 (1988) pp. 83-107.

However, as of 1915, cholera was also introduced from Russia though Russian troop movements. In 1917, cholera occurred in Mazandaran and from there spread to Mashad (total deaths 900). In 1918, cholera was again introduced from Russia. The outbreak remained limited to the northern part of the country and it appeared that it was not a major outbreak. In 1923, there was an outbreak of cholera in Baghdad, but quarantine measures prevented its spread into Persia. In Abadan, nevertheless, 911 people died.[23] In addition to improve public and personal hygiene in Persia, which was easier said than done, the only effective method to stop outbreaks of cholera was, of course, to stop it from being introduced into Persia. This required, amongst other things, a strong quarantine service, which only came only into being after 1904, and also preventive measures of the countries where the disease was endemic, such as India and Russia.

However, the required public health measure, as known at the time, was not the response of the Persian medical community or the government for that matter. For cholera fitted nicely in the hot-cold dichotomy of diseases, according to traditional Persian medical lore. "It appears that the natives have imbibed a notion that the disease [cholera] is of a *hot* nature, and must be counteracted by *cold* remedies; it is therefore that they drench those who are taken ill with cold water, and give them of that and of a sort of verjuice to drink; means which, according to our theory, are calculated rather to accelerate death, than to promote recovery. But with all the respect they have in general for European science in medicine, we could not persuade them of the danger of their practice, or induce them to change it."[24] Rich reported the same information, which is not surprising because he and Fraser were together in Shiraz at that time, where, ironically and tragically, Rich succumbed to the cholera. Rich elaborated that "they made him swallow quantities of grape verjuice, called kora soo, mixed with salt, which they said was good to cut the bile

---

[23] Gilmour, *Rapport*, pp. 42-43; Neligan, "Public Health," part II, pp. 691-92 (like Gilmour with a detailed table of cholera outbreaks between 1914 and 1924); Mullen, T. F. "Cholera in Persia," Appendix C to Part I of Government of India, *Administration Report of the Persian Gulf Political Residency and Muscat Political Agency* for the Year 1889-90, pp. 15-18; Seyf, Ahmad. "Iran and Cholera in the Nineteenth Century," *Middle Eastern Studies* 38 (2002), pp. 169-78; Schlimmer, *Terminologie*, pp. 130-35 (q.v. choléra), 282 (q.v. fièvre cholérique); Polak, *Persien*, vol. 2, pp. 314-15, 345; Gilbar, "Demographic Developments," pp. 137-38; Baker, "A few remarks," p. 325; Fowler, *Three Years in Persia* 2 vols. (London: Colburn, 1841), vol. 1, pp. 31-32 (eye-witness account of the 1830 epidemic), 276; Tholozan, J.D. *Prophylaxie du choléra en Orient. L'hygiène et la réforme sanitaire en Perse* (Paris: Masson, 1869); Khan Ali, *Choléra en Perse. Prophylaxie et traitement* (Paris: thesis, 1908); Nateq, Homa. "Ta'thir-e ejtema'i va eqtesadi-ye bimari-ye vaba dar doureh-ye Qajar," *Tarikh* 1/2 (2536/1977), pp. 30-62; Ibid., "Mosibat-e vaba va bala-ye hokumat," (Tehran, 2536/1977); Lorimer, J. G. *Gazetteer of the Persian Gulf* (Calcutta, 1915 [Gregg: Westmead, 1970]), pp. 2517-30; Sayyah, Hajj. *Khaterat-e Hajj Sayyah ya Dowreh-ye Khowf va Vahshat* ed. Hamid Sayyah (Tehran: Ebn Sina, 1347/1968), p. 450; Larbey, "Notice," p. 6; Dequevaullier, "Notice," pp. 16, 19-20; Burrell, R.M. "The 1904 epidemic of cholera in Persia: Some aspects of Qadjar society," *BSOAS* 51 (1988), pp. 258-70; Government of Iran, *Ettefaqiyeh-ye Vaqaye`*, Index q.v. *vaba*; Colvill, W.H. "Sanitary Report on Turkish Arabia," *Transactions of the Bombay Society* 11 (1872), pp. 56-66 (I thank Mr. Farhad Hakimzadeh for bringing this reference to my attention as well as for sending me a copy of it).

[24] Fraser, J.B. *Narrative of a Journey into Khorasan in the Years 1821 & 1822* (London, 1825 [Delhi: Oxford UP, 1984]), pp. 58-59, 62 (some concrete cases of people who were drenched and died), 96 (Bushire).

and strengthen the stomach, and kept sousing him over head and ears in the coldest water they could procure. If a poor man, they tumbled him headlong into the first tank or pool; if a rich one, they cooled the water first with snow. Numbers died under the operation, and a great many more from the effects of it, which, added to those who died from neglect, and those who killed by terror, will reduce the real deaths by cholera considerably."[25]

Fraser and others reported that nevertheless this treatment was applied all over Persia, whether in Bushire or Tabriz. The patient was drenched in cold water, had to swallow verjuice, and ice was applied to the stomach. The idea behind the treatment was that "A chill was thus given which probably aided the disease, the nature of which is to drive the circulation from the surfaces and extremities."[26] Because many people died as the result of this cold treatment, it "occasioned some doubts as to its efficacy, and these remedies were at length prohibited by proclamation."[27]

In addition to the application of cold medicines, other remedies also were tried. Fraser reported that, "At Cauzeroon, they had been firing guns, and making a great noise, to drive away the distemper. The inhabitants had commenced the same at Sheerauz, with a view to prevent its arrival there; but the prince, on hearing the noise, sent to put a stop to it, declaring they were fools to act in such a manner before the enemy had reached them."[28] The reason for the supposed effectiveness of this therapy was the following, as reported by Fraser. "The natives, we heard, with their usual superstitious belief in the powers of the celestial bodies, attributed the ravages of this disease to the influence of the star Canopus, which became visible at this time above the horizon, a little before sunrise."[29] In the same way, Holmes reported that in the 1840s people were engaged in a lot of noise making to chase away an eclipse.[30] The link between these seemingly unrelated events is the belief propagated by some Persian doctors that the cholera outbreak had been caused by a specific constellation of the planets. Other doctors also held the view that the epidemic was the expression of God's will to punish the people for their sins. In

---

[25] Rich, Claude James. *Narrative of a Residence in Koordistan ... and of a visit to Shirauz and Persepolis*. 2 vols. (London: James Duncan, 1836), vol. 2, p. 235; Schlimmer, *Terminologie*, p. 550 (verjuice: *ab-e ghoureh* or *ghoureh-su*).

[26] Fraser, James B. *Travels and Adventures in the Persian Provinces and the Southern Banks of the Caspian Sea* (London: Longman, Rees, Orme, Browne and Greene, 1826), p. 317; Sheil, Lady. *Glimpses of Life and Manners in Persia* (London, 1856 [New York: Arno, 1973]), p. 213.

[27] Fraser, *Narrative*, p. 96.

[28] Fraser, *Narrative*, p. 63.

[29] Fraser, *Narrative*, p. 64 ("this star has very extraordinary powers, good and malignant").

[30] Holmes, W.R. *Sketches on the Shores of the Caspian, Descriptive and Pictorial*. (London: Richard Bentley, 1845), p. 108. When referring to an eclipse, Persians said *Mah gereft* (the Moon has been seized), i.e., by Satan. According to Collins, Henry. W. *From Pigeon Post to Wireless* (London: Hodden and Stoughton, 1925), p. 207, "no eclipse ever takes place without the continuous firing of guns to frighten his Satanic Majesty away, always, presumably, with greater or lesser success, according to the degree and length of the period of obscuration!" See also Chodzko, Alexandre. "Le Ghilan ou Les marais Caspiens," *Nouvelles Annales des Voyages*, N.S. 2 (1850), p. 294. This type of apotropical rite also occurred in other cultures and religions (*e.g.*, Christianity, Bhuddism), see Heiler, *Erscheinungsformen*, pp. 177-78 and Donaldson, *The Wild Rue*, pp. 102-07.

either case, recitation of Koran verses or of the Imams' sayings was prescribed, in addition to the making of much noise.[31]

The cholera in Shiraz in 1821 created a bizarre situation, and, at the same time, shows how desperate people were in the face of this dreaded disease. According to Fraser, although the disease ravaged the town, it had not yet reached the quarters inhabited by the Jews and Armenians, "and as these people are in the habit of drinking strong liquors, many were disposed to attribute their exemption from the disease to this practice, and accordingly got furiously drunk. Several, under the joint operation of the brandy and their fears, ran raving about the streets in paroxysms of terror; while others, rendered bold by their potations, imagined to themselves a tangible foe, and called wildly aloud 'where is this disease, this dreadful malady, let him shew himself, that I may fight and kill him.'"[32] A similar occurrence took place in Urumiyeh in 1905. The Christians in that town had followed the advice of the American missionaries and boiled their water, Moslems did not and had faith in God. When, as a result, 4,000 Moslems died and only five Christians, Moslems "held that Azrael was showing undue partiality to infidels, and many of them even put the Cross over their doors to deceive him!"[33]

Although the application of cold water and ice was still the main treatment around 1850, by the 1880s, according to Bassett, "this treatment is, I think, quite out of use in these times." He believed that this change had been brought about, because people realized there was no hope, and that little could be done.[34] Eastwick, some 20 years earlier, seems to bear out Bassett, because he reported that, when cholera or "*tab-e ghash* or fainting fever" had broken out, "bleeding is the only remedy."[35] People also had resource to drugs, and, in 1886, when cholera had broken out and allegedly 90% of the population was affected there were long queues in front of the druggist shops. In the case of Pirzadeh, a senna leaf purgative (*dava va moshel-e senna*), manna (*shirkhesht*) with watermelon liquid was given. He was kept on this regime for two days after which he slowly recovered. An acquaintance of Pirzadeh who also got cholera was given glasses of a quinine concoction and various unnamed drugs prescribed by the doctors, but he did not get better. Even the pill, made from rats bane (*samm al-far*), that Mirza Kazem Hakim-bashi had given him several times did not help.[36] Schlimmer reported that Persian physicians had no remedy against cholera. He rhetorically asked what good can overdoses of corn poppy, or purgatives with bad castor oil, or rice boiled in water with egg yolk do? He himself claimed some success, as long as there was not as yet diarrhea,

---

[31] Ebrahimnejad, Hormoz. "Theory and Practice in Nineteenth-Century Persian Medicine: Intellectual and Institutional Reforms," *History of Science* 38 (2000), p. 175.

[32] Fraser, *Narrative*, pp. 84, 96.

[33] Wigram, W.A. and Wigram, T.A. *The Cradle of Mankind. Life in Eastern Kurdistan* (London: A&C Black, 1936), p. 207.

[34] Basset, James. *Persia, the Land of the Imams* (New York: Charles Scribner's Sons, 1886), pp. 34-35.

[35] Eastwick, Edward B. *Journal of a Diplomate's Three Years' Residence in Persia*. 2 vols. (London, 1864 [Tehran: Imp. Org. f. Soc. Services, 1976]), vol. 1, p. 188.

[36] Pirzadeh, *Safarnameh-ye Hajji Mohammad `Ali Pirzadeh*. 2 vols. Hafez Farmanfarmayan (Tehran: Daneshgah, 1343/1964), vol. 1, pp. 40-42. In case of cholera a wine enema (*emaleh-ye sharab*) was a popular remedy. Polak, *Persien*, vol. 2, p. 218.

with a concoction of his own. Schlimmer also described the unclear result with the use of creosote, and had to admit that more often than not he was usually called too late and just in time to assist at the funeral.[37] Those who could afford to would just flee from the town and village where they were; those that stayed had resource to constant chanting praying and reading from the Qoran.[38]

PLAGUE

According to Tholozan, Naser al-Din personal physician and head of the national Sanitary Council, who had made a special study of the occurrence of this disease in Persia, the plague (ta'un) never acquired endemic proportions in Qajar Persia. He only classified the outbreak of 1829-1833 as an epidemic. Its occurrence remained limited to the Caspian littoral and the province of Khorasan. The second time that the plague occurred in the nineteenth century was in 1871, although it remained mainly restricted to Kurdistan.[39] In 1877, it once again struck the Caspian littoral and Khorasan. There also were some epidemics of local importance, the most important one occurred in 1906 in Seistan. It remained limited to the semi-nomadic population that lived around Lake Seistan, and probably had been imported by goods (old clothing) imported from India.

In Bushire the plague had been unknown until 1910. In April of that year, however, Bushire was struck by the plague, followed by a more severe outbreak in the spring of 1911. This led to flight of people, which had a downward effect on trade. In 1910, 66 people died of the plague and 98 in 1911. The total number of other deaths was 637 in 1910-11 as against 965 in 1909-10, of which almost 25% were children.[40] The plague appeared again in February 1912 and led to large-scale flight of the population. The authorities urged the inhabitants to inoculate themselves and 4,000 vaccinations took place, which was mostly very effective for that group, according to the British consul. The epidemic lasted till June, and the number of deaths was 725 or 75% of the 965 reported cases. This represented 3% of the island's population and this mortality rate brought business to a standstill and over 8,000 people left the island between February-June. From April to May the bazaars were closed, and only life necessities were sold. Manual labor was unavailable and ships could hardly be unloaded. The plague also

---

[37] Schlimmer, *Terminologie*, pp. 134-35.
[38] Rich, *Narrative*, vol. 2, pp. 232-33 (for a graphic description of the panicky flight of the governor and the elite from Shiraz); Taj al-Saltaneh. *Crowning Anguish. Memoirs of a Persian princess from the Harem to Modernity*. Tr. Anna Vanzan and Amin Neshati (Washington, DC: Mage, 1993), p. 280.
[39] Tholozan, J. D. *Histoire de la peste bubonique, 1er Mémoire- en Perse* (Paris: G. Masson, 1874); Ibid., *Note sur le développement de la peste bubonique dans le Kurdistan en 1871* (Paris, 1871); Ibid., *Sur deux petits épidémies de peste dans le Khorassan* (Paris: Gauthiers-Villars, n.d.); Polak, *Persien*, vol. 2, p. 346. See also Alamol-Mulk, Mirza Abbas Khan. *Taoun, Étude sur la peste en Perse* (Paris: thesis, 1908); Nazare-Aga (Ardachir Khan), *Contribution à l'étude de la peste* (Paris: thesis, 1903); "Die Pest in Persien," *Das Ausland* 4 (1831), pp. 959-60; Mahé, "Épidemies de la peste," *Gazette médical d'Orient* 1887; Government of Iran, *Vaqaye'-ye Ettefaqiyeh*, vol. 1, pp. 94, 235; vol. 2, p. 914; Colvill, "Sanitary Report," pp. 43-56. See also Reza Ostadi ed. "Marg va Mirgozaresh-e Ta'un dar Sal-e 1246 Karbala," in *Mirath-e Eslami-ye Iran*, vol. 3, pp. 439-844.
[40] Government of Great Britain, *Trade Report 1910-11*, p. 6. There had been a minor, short-lived outbreak of plague in Bushire in 1899 with two deaths, see Lorimer, *Gazetteer*, pp. 2538, 2548.

penetrated to villages 30 miles inland.[41] The plague reappeared in April 1913, but in a mild form only, and there were only 30 cases of which 25 died.[42] Bushire would remain free from the plague till 1924, when the disease struck once again.

Table 2: The incidence of mortality in Bushire during 1910-1917

Year	Plague	Other causes	Total deaths
1909-10	66	965	1031
1910-11	98	637	735
1911-12	729	599	1328
1912-13	678	518	1196
1913-14	25	525	550
1914-15	-	436	436
1915-16	-	571	571
1916-17	-	1149	1149

Source: Government of Great Britain, *Trade Report 1913-14*, p. 7 (262 of the deaths were children); Ibid., *Trade Report 1914-15*, p. 4; Ibid., *Trade Report 1915-16*, p. 5. The higher figure of deaths for 1916-17 is due to the heat that prevailed and the 5,000 temporary workers (poor peasants) that migrated to Bushire for the unloading of ships at Basrah. Ibid., *Trade Report 1916-17*, p. 5.

However, there occurred several localized outbreaks of the plague elsewhere in the Persian Gulf littoral:

Table 3: Occurrence of localized outbreaks of the plague during 1917-1924

Location	Year	Cases	Deaths
Mohammarah	1917	-	-
Mohammarah	1923	79	43
Abadan	1923	481	409
Mohammarah	1924	-	-
Bushire	1924	-	-
Bandar `Abbas	1924	-	-
Abadan	1924	-	-

Source: Gilmour, *Rapport*, p. 40; Neligan, "Public Health," part II, p. 691.

As is clear from Table 3, all cases of the plague occurred in the Persian Gulf littoral in the first quarter of the twentieth century. Most likely, the disease was inadvertently imported from India.[43] One of the reasons that the plague was not endemic was that, apart from the

---

[41] Government of Great Britain *Trade Report 1911-12*, p. 6. Waters, Lieut. Col. Geo. *Travel Reminiscences* (n.p., n.d.), p. 25, reports that "he was one of the five out of the hundred plague suffered as recovered." This occurred around 1870, and it may have been due to the fact that he was shipped out from plague-stricken Masqat to plague-free Bushire.

[42] Government of Great Britain, *Trade Report 1912-13*, p. 12.

[43] Gilmour, *Rapport*, p. 40; Polak, *Persien*, vol. 2, p. 346; Schlimmer, *Terminologie*, pp. 433-55 (q.v. peste) for a detailed account of the 1871 plague; Gilbar, "Demographic Developments," p. 139; Baker, "A few remarks," p. 325; Neligan, "Public Health," part II, pp. 690-91 (like Gilmour with a detailed list of local outbreaks of the plague between 1914-24); Lorimer, *Gazetteer*, pp. 2531-44.

Caspian littoral and the southern ports, rats did not occur in Persia, and there were no other non-human carriers.[44]

Because most of the outbreaks of the plague in the twentieth century occurred in the area where the Anglo-Persian Oil Company (APOC) operated, its medical service took effective measures to prevent its future occurrence. The APOC asked its staff to identify the location of dead rats, while it also tried to kill as many rats as possible. Inoculations were also started in 1924 and 4,553 persons were effected. Houses were fumigated, while public health measures were taken when new cases were signaled (disinfections of clothes, isolation of the person, destruction of the home with indemnity, ban to construct a home on the same site). The APOC further introduced a water-borne system of lavatories, clean piped water, regular inspection of food and milk supplies, and a clean vegetable bazaar. Hygienic staff housing was also supplied.[45]

TYPHUS

Typhus fever was another endemic disease that was national in its reach, although epidemics were rare. Exanthematic typhus (*asba*; *homay-e hesbeh'i*) occurred throughout the country, and although no data are available, it is believed that during the 1917-18 famine this illness contributed much to the high number of deaths.[46] Typhus often assumed epidemic forms during fall and wintertime, especially among children. It was not common among adolescents, but would recur among people at an advanced age. It was considered a second attack of the same illness. The main cause was polluted drinking water. Depending on the benign and the malignant character of the illness it was referred to as *motbeqeh* (febris mucosa) and as *mohreqeh* (febris septica). Persian doctors treated *motbeqeh*, which was translated as typhoid in the twentieth century, with bleeding, light purging, and clysmas. In case of *mohreqeh*, which was translated as typhus in the twentieth century, they considered bleeding dangerous and only prescribed lavements and *Nardostachys grandiflora DC.*, but for internal use only.[47] Paratyphoid fever also was prevalent, but was not a major public health problem. It was believed that this was due to immunity acquired during infancy. This seems unlikely, however, due to the prevalence of the many kinds of Salmonella that may cause the disease.[48]

---

[44] Neligan, "Public Health," part II, p. 691. The plague is caused by *Pasteurella pestis* (*Yersinia pestis*), discovered independently by Shibasaburo Kitasato and Alexandre Yersin in 1894, a bacterium that is transmitted to people by fleas from rats. Therefore, rodent control is important in areas of known infection.

[45] Gilmour, *Rapport*, pp. 40-41; Williamson, *In A Persian Oil Field*, pp.139-44. On vaccinations and inoculations agaist the plague see Sir Philip H. Manson-Bahr, with the editorial assistance of Charles Wilcocks, *Manson's Tropical Diseases* 16th edition (London: Bailliere, Tindall and Cassell, London, 1966), p. 239.

[46] Gilmour, *Rapport*, pp. 43-44.

[47] Gilmour, *Rapport*, p. 46; Schlimmer, *Terminologie*, pp. 197-202 (q.v. dothinnenterie); Polak, *Persien*, vol. 2, pp. 238, 343-45; Ibid., "Medicinische Briefe aus Persien," *Zeitschrift der k.k. Gesellschaft der Aerzte zu Wien* 9 (1859), pp. 138-39; Baker, "A few remarks," p. 324; Neligan, "Public Health," part II, p. 692 (like Gilmour with a detailed table of typhus fever outbreaks between 1914-1924); see also Government of Iran, *Vaqaye`-ye Ettefaqiyeh* (Index q.v. *mohreqeh* and *motbeqeh*).

[48] Neligan, "Public Health," part II, pp. 692; Government of Great Britain, *Geographical*

ANTHRAX

Human cases of benign anthrax (*kefgirek, gondeh tavol*) frequently occurred, primarily among the wealthy class, according to Schlimmer. However, Neligan reported that it generally occurred in the villages. Not much is known about the treatment. Malignant anthrax (*khoraj-e radi*) also occurred, but in small numbers. The animal variety was endemic. One of the main sources of the disease was the custom of killing animals and allows their blood to soak into the soil.[49]

TUBERCULOSIS

Tuberculosis, which Baker said hardly occurred in Persia, and which Schlimmer did not even list in his *Terminologie*, had become quite prevalent by the end of the Qajar regime. According to Dieulafoy, writing two years later than Baker, phthisis was one of the main diseases. It not only prevailed in densely populated Tehran, but also in the villages and among the nomads. In Tehran it was the leading cause of death in the 1920s. Neligan ascribed its spread to bad hygienic housing conditions, the use of wadded quilts, which were shared in an unwashed state, bad health condition of the people, and late diagnosis.[50]

In this connection it is of interest to note that around 1850, some very clever persons among the Jewish population of Baghdad concluded after careful observation that phthisis, which was on the increase among them, was a contagious disease. This was long before in Europe physicians came to the same conclusion in 1882. The entire Jewish community then decided to isolate each infected person. The community leaders told Dr. Coville that since then the illness was on the decrease. Coville reported this in 1872, but he was not convinced that contagion was a factor in the spread of the disease.[51] It would be of interest to know whether the Jews in Kermanshah and Hamadan, who had very close ties with their co-religionists in Baghdad, knew about this and applied the same system.

Handbook, p. 421. It was only in 1850, that typhus and typhoid fevers were accepted to be two different diseases. In 1880, Eberth discovered *B typhosus*, while in 1884 Graffke and Virchow showed that the disease was waterborne and not airborne. Although typhoid vaccines already existed in 1896-97, they were only applied on a large-scale and with great success during the First World War.

[49] Gilmour, *Rapport*, p. 14; Schlimmer, *Terminologie*, p. 43; Polak, *Persien*, vol. 2, pp. 294-95; Jozani, Niloufar. *La Beauté Menacée* (Paris-Tehran: IFRI, 1994), pp. 198-99; Neligan, "Public Health," part II, p. 694.

[50] Dieulafoy, *La Perse*, p. 94; Neligan, "Public Health," part II, pp. 693; Gilmour, *Rapport*, pp. 65-66; Rice, *Persian Women*, p. 256 ("in particular tubercular bone trouble is common."); Linton, J.H. *Persian Sketches* (London: CMS, 1923), p. 107; Wood, *Glimpses*, p. 70; *Turbiyat*, Index q.v. *Sel*.

[51] Colvill, "Sanitary Report," pp. 38-40. It was a centuries-old belief that consumption arose spontaneously in each affected organism. However, it was only in 1882 that Robert Koch discovered a staining technique that enabled him to see *Mycobacterium tuberculosis*, thus proving the theory that a specific microorganism was the cause of the disease, and enabling the development of effective treatment of the disease, which included the isolation of the sick from the general population.

INFLUENZA

Influenza was little known in Persia.[52] At least that is the impression one gets from Gilmour's observation that influenza also struck Persia in 1918, implying that it had not before that time. The disease, Gilmour referred to, was, of course, the worldwide Spanish influenza pandemic, which penetrated the country from three sides (Kermanshah; `Ashqabad, Bushire). It seemed that villagers and pastoralists were more affected than the urban population.[53] Gilmour's assessment is also confirmed by a report from the British consul in Bushire, who reported that in 1918-19, an influenza epidemic had broken out, which was not a disease known before in Fars. It led to great mortality, whole families being wiped out. It was estimated that the Qashqa'i tribal forces collected outside Shiraz lost 30% of their numbers.[54] According to Sykes, 10% of the population of Shiraz succumbed to the illness.[55] Referring to a situation of two decades earlier, Ella Sykes recorded that, "Persians say it is a good thing to get influenza, but that if the complaint attacks the head it turns the hair white, and they also affirm that those who have never been victims to *mesh mesh* as they call it, get grey very early in life."[56] This means, if this information is correct, that influenza already occurred in Persia around 1900. Its even earlier occurrence is further suggested by its listing in Schlimmer's 1874 medical lexicon, although this may have been for other purposes, *i.e.*, to make Persian physicians aware of the existence of this disease.[57]

Relapsing fever or recurrent fever was endemic, but due to low population density, posed no major public health problem. Because it occurred mostly among travelers in the northwestern provinces, where it was endemic, it was believed that the *Argus Persicus* insect probably caused it. This insect, the fowl tick, also known as the "blue bug," was found on the Tabriz-Zenjan road, and also occurred in Khorasan (Shahrud, Bestam), where it was known as *shabgaz*, and at Musreh, on the road from Resht to Tehran. According to Baker only non-locals were affected by its bite. Later it was established that the infection was louse borne and that the insect transmitted certain forms of relapsing fever. However, no link could be established between the Miyaneh bug and relapsing fever. There was a serious outbreak of relapsing fever in 1924 in Tehran and in several districts of Khorasan.[58]

---

[52] Elgood, Cyril. *Medical History of Persia, and the eastern caliphate* (Cambridge: CUP, 1951), p. 466 mentions a possible influenza epidemic in Tehran in 1833.

[53] Gilmour, *Rapport*, p. 45; Sykes, P.M. *The History of Persia* 2 vols. (London: Routledge-Kegan Paul, 1969), vol. 2, p. 515; Ghani, Qasem. "Tavallod va Kudaki," in *Yaddashtha-ye Doktor Qasem Ghani* 9 vols. ed. Sirus Ghani (Tehran: Zavvar, 1367/89), vol. 1, p. 188.

[54] Government of Great Britain, *Trade Report 1918-19*, p. 2.

[55] Gilmour, *Rapport*, p. 45; Sykes, P.M. *The History of Persia* 2 vols. (London: Routledge-Kegan Paul, 1969), vol. 2, p. 515.

[56] Sykes, Ella. *Persia and its People* (London: MacMillan, 1910), p. 339. According to Bird, *Journeys*, vol. 2, p. 74, "for fever they use an infusion of willow bark, which is not efficacious."

[57] Schlimmer, *Terminologie*, p. 306 (q.v. grippe or *nazaleh-ye vaba'i-ye qasabeh al-riyeh*). Schlimmer, indeed, just listed the disease, but neither discussed its diagnostic nor its therapeutic issues. The Persian term for the disease clearly is descriptive and one coined by Schlimmer or one of his colleagues at the *Dar al-Fonun*.

[58] Gilmour, *Rapport*, pp. 44, 52; see for further details Schlimmer, *Terminologie*, pp. 50-51 (q.v. Argus persicus), 283; Baker, "A few remarks," p. 326; Olivier, G.A. *Voyage dans l'Empire*

The traditional Persian treatment for the bite of the *Argus Persicus* bug or other ticks could be rather unsettling. An unspecified bug had bitten the British journalist O'Donovan. This resulted in a swollen skin that became a tumor, and he became ill. People at Shahrud recommended treatment.

> By one I was advised to eat some clay of the place. Another recommended making up a few of the insects themselves in bread and swallowing them; and a third counseled standing on my head frequently and then rolling rapidly on the floor. But the oddest remedy of all was that proposed by a moullah, or priest, who also practiced the healing art. He brought with him a large net like a hammock, in which he proposed to envelop me. My head was allowed to protrude, and I was then to be hung up from the branch of a tree in the garden. When I had swallowed a large quantity of new milk I was to be turned round until the suspending cords were well twisted, and then, being let go, to be allowed to spin rapidly round. This operation was to be repeated indefinitely until sickness was produced, when other measures were to follow. I declined, however, to allow myself to be bagged in the proposed manner, especially as I had previously heard from my friend General Schindler, at Teheran, that he once saw this method of cure tried on an old woman, who, when taken down for supplementary treatment, was found to be dead. The bite of this villainous insect has often proved fatal.[59]

O'Donovan's description of the treatment is quite similar to the regular cure applied at Mashad for having been bitten by the poisonous bug at Deh Mulla. According to Eastwick, this was to "go to a house at Meshed, where bowls of curds are served out to them. After they have drunk the contents, they sit down in a seat suspended from ropes, which are then spun violently round, till it acquires a motion like a top. The effect of this movement acting on the curds is to produce vomiting to such an extent that seasickness is a pleasant pastime in comparison. Of source the patient is so weakened that no more life remains in him, and he faints."[60]

EYE DISEASES
Cataract (*nozul-e ab-e marvarid, abshar-e bozorg* or *tufan*) was most common, "even in comparatively young persons."[61] Ophthalmia also was very common.[62] Keratitis and

---

Othoman, l'Egypte et la Perse. 6 vols. (Paris: Agasse, 1802-07), vol. 5, p. 170; Government of Great Britain, *Geographical Handbook*, p. 416; Neligan, "Public Health," part II, p. 692; O'Donovan, Edmond. *The Merv Oasis*. 2 vols. (London: Smith, Elder & Co, 1882), vol. 1, pp. 327-29, 370, 454. European travelers generally referred to it as the Miyaneh bug and gave it much attention, including in the European scientific literature, see, for example, Heller, Camil. "Anatomie von Argas persicus," *Sltz. Ber. d. Akad. d. Wiss., Math.-Nat. Kl* 30 (1858), pp. 297-326.

[59] O'Donovan, *Merv Oasis*, vol. 1, p. 393-94. For a similar description see Ts., S. "Persidskie Doktora," pp. 168-89 (eating several of the bugs was recommended to prevent the disease).

[60] Eastwick, *Journal*, vol. 2, p. 215 (he recovered and thanked Imam Reza, p.216).

[61] Landor, *Across*, vol. 2, 180; Polak, *Persien*, vol. 2, p. 346 (gray cataract especially occurred among women); Schlimmer, *Terminologie*, p. 115; Stirling, Edward. *The Journals of Edward Stirling in Persia and Afghanistan 1828-1829* ed. Jonathan L. Lee (Naples: Instituto Universitario

bleared eyes (*varam-e qarniyeh*) were universal among the Turkmen because of the creosote produced by the constant fires in their tents.[63] According to Hume-Griffith, glaucoma (*yobusat-e rotubat-e zojajiyeh*; *nozul-e ab-e sabz*) was also referred to in Persian as black cataract.[64] Trachoma (*gusht zadeh*, granulation), spots on the cornea and web in the eye or pannus (*sabal*) and bacterial conjunctivitis was endemic and was spread by human contact and the absence of hygiene. Iritis was often epidemic during the fall.[65] There were "more operations needed for trachoma and inturned eyelashes than for anything else," according to Rice.[66] Dr. Morton argued that, "In the case of women these infections, as well as those of the skin, are aggravated as well as caused by the wearing of the dust-infiltrated veils and *chadars*, and the lending of these to other women. Abscesses and inturned eyelashes are frequent. These, being obvious, caused the afflicted to seek prompt relief."[67]

Trachoma, glaucoma, and cataract were horrible afflictions, due to its widespread occurrence and its consequence, blindness. Most cases of trichiasis and distichiasis also often ended in blindness. If operated then eyesight could be restored, as Polak showed in hundreds of cases.[68] In the case of trachoma, Persian doctors would rub the granulation away with a piece of sugar. In case of pannus, they removed a thin circle-formed part of the conjunctiva around the cornea. Iritis and ophthalmia were vigorously treated with eye rinses and mercury.[69] Infantile conjunctivitis was treated "with fresh mother's milk squirted directly into the eye (good, sensible treatment this, for it is sterile, convenient, mild antiseptic)."[70]

Orientale, 1991), p. 43 (caligo cornea, cataract).
[62] Landor, *Across*, vol. 2, 180.
[63] O'Donovan, *The Merv Oasis*, vol. 1, p. 223.
[64] Hume-Griffith, M.E. *Behind the Veil in Persia and Turkish Arabia* (Philadelphia, J.B. Lippincott, 1909), p. 144; Schlimmer, *Terminologie*, p. 302.
[65] Polak, *Persien*, vol. 2, p. 346.
[66] Rice, *Persian Women*, p. 256.
[67] Morton, *A Doctor's Holiday*, p. 216.
[68] Polak, *Persien*, vol. 2, p. 346. See Schmidt-König, Fritz. *Ernst J. Christoffel: Vater der Blinden im Orient* (Giessen & Basel: Brunnen-Verlag, 1969) amongst other things, about the opening of an institution for blind people at Tabriz (1925) and Isfahan.
[69] Polak, *Persien*, vol. 2, p. 346; Ts., "Persidskie Doktora," p. 167 (a syrup made, preferably with Russian sugar, was applied to the eyes and then washed away with warm water).
[70] Lichtwardt, "Ancient Medicine," p. 84; Ts., "Persidskie Doktora," p. 167 (preferred was the milk of mother of a baby girl).

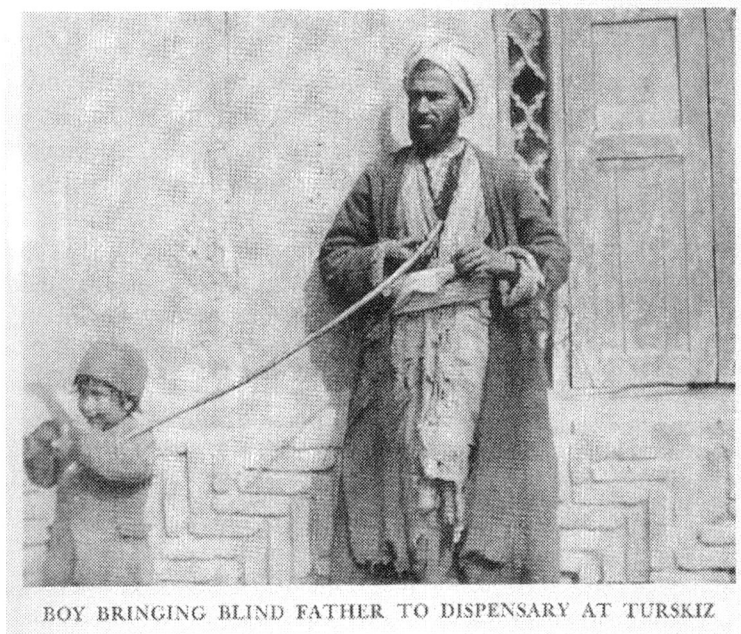

Figure 1: Boy bringing blind father to dispensary at Turksiz

RHEUMATISM

Although rheumatism allegedly did not occur as much as in Europe, according to Baker, there were nevertheless many people who suffered from that ailment.[71] In the Caspian littoral rheumatism occurred quite frequently in the 1850s, according to Häntzsche.[72] Rheumatism also occurred among the Bakhtiyari nomads. Isabella Bird maintained that it "doubtless comes from sleeping in cotton clothing, and little enough of it, on the damp ground."[73] The person to turn to for treatment was the barber. Cautery (*dagh*) was his only form of treatment. The barber would heat a small iron (*daghineh* or *dagh-e ahan-e dagh*) in "his earthen fire-pot, the patient lies down, and the barber, previously invoking the name of Mahommed, the Apostle of God, and the blessed saints, Hussain and Hassan, calmly inflict three severe burns on the man's loins. The sufferer pays his pence and goes his way."[74] In Bandar `Abbas, a different method was applied to cure rheumatism. Brittlebank witnessed while walking in that town a man leaning against "a wall in an almost perfectly nude state. His head rested on his arms, and behind him sat a little boy gently rubbing the

---

[71] The illness was important enough to be discussed in the weekly *Danesh*, p. 304 (nr. 3, October 14, 1910).

[72] Häntzsche, "Physikalisch-medicinische Skizze," pp. 562, 568. According to Polak, *Persien*, vol. 2, pp. 327-28 various types of rheumatism occurred in Persia, in partcular in the littoral of the Caspian Sea.

[73] Bird, *Journeys*, vol. 2, p. 75 ("For rheumatism headache, and debility they have no remedies"). According to Polak, *Persien*, vol. 2, pp. 327-28 various types of rheumatism occurred in Persia, in partcular in the littoral of the Caspian Sea.

[74] Wills, *Persia*, p. 137; Schlimmer, *Terminologie*, p. 117 (q.v. cautere); Polak, *Persien*, vol. 2, p. 241.

calves of his legs, which were stretched to their greatest tension, with rough grass. When we drew nearer we noticed that he was covered with blood, the rough 'shampooing' to which he was being subjected having frayed and torn away the skin at different parts of the legs."[75] Among the Armenians of Azerbaijan rheumatism was "cured by bathing the affected member three times in warm water, rubbing it with salt, and finally passing over it the blade of a knife with the words: 'As this salt melts, so may the evil melt.' The house is then swept with a new broom, the sweeper saying as the dust is swept out, 'So may all evil be swept away.'"[76] Moslems in Azerbaijan used pork as a remedy to cure rheumatism.[77] Another remedy was a diet of "a teacupful of honey, without bread, and soup made of lentils, beetroot, barley flour, mint, asparagus, and plenty of vinegar."[78]

In addition, hot or cold mineral springs (*ab-e garm*; *ab-e ma`dan*) were touted as one of the most effective remedies against rheumatism. Some of the springs also were believed to be effective treatment for other diseases such as skin diseases. In the mountainous areas of Persia there were many sulfurous pools and springs that attracted a large number of people afflicted with rheumatism. The British consul Lovett noticed various hot springs in the Elburz Mountains. "The sulphur baths at this place [the village of Ask] are much resorted to by patients suffering from rheumatism." This was not the only location, for there were "also the mineral springs, especially at Surt, where sulpherous sources exist, resorted to by rheumatic patients." These were also hot springs near Sir Derwazeh (Astarabad). "The water from the spring is conducted into shallow reservoirs in which patients bathe, the water having been warmed by means of stones highly heated and thrown in."[79] In Mazandaran, there are a number of hot springs called Ab-e Garm-e Bozorg, near Sakhtsar that contain much sulfur. "There are likewise iron and lime with a small admixture of salts. The people of the country only use them externally and follow no diet; they go there for skin diseases, rheumatisms, and the after effects of fever."[80] These hot springs also existed in Darzin (Kerman), where Vakil al-Molk had built a facility for the sick who frequented the springs, as well as near Mahallat where Mohammad Shah had built a bathhouse that was frequented by the sick.[81]

---

[75] Brittlebank, William. *Persia During the Famine* (London: Basil Montague Pickering, 1873), p. 83.

[76] Shabaz, Absalom D. *Land of the Lion and the Sun* (Madison, Wis., 1901), p. 137.

[77] Adams, Isaac. *Persia by a Persian* (n.p., 1900), p. 59.

[78] Rice, *Mary Bird*, p. 111.

[79] Lovett, Lieut. Col. Beresford, "Itinerary Notes of Route Surveys in Northern Persia in 1881 and 1882," *Proceedings of the Royal Geographical Society* II 1883, pp. 65, 72, 76; Stark, *The Valley*, p. 182 (Alamut region); Polak, *Persien*, vol. 2, pp. 226-30 (for a long list of mineral springs). For pictures of the healing hot springs at Cheshmeh-`Ali, visting pilgrims as well as its amenities see Heinrich, Gerd. *Auf Panthersuche durch Persien* (Berlin: Reimer/Vohsen, 1933), pp. 121-22, 130, 135.

[80] Rabino, H. L. "A Journey in Mazanderan (from Resht to Sari)", *Geographical Journal* 42 (1913), pp. 438-40; Orsolle, E. *Le Caucase et La Perse* (Paris: Plon, Nourrit et Cie., 1885), p. 346 (considered to be efficacious against various maladies). These 'spas' also existed elsewhere, see, for example, Alexander, James Edward. *Travels from India to England* (London: Parbury, Allen, and Co., 1827 [New Delhi, 2000]), p. 196, Porter, *Travels*, vol. 1, p. 121 (Tiflis).

[81] Farmanfarma, Firuz Mirza. *Safarnameh-ye Kerman va Baluchistan*. ed. Mansureh Ettehadiyeh (Nazem-Mafi) (Tehran: Babak, 1360/1981), p. 6; Pirzadeh, *Safarnameh-ye Hajji Mohammad `Ali*

But not only hot sulphurous water was believed to be beneficial to sufferers of rheumatism and other diseases. In Ab-e Anderman, a village to the west of Shah `Abdol-`Azim, for example, there is a pool with cold water. People came there to find healing for some unnamed diseases. The reason for coming there probably was because next to it there was an Imamzadeh of Abu'l-Hasan.[82] In Damghan there is a source, called Baqer Khani, a.k.a. Gondiyab, with reddish water in which people bathed to be rid of some unnamed diseases, and the same happened in the warm water source in Shuriyab, near Nishapur.[83] The Imamzadeh BiBi Sakineh (near Kahrizak-Tehran) had a well, which was said to heal most skin diseases (*amraz-e jeldi*).[84] It would seem that often, like the last mentioned one, these water sources derived their alleged healing powers from the nearby Imamzadehs. For example, in the Shah Rud valley there was the shrine of Sitt Zeinabar, which was good for cures. There was a little well of water that the local population called the Spring of Healing.[85]

INTESTINAL DISEASES

There were various intestinal worms (*didan, kerm*) that inconvenienced the life of many Persians. "Half the population has round worms, as the result of raw food and water infection."[86] Tapeworm was widespread, and so were other kinds of worm, which kept children weak and anemic. However, before 1870, its incidence must have been much lower than later in the century. According to Polak, referring to the 1850s, tapeworm was no major issue in Persia, because the mainly Moslem population did not eat pork, little fish, and their meat was well cooked. It only occurred among imported black slaves. Schlimmer mentioned that among the Armenian population of Khereganeh (Isfahan) the occurrence of tape worm was quite common, while the Moslem population in the same area did not have it, thus confirming Polak's finding. Nevertheless, among the population of the Caspian littoral the tapeworm (Taenia lata; *hobb al-qar`, kadudaneh*) had infected almost the entire population, according to Häntzsche. This implies that tapeworm must have been more prevalent than suggested. This, indeed, was the case. In 1902, Landor reported that, "The tape worm, so common in many other parts of Persia, is absolutely unknown in Sistan," due to the good water.[87] This implies that its occurrence had become more widespread than in earlier periods.

The maw worm (Oxyurus vermicularis; *kermak* or *dud ol-khall*) seldom occurred in the arid areas, according to Polak. However, practically all breast-fed children had it, while,

---

Pirzadeh. 2 vols. Hafez Farmanfarmayan (Tehran: Daneshgah, 1343/1964), vol. 1, p. 8.
[82] Mohandes, Hajji Mohammad Mirza-ye. "Raport-e Mamlekat-e Khorasan ba ba`zi molheqat-e an. ed. Qodratollah Rowshani," *Mirath-e Eslam*, vol. 6, p. 507.
[83] Mohandes, "Raport," pp. 517, 540.
[84] `Eyn al-Saltaneh, Qahraman Mirza Salur. *Ruznameh-ye Khaterat*. 10 vols. eds. Mas`ud Salur and Iraj Afshar (Tehran: Asatir, 1376/1997), vol. 1, p. 547.
[85] Watelin, *La Perse*, p. 40; Stark, *The Valley*, p. 209.
[86] Morton, *A Doctor's Holiday*, p. 215.
[87] Landor, *Across*, vol. 2, p. 181; Schlimmer, *Terminologie*, p. 549 (q.v. ver solitaire); Polak, *Persien*, vol. 2, pp. 315-16; Baker, "A few remarks," p. 325; Häntzsche, "Physikalisch-medicinische Skizze," pp. 563; Saad, *Sechzehn Jahre*, p. 184.

in case of girls it caused vaginal slime secretions. The Guinea worm (Filaria medinenses; *reshteh*, *`arq-e madani*, *poyuk*) occurred in the Persian Gulf littoral, in particular in the area from Bandar `Abbas up to Lar.[88] "In the low land around Resht, hookworms reduced the vitality of thousands."[89] In Kerman province there was a worm called *piyu*, and which was unlike the Guinea worm. The afflicted person's forehead would get hot and cause an itch, after which he started to scratch and thus caused swellings. If this disorder were not treated immediately, the swellings would grow worse on the head, breast, and throat and would suffocate a person. The only treatment was surgery, in which people from Bam were very expert. If the swellings continued to grow they would put the flat head of a gun-stick (*sonbeh-ye tofang*) into a fire, then put it onto the affected spot and hold it there for a moment so that it would scorch it till it reached the bone. Then ointment was pot on the burnt spot. Twice per day they would pull a warm skin of a red goat over the head of the patient till it reached his waist, and to enable him to breathe they made an opening for his mouth. In two to three days, having been treated in the same manner, the patient would be healed and cured.[90]

Clay eating (*gel khordan*) was quite common among Persian women, even when they were not pregnant. According to Persian doctors, women had adopted this habit to be rid of intestinal worms, for which Schlimmer could not find any evidence. However, the same habit also prevailed among young children where the reason indeed was to get rid of an unidentified worm.[91]

<u>Scabies and fungus diseases</u> were also endemic. Their cause was the absence of hygiene and they were spread by human contact. Fungus diseases of the scalp (ringworm, favus) were widespread due to lack of hygiene and spread through public baths. Scabies and pediculosis were common among the poor. Scabies (*kachali* or *hozaz*) often occurred, because the heads of young children, including their eyebrows, were always covered. Moreover, newborn babies were swaddled tightly. "A wretched superstition exists amongst the Persian women, that a baby's head must not be washed until it is several weeks old. No man is allowed to attend a woman in her confinement, and when the infant is born the midwife plasters its head with a mixture of clay and rancid butter. This is allowed to remain until the first hair falls off, when this foul compound comes away with it. Even then, the head is smeared with oil rather than washed in soap and water," which contributed to the high mortality rate among infants.[92]

---

[88] Polak, *Persien*, vol. 2, pp. 315-16; Schlimmer, *Terminologie*, pp. 422 (q.v. Oxyurus), 549 (q.v. ver solitaire), 203-216 (q.v. dragonneau); Jozani, *La beauté*, pp. 202-03; Saad, *Sechzehn Jahre*, p. 184.

[89] Morton, *A Doctor's Holiday*, p. 215.

[90] Farmanfarma, *Safarnameh*, pp. 15-16.

[91] Schlimmer, *Terminologie*, pp. 299-300 (q.v. géophagie); Polak, *Persien*, vol. 1, p. 219, vol. 2, pp. 235-36; Binder, *A Journey*, vol. 1, p. 165 ("In certain parts of the country, a kind of reddish clay, having a sweet and slightly acid taste, is found; and this, some imprudent persons become passionately fond of eating. The practice is a most pernicious one: the clay eater invariably becoming emaciated and sickly: but when the habit has once been formed, it is very difficult to relinquish it; and some kill themselves by it. It is a singular that this custom prevails in some parts [Georgia, Carolinas] of the United States of America, and the same clay is to be found there.")

[92] Forbes-Leith, A.C. *Checkmate and Fighting* (London, 1927 [New York: Arno, 1973]), p. 95;

Forbes-Leith, when he was 'forced' to provide medical services, bought amongst other things some drugs and powdered brimstone for a campaign against scabies. He handed out pounds of sulphur ointment, but the treatment was useless unless accompanied by continual baths and change of clothes. He therefore insisted that they boiled their clothes, came to his clinic in a towel and submitted their clean clothes for inspection. He explained that small bacteria caused scabies, but people did not believe it. They had looked for hours for small bugs, but had not seen anything. Still there was improvement and with the help of the village mullah the water of the village bath (Latgah) was changed every week. "The only impression that I created by doing this was that I was making myself a party to a shocking waste of water, which is very valuable commodity in this part of Persia."[93]

VENEREAL DISEASES

"Skin diseases are not often met with, and are generally of syphilitic origin," according to Baker,[94] which was rather an understatement. In fact, venereal disease (*bimariha-ye jeldi*) was rampant in the cities.[95] It was estimated that 20-40% of the entire population of Tehran, for example, was affected. It may have been less prevalent in the rural areas, although it occurred there as well in large numbers. Shanker (*kufti, taqereh-e solb-e kufti, akaleh*) the primary lesion of syphilis was treated with a sulphuric arsenic powder.[96] The secondary symptoms (*ateshak, kuft-e jeldi*) would manifest themselves already soon after the first stage, in 6-8 weeks. European physicians considered the Persian variety of syphilis (*marz-e mashur, kuft, akaleh*) much more benign than the European one. In contrast to Europe, the tertiary stage of the syphilis rarely manifested itself in Persia. The stigmata of congenital syphilis on the face or in the mouth were rare. Persians did not consider syphilis as being infectious and it was not something to be ashamed of. In fact, the disease was discussed in polite society, even in the presence of women and children.[97] According to Landor, "Siphylitic [sic] tonsillitis is almost the only throat complaint noticeable in Sistan, but inflammation of the palate is not rare, and there are but very few lung affections."[98] In consonance with the prevalence of syphilis, gonorrhea (*suzanak, harqat al-bowl, komsuzak*, and in Isfahani idiom, *suzak*) also was widespread and was the

---

Polak, *Persien*, vol. 2, p. 308; Schlimmer, *Terminologie*, pp. 529-30 (q.v. teigne). For a discussion of this disorder from the point of view of a person's appearance, see Jozani, *La beauté*, pp. 186-94; for Persian remedies to cure scabies see Ibid., pp. 194-97. "The flower of the hollyhock is made into a wash for the hair, and is also taken as cooling medicine." Stack, Edward. *Six Months in Persia*. 2 vols. (New York: G.P. Putnams, 1882), vol. 2, p. 58.
[93] Forbes-Leith, *Checkmate*, pp. 89-91.
[94] Baker, "A few remarks," p. 325.
[95] Government of Great Britain, *Trade Report 1920-21*, p. 1-2 ("venereal disease is rampant" in Bushire); Landor, *Across*, vol. 2, p. 181 ("Venereal complaints are almost as common."); Morton, *A Doctor's Holiday*, pp. 219-20 ("a menace to the nation."); Rice, *Persian Women*, p. 256.
[96] Schlimmer, *Terminologie*, p. 123 (q.v. chancre).
[97] Polak, *Persien*, vol. 2, p. 308; Schlimmer, *Terminologie*, p. 527; Jozani, *La beauté*, pp. 214-16; Neligan, "Public Health," part II, p. 693; Wood, *Glimpses*, p. 70.
[98] Landor, *Across*, vol. 2, p. 181. In the 1960s, syphilis, locally known as *azar*, was a hereditary disease and very common. Afshar, Iraj. "Kerman va Seystan," in Afshar, Iraj. ed. *Savad va Bayaz* 2 vols. (Tehran: Dehkhoda, 1349/1970), vol. 1, p. 313.

case of much infertility. The term *suzanak* also referred to other mucous membranes. If not interfered with and the patient kept to the prescribed regime, syphilis healed, otherwise it became chronic and a long-term disorder.[99]

The disease was spread through the promiscuous behavior of the males either through frequenting male and/or female prostitutes and/or the contracting of temporary wives in the major pilgrimage and trading towns. The prevalence of sodomy and pederasty (*bachchehbazi*) either in cabarets and coffeehouses or in people's homes through the contracting of musicians and their dancing boys (*geda*s) also contributed to the transmission of this disease.[100] Many 8-10 year old boys had syphilis, because of the widespread occurrence of pederasty.[101]

Although venereal diseases were widespread in Persia, European sources do not report much about the actual treatment given to sufferers of these diseases.[102] Landor reported that, "the most terrible form of syphilis, curiously enough, being treated even by Persian doctors with mercury-a treatment called the *Kalyan Shingrif*-but administered in such quantities that its effects are often worse than the ailment itself."[103] E'tesam al-Molk suffered himself from a gonorrhea (*herqat al-bowl*). When he was in Mashad, he asked a doctor for medicine. The physician told him to bring a glass with urine, after which he would make him a remedy. When E'tesam al-Molk got the medicine, he took an enema (*hoqneh*); it burnt sharply. He later took another dose, and later another one, but not the right quantity. Although he did not understand its effect, it gave some solace. Later he contacted another physician, who prescribed a pill of winter cherry (*kakonj*). E'tesam al-Molk took the pill each morning with tea or warm water, but it was not clear to him whether it really helped.[104] Old women specialized in syphilis treatment "by calomel

---

[99] Gilmour, *Rapport*, p. 49; Polak, *Persien*, vol. 2, pp. 308-09; Ibid., Ueber die Syphilis in Persien," *Zeitschrift der Gesellschaft der Aertzte in Wien* (1857); Schlimmer, *Terminologie*, pp. 79 (in case of women, syphilis was known as *suzanak-e mozmen-e gheyr-e mosri-ye anath*), 527; Jozani, *La beauté*, pp. 217-18; Neligan, "Public Health," part II, p. 693; Elgood, Cyril. "Translation of a Persian monograph on syphilis," *Annals of Medical History* 3/5 (1931), pp. 465-486.

[100] Floor, Willem. "Some Notes on Mut'a," *ZDMG* 138 (1988), pp. 326-31; Dupré, A. *Voyage en Perse fait dans les années 1807, 1808, 1809*, 2 vols. (Paris: Dentu, 1819), vol. 1, p. 464; Shamissa, Sirus. *Shahedbazi dar Adabiyat-e Farsi* (Tehran: Ferdows, 1381/2002).

[101] Polak, J.E. "Ueber den Gebrauch des Quecksilbers in Persien," *Wiener Medizinische Wochenschrift* 10 (1860), pp. 567.

[102] For the treatment according to Persian sources see, for example, Jozani, *La beauté*, pp. 216-17 and Polak, "Ueber," pp. 566-67.

[103] Landor, *Across*, vol. 2, p. 181. Since 1496, syphilis had been treated in Europe with mercury. The next chemical treatment to be developed specifically for syphilis was Potassium Iodide in the 1840's. The treatment was amazingly effective, even on patients with later stages of the illness. Mercury had been only moderately effective on late stages of syphilis and was not effective on very deep lesions. The introduction of Potassium Iodide gave people new hope that there could be a better cure in the future. It set the stage of the introduction of Salvarsan (an arsenic compound) in 1910, and later penicillin (1929).

[104] E'tesam al-Molk, *Safarnameh*, pp. 115-17, 133, 139, 142-43, 145, 148. For other treatments prescribed or dissuaded by Persian physicians see Jozani, *La beauté*, pp. 218-19 and Shahri, *Tarikh*, vol. 2, pp. 696-97; Polak, *Persien*, vol. 2, p. 233-35.

fumigations, but since the introduction of salvarsan less has been seen of their results."[105] There also were other methods of treatment, such as one, prescribed by a village barber. Forbes-Leith described the case of a man who came to see him; his wife had developed signs of secondary syphilis soon after their marriage three years ago. The village barber whom she had consulted had told her "to catch a small snake of a particular breed, to kill it, and eat it. He said that she had followed his advice, and had been cured of her complaint by this remedy, but that the snake had not been properly killed and was still living in her stomach, and as it was a female snake it had bred a large family. A large dose of powdered Arica [sic; areca] nut, followed by a copious draught of sulphate of magnesia, soon cured this severe case of thread worm, and the couple went on their way rejoicing."[106]

LEISHMANIASIS

The cutaneous form caused by Leishmania tropica, generally known as *salek* (literally, the little year) or as the oriental sore, had acquired endemic proportions in certain regions of Persia. "Every one has one or more flattish depressions on her face-scars in fact-the size of a large date stone. Nearly the whole population is thus disfigured."[107] It was also known as *köpöj* (dog in Chagatay Turkish), *khormachibani* (date boil or mark, Turkish), *yelchibani* (Turkish) and *godovnik* (Russian). The infection was transmitted by sand flies, and street dogs were an important reservoir of infection. Despite that both sand flies and street dogs were found all over Persia, *salek* was absent from certain areas, for unexplained reasons. From northwestern Persia downwards, along the border, to Kermanshah, those who had never moved from their place of residence were not infected, nor were those in the Caspian region. However, in Tehran, Isfahan and Mashad it was rare to see somebody whose face had not been scarred by this disorder. According to Polak, it was quite prevalent in Qom, Kashan and Isfahan. Towards Shiraz it slowly disappeared. In most villages that did not dot the major trade arteries it was seldom seen, so Polak alleged. However, in remote Seistan the disorder also occurred. According to Landor, "The most common complaint is the 'Sistan Sore,' which affects people on the face or any other part of the body. It is known by the local name of *Dana-i-daghi*. It begins with irregularly-shaped pustules-very seldom circular-that come to suppuration and burst, and if not checked in time last for several months, extending on the skin surface, above which they hardly rise."

Salek developed on the exposed parts of the body, mostly on the face, then the arms, and rarely on the legs. It was rare to find it on the covered parts of the body, except among children. *Salek* effected all ages, but in particular young people. There could be only one sore, there could be more, and even several groups of boils. If the boils occurred on the eyelids, nose, or lips the scars really disfigured a person. Therefore, as reported by Polak, it was said that the girls of Isfahan only wanted to be looked at *en profil*. However, Mrs. Bishop reported that in Baghdad among "Armenian girls, that so far from being regarded as a blemish, it is viewed as a token of good health, and it is said that a young man would hesitate to ask for the hand of a girl in marriage if she had not a 'date mark' on her face."

---

[105] Neligan, "Public Health," part III, p. 742.
[106] Forbes-Leith, *Checkmate*, p. 93.
[107] Bird, *Journeys*, vol. 1, p. 38.

The boils reached their maximum size at the end of summer, *i.e.*, from September till December, after January it was rare. People also tried through inoculation on the leg to obtain immunization. Once the sore showed people would allow it to develop, because it was believed that it needed several months before immunity could be obtained.[108]

LEPROSY

Leprosy (*jezam*; *pis*) also occurred. According to Polak it was mainly concentrated in the Khamseh province with its center at Zenjan, and in the districts of Khalkhal and Qaradagh, but Dr. D'Vaume also found it to be prevalent in parts of Kurdistan[109] In 1857, Polak had been able to convince the Persian government to second one of his students to Khamseh district and in particular the town of Zenjan to treat the lepers there.[110] Neligan, however, reported that leprosy prevailed in Khorasan, Azerbaijan, Gilan, Kermanshah, and Kurdistan.[111] Sometimes mistaken for, but not related to leprosy, was vitiligo or *baraz*.[112] Alphos (*pis* or *beres*) was an endemic disorder, also sometimes mistaken for leprosy, about which little was known at that time.[113] Likewise, sphacelus, described as a dry gangrene, occurred in some towns, and it was feared as much as leprosy.[114]

Although a not very prevalent disease, those unfortunates suffering from leprosy (*jezam*) had to fend for themselves. Many frequented the roads, on the outskirts of villages and towns, eking out a miserable existence by begging. They were not permitted to enter the towns and in Azerbaijan and Khorasan they were encouraged to live in villages by themselves. "There is a village of them about six miles from Tabriz. Their hamlet is called Payon, or the 'Village of the Sick,' and there are about five hundred of them, little, if at all, segregated."[115] It was the only leper village in Persia. In the late 1850s, `Aziz

---

[108] Gilmour, *Rapport*, p. 50; Neligan, "Public Health," part II, p. 694; Polak, *Persien*, vol. 2, pp. 296-305; Schlimmer, *Terminologie*, pp. 84-92; Landor, *Across*, vol. 2, 180; Bird, *Journeys*, vol. 1, p. 39; Loghman ed-Dowleh, Mohammed Hussein Khan Moïn ol-Atebba. *"Salek" Etude du bouton d'Orient*. (Thesis Paris faculty of medicine, 1908); Grothe, Hugo. *Wanderungen in Persien* (Berlin, Alg. Verein f. Deutsche Literatur, 1910), pp. 80-81; Jozani, *La beauté*, pp. 181-84; Elgood, Cyril, "The early history of the Bagdad Boil," *Journal of the Royal Asiatic Society*, July 1934, pp. 519-533; Colvill, "Sanitary Report," pp. 40-43 (also a description of an experiment of inoculation by the Jews in Baghdad); Häntzsche, "Physikalisch-medicinische Skizze," p. 565; Saad, *Sechzehn Jahre*, pp. 183-84 (often occurred when the datetrees flowered).

[109] Polak, *Persien*, vol. 2, pp. 305-07, vol. 1, pp. 311-12; Ibid., "Lepra in Persien," *Virchows Archiv* 27 (1863), pp. 175-80; Häntzsche, J.C. "Lepra in Persien," *Virchows Archiv* 27 (1863), pp. 180-83; D'Vaume, Dr. "La Lèpre Dans Le Kurdistan Persan," *Bulletin de la Société d'Anthropologie de Lyon* 5 (1886), pp. 158-62; Schlimmer, *Terminologie*, pp. 228-254. Polak also tried to treat the illness and showed a case to his medical students in the *Dar al-Fonun*. Government of Iran, *Vaqaye`-ye Ettefaqiyeh*, vol. 2, p. 1235 (nr. 193, 19 Moharram 1271/March 8, 1856).

[110] Polak, "Medicinische Briefe," p. 140.
[111] Neligan, "Public Health," part II, pp. 694.
[112] Polak, *Persien*, vol. 2, p. 307.
[113] Schlimmer, *Terminologie*, pp. 28-31, 365-66 (q.v. melas); Polak, "Lepra," pp. 178-79.
[114] Polak, "Lepra," p. 179.
[115] Wilson, *Persian Life*, pp. 140-41; Cochran, "Treatment," pp.105; de Gobineau, A. *Trois Ans en Asie (de 1855 A 1858)* 2 vols. (Paris, Bernard Grasset, 1923), vol. 2, p. 259 (deformed beggars at Miyaneh); Watelin, Louis-Charles. *La Perse Immobile* (Paris: Chapelot, 1921), p. 6; Ussher, John.

Khan Sardar, then governor of Tabriz, ordered to bring all the lepers from Azerbaijan at one location. He assigned a piece of land to them, "furnished them with oxen and farming implements, and established them as a separate community. At first they were given charity, month by month from the public treasury. If it was delayed beyond the regular time they came trooping down to the city. Now, on the contrary, it is said that they pay taxes to the government."[116] By 1920, there were three leper colonies, one at Arpadarassi, another at Khalkhal, and finally a third one near Mashad.[117] There also seems to have been one near Senneh.[118] The British government in India, in the absence of effective treatment, also isolated lepers from the population at large and forced them into segregated leper colonies.[119]

If one of the high and mighty was infected with leprosy a different approach was taken, because of the person's political influence and his wealth. The British ambassador Jones-Brydges related an event, which he witnessed in Shiraz, at the time when he was the agent for the English East India Company visiting the Zand court in the 1780s.

> Ja'far Khan asked royal physician to help a great khan, who was afflicted with the leprosy. The learned person recommended that the patient should daily be made to swallow a certain quantity of china-ware broken fine. The disease, however, was obstinate, and did not yield to the prescription. The King took it into his head that the fault lay in the insufficiency of the dose, and so ordered the patient to swallow a double one. This, however, produced no alteration in the state of the leper. The Hakim Bashi was consulted again, and he laid the failure of success to the account of the china administered *not being sufficiently old*. In consequence, the oldest and finest china in the Palace was broken up, ground to powder in quantities, and given to the afflicted Khan, with just the same success that the les valuable china had been. The Hakim Bashi now delivered it as his opinion that the disease was occasioned by *impurity of blood*; the only sure way to remedy which was, to draw blood from the patient and put it back again, *i.e.* cause him to drink it. This last prescription, aided, perhaps, by the *very old china*, certainly cured the poor man's leprosy, and, indeed, all his other complaints, if he had any; for before I left Schyras, I saw his corpse carried to the grave."[120]

Whooping cough (Pertussis) or *siyah sorfeh* was very widespread and sometimes assumed epidemic proportions. Most of the Persian physicians were of the opinion that

---

A Journey from London to Persepolis (London: Hurst and Blackett, 1865), p. 652 ("The whole of north-west Persia would seem to be afflicted with this frightful scourge of humanity.").

[116] Wilson, *Persian Life*, pp. 140-41; Neligan, "Public Health," part II, pp. 693; Brugsch, Heinrich. *Im Lande der Sonne. Wanderungen in Persien* (Berlin, 1886), p. 170.

[117] Gilmour, *Rapport*, p. 30

[118] Rasooli, Jay M. and Allen, Cady H. *The Life Story of Dr. Sa'eed of Iran* (Grand Rapids: Grand Rapids International Publications, 1958), pp. 22-23; D'Vaume, "La Lèpre, pp. 158-59.

[119] In 1925, at the initiative of a number of Moslem Mashadi citizens the American Christian Hospital established the 'Society against Leprosy' for lepers in Persia. Lichtwardt, A.H. "Western medicine in Iran," *Muslim World* 32/3 (1941), pp. 236-37; Ibid., "Leprosy in Iran," *Leper Quarterly* 14 (1940), pp. 12-18.

[120] Brydges-Jones, *An Account*, pp. 436-36 note.

the disease had to run its course without medical intervention. According to Rice, however, it had many young victims.[121]

SKIN DISEASES

Erythema or rash (*sahaj-e jeld*) occurred frequently in spring, but for a short while and of no major import.[122]

Erysipele or red-fire (*homreh, bad-e sorkh* or *bad-e mobarak*) occurred sporadically, but assumed epidemic proportions at times. Most of the cases were benign in nature; seldom did it end with death due to infection. Due to excessive use of leeches, laxatives, and Armenian bolus prescribed by native doctors convalescing patients suffered from lengthy anemia.[123]

SMALLPOX

Smallpox (*abeleh, joderi, sherk*) was endemic and although there were no major national outbreaks, there were frequent local epidemics. It was a main cause of death among children. Also, many new army recruits, Negro slaves and Baluchis succumbed to it, according to Polak. There were in particular several outbreaks in the south in 1871-72 and to a lesser extent in 1898-1903 in Khuzistan and in 1906 in Khorasan.[124] Smallpox was endemic in Bushire, usually in early spring. Nevertheless, people in general were not in favor of vaccination, even during an epidemic.[125] Since the beginning of vaccinations in 1909 the incidence of this malady was reduced significantly, according to Gilmour. However, Neligan commented that, "unfortunately there are no statistics to support this statement."[126]

Despite the fact that smallpox was a disease that regularly ravaged the population little was done about it either by Persian physicians or by the Persian government. This was surprising because the vaccine existed and had been known in Persia for ages. For example, inoculation against small-pox was practiced in Georgia, which Mme. de Freygang ascribed to the need to keep the Georgian girls free from blemish for sale to Turkish harems.[127] But at the diagonal other end of the country it was equally well-known and also for ages. Schlimmer reported that in Baluchistan, both among the tribes and

---

[121] Schlimmer, *Terminologie*, p. 156 (q.v. coqueluche); Rice, *Persian Women*, p. 256; Knanishu, *About Persia*, p. 185 ("When children have whooping-cpough they say, 'Give them donkey's milk to drink.'"); Saad, *Sechzehn Jahre*, pp. 183, 187 (for coughing blood of a freshly killed chicken had to be drunk; the next morning the patient had to eat the chicken).
[122] Polak, *Persien*, vol. 2, p. 292; Schlimmer, *Terminologie*, p. 266.
[123] Polak, *Persien*, vol. 2, p. 292; Schlimmer, *Terminologie*, p. 266.
[124] Polak, *Persien*, vol. 2, pp. 292-93; Schlimmer, *Terminologie*, p. 546; Gilbar, "Demographic Developments," p. 139; Sepehr, `Abdol-Hoseyn. *Mer'at al-Vaqaye`-ye Mozaffari va Yaddashtha-ye Malek al-Mo'arrekhin* ed. `Abdol-Hoseyn Nava'i (Tehran: Zarrin, 1368/1889), p. 149.
[125] Government of Great Britain, *Trade Report 1920-21*, pp. 1-2.
[126] Gilmour, *Rapport*, p. 44. Neligan, "Public Health," part II, pp. 693. Neligan was the physician of the British legation (1906-26) and for many years vice-chairman of the Sanitary Council of Persia.
[127] De Freygang, Madame. *Letters from the Caucasus and Georgia* (London: John Murray, 1823), p. 176.

sedentarized population, inoculation took place in a simple manner. A child that had been wounded by accident would be taken to milk an infected cow. The Baluchis called the vaccine, *potogav*. It was no use to try to convince the Baluchis of the advantage to vaccinate by lancet. The Baluchi white-beards, who at the same time were the healers, maintained that the wound had to be accidental. A warrior who wounded himself on purpose did not merit the name of a warrior. An unnamed English traveler reported the occurrence of an analogous vaccine among the camels of Baluchistan. Several Baluch chiefs told Schlimmer that this was indeed the case. However, this eruption was rare and he was not able to confirm it himself. The vaccine was known as *potoshotor*.[128] Among the Narui Baluchis there was an official smallpox inoculator, an important function that was passed from father to son. In the Malek Shah Khan region he was the only one who held this function, which was not known among the neighboring Baluchi groups. If among the latter smallpox would break out they would ask for the Narui 'doctor' and inoculate those who needed to.[129]

It is, of course, possible that neither Persian physicians nor Persian government were aware of the existence of the smallpox vaccine within its borders as well as with the experience of inoculation as practiced in both provinces mentioned, although that seems very unlikely. For when Binning reported on the British effort to introduce vaccination, the Persians, he wrote, were not interested. "Many years ago British physicians tried to introduce vaccination, but Persians neutralized it. Claimed they had discovered this prophylactic already."[130] The discovery referred to probably was inoculation as practiced by certain communities. According to Malcolm, referring to the situation in the first decade of the nineteenth century, "Persian physicians are acquainted with inoculation for the smallpox, but it is little practiced."[131]

In 1804, Dr. Jukes vaccinated a number of children in Bushire at the request of their mothers, but the governor and others in town were alarmed by his activities. It is not known whether he continued his vaccinations in Bushire, which he left in 1808.[132] In 1809, Dr. Jukes was able to vaccinate a number of Armenian children, but he was not allowed to do the same for Moslem children.[133] The efforts initiated by the Ouseley embassy to introduce

---

[128] Schlimmer, *Terminologie*, pp. 544-45 (q.v. vaccine).

[129] Gabriel, Alfons. *Weites Wildes Iran* (Stuttgart: Strecker und Schröder, 1940), p. 55.

[130] Binning, R.B.M. *A Journal of Two Years' Travel in Persia, Ceylon, etc.* 2 vols. (London: Wm. H. Allen & Co, 1857), vol. 2, p. 220. See also See Richter-Bernburg, Lutz. "Avicenna gegen Pockenimpfung. Iranische Reaktion auf die Einführung westlicher Medizin im 19. Jahrhundert," in: Tilman Nagel ed., *Asien blickt auf Europa. Begegnungen und Irritationen* (Beirut, 1990), pp. 73-87.

[131] Malcolm, John. *The History of Persia.* 2 vols. (London, 1820 [Tehran: Imp. Org. f. Soc. Services, 1976]), vol. 2, p. 532.

[132] Kotobi, Laurence-Donia. "L'émergence d'une politique de santé publique en Perse Qâdjâre (XIX-XXe siècles)," *Studia Iranica* 24 (1995), pp. 278. Von Gardane, Ange. *Tagebuch einer Reise durch die asiatische Türkei nach Persien, und wieder zurück nach Frankreich. In den Jahren 1807 und 1808*(Weimar, 1809), p. 69 related that Dr. Salvatori of the 1807-08 Frenchmission led by general Gardane proposed to the grand-vizier, Mirza Shafi`, to initiate vaccinations against smallpox. The grand-vizier who did not like the idea referred him to the royal physician.

[133] Wright, Denis. *The English Amongst the Persians* (London: I.B. Tauris, 2001), p. 123.

smallpox vaccination in Tehran in the winter of 1811-12 were not supported by either the Persian medical profession or the government. According to Morier, the secretary of the embassy:

> During the winter, the surgeons of the Embassy endeavoured to introduce vaccination among the Persians, and their efforts at first were very successful; but owing to the opposition of the Persian doctors, and to the little countenance which they received from men in authority, their labours had nearly proved abortive. The surgeons, having procured the cow-pock from Constantinople, commenced their operations at Teheran with so much success, that in the course of one month they had vaccinated three hundred children. Their houses were constantly thronged with women, bringing their offspring to them; and there was every appearance of a general dissemination of this blessing throughout Teheran, when of a sudden its progress was checked by the Government itself. [*Farrash*es were put at the British mission's gate, who] said, that if the people wanted their children to be vaccinated, the fathers and not the mothers were to take them to the surgeons, by which means the eagerness for vaccination was stopped; for we soon discovered that the males did not feel one half the same anxiety for their offspring as the women. [...] Almost all the children vaccinated by our surgeons belonged to the poor, who were glad to their medical assistance gratis.[134]

Morier, in his fictional account of Qajar Persia, describing the *Adventures of Hajji Baba*, has the royal physician make the following comment to Morier's hero, making it explicit that Morier believed that opposition to vaccination was a monetary and not a medical issue.

> Hajji, you must know that an ambassador from the Franks is lately arrived at this court, in whose suite there is a doctor. This infidel has already acquired considerable reputation here. He treats his patients in a manner quite new to us, and has arrived with a chest full of medicines, of which we do not even know the names. He pretends to the knowledge of a great many things of which we have never yet heard in Persia. He makes no distinction between hot and cold diseases, and hot and cold remedies, as Galenus and Avicenna have ordained, but gives mercury by way of a cooling medicine; stabs the belly with a sharp instrument for wind in the stomach;[135] and, what is worse than all, pretends to do away with the small-pox altogether by infusing into our nature a certain extract of cow, a discovery one of their philosophers has lately made. Now this will

---

[134] Morier, James, A. *A Second Journey through Persia, Armenia, and Asia Minor ... between the years 1810 and 1816* (London: Longman, Hurst, Rees, Orme, and Brown, 1818), p. 191; Malcolm, *The History*, vol. 2, p. 532. In 1798, Jenner had successfully demonstrated that skin injection with cowpox virus provided protection against a much more deadly smallpox, and British doctors wanted to transmit their compatriot's discovery to stop further outbreaks of the disease. This followed the successful vaccination introduced in Baghdad and Basra in April 1802, see Lorimer, J. G. *Gazetteer of the Persian Gulf* (Calcutta, 1915 [Gregg: Westmead, 1970]), p. 2254; Colvill, "Sanitary Report," p. 68; see also Ebrahimnejad, Hormoz. "Introduction de la médecine européenne en Iran au XIXe siècle," *Sciences Sociales et Santé* 16/4 (décembre 1998), p. 72.
[135] "This alludes to tapping in cases of dropsy; an operation unknown among the Persians, until our surgeons taught it them." (note in the original, see next footnote)

> never do, Hajji. The small-pox has always been a comfortable source of income to me; I can not afford to lose it because an infidel chooses to come here and treat us like cattle. We can not allow this him to take the bread out of our mouths.[136]

In 1812, Dr. James Campbell won the gratitude of `Abbas Mirza, whom he cured of a venereal complaint, while he also vaccinated his entire family.[137] This success led to the employment of Dr. John Cormick by `Abbas Mirza as his personal physician, whom he instructed to start a vaccination campaign against smallpox. Although children in some villages were vaccinated the campaign was stopped, due to popular opposition.[138] His older brother and rival, Mohammad `Ali Mirza, governor of Kermanshah also had a smallpox vaccination campaign carried out in the border area with Iraq. Jean de Murat, a French trader, carried out the vaccination campaign in Kermanshah. According to his own account, he had introduced smallpox vaccination in Baghdad in 1809. Only through the intervention of Grand Mufti, Ahmad Effendi, had he been able to actually perform the vaccinations. He then trained natives of Mosul and Erevan so that they might do the same in their hometown. His wife trained a few Christian women in the vaccination technique, one of whom continued vaccinations in Basra after de Murat and his wife had left Iraq. De Murat declared that he had vaccinated more than 4,500 children by 1819. In that year, the governor of Kermanshah invited him to become his chief interpreter. In that town he vaccinated more than 500 people, amongst which 25 Qajar princes and princesses. When the prince-governor died in 1822, de Murat wandered from Kermanshah to Hamadan, Tehran, Kashan, on to Isfahan and finally Jolfa, where he still resided in 1828. "He vaccinated at all those towns and kept up vaccination at Julfa," about which he regularly sent reports to Dr. McNeil, the surgeon of the British Legation. It would seem that de Murat "got his lymph from Dr. Milne at Busreh."[139] According to Polak, practically all members of the royal family, some 10,000 persons, had been vaccinated. Because of this the royal family was growing while other important families lost many to smallpox epidemics.[140] The manner in which vaccination took place "was to prick the skin with a sharp piece of silver and afterwards to introduce the lymph with a quill." Later unarmed bone points were used.[141]

It took another 30 years before the Persian government actively pursued smallpox vaccination again. The reformist grand vizier, Amir Kabir (1848-51), to improve the lot of the population took various public health measures, amongst which a vaccination campaign. Amir Kabir also had Dr. Cormick's book on smallpox vaccination reprinted.[142]

---

[136] Morier, James. *The Adventures of Hajji Baba*, chapter XIX.
[137] Wright, *The English*, p. 123.
[138] Ebrahimnejad, "Religion and Medicine," pp. 99-100.
[139] Colvill, "Sanitary Report," pp. 68-69. In Persian sources de Murat's name was Armenianized. For example, they noted that in 1234/1818, Hovannes Moradiyan carried out vaccinations in Kermanshah province. Soltani, *Joghrafiya*, vol. 1, p. 531; Eqbal, `Abbas. "Abeleh-kubi," *Yadgar*, vol. 4/3, pp. 69-71; Adamiyat, Fereydun. *Amir Kabir* (Tehran: Khvarezmi, 1348/1969), p. 324.
[140] Polak, *Persien*, vol. 2, p. 203.
[141] Colvill, "Sanitary Report," p. 70.
[142] E`temad al-Saltaneh, Mohammad Hasan Khan. *Montazam-e Naseri*. 3 vols. (Tehran, 1300/1883), vol. 3, p. 207; Polak, *Persien*, vol. 1, p. 298.

Already in the third issue of the *Vaqaye`-ye Ettefaqiyeh* newspaper an article appeared describing the ravages caused by smallpox and the need to take action.[143] At that time, according to Binning, smallpox prevailed in the northern provinces. The shah therefore "ordered the vaccinators to go there to inoculate the children."[144] Amir Kabir used barbers and surgeons to do the vaccination, whom he paid well. They applied the lymph in the center of the lower part of the forearm; after light scratching of the skin and the stopping of the blood the powder of ground lymph crusts were rubbed into the wound. The adhesion was practically always successful, but left quite distinct scars. It was not customary to vaccinate using fresh lymphs, because no mother would make her children available, although there was no opposition against vaccination per se. Often there was a lack of the vaccine, so that often smallpox puss had to be used. In Tehran most children were vaccinated during that period so that smallpox outbreaks were less serious than before, according to Polak.[145]

According to the government newspaper, the people in Gilan, Mazandaran and Yazd brought their children gladly to be vaccinated. In Mazandaran already 300 children had been vaccinated by July 1851.[146] The government took a five tomans fine from the parents, in case of refusal as happened in, for example, Isfahan and Kashan. The refusers claimed that they had acted out of ignorance, because they could not read. They also claimed that they feared that the vaccination would be like the puncture of the skin by a jinni, which, in traditional medicine, was one of the causes of disease. However, the order had also been cried out loudly in the streets. The men were given the bastinado and had to pay the fine. Because they had no money, Amir Kabir gave them the money out of his own pocket to pay the fine.[147]

After the fall of Amir Kabir in 1851, the entire public health program was cancelled or rendered ineffective. In the second half of the 1850s, Polak, who taught at the *Dar al-Fonun* (Persia's only Polytechnic School) since 1852, and later was the shah's private physician, argued that the high mortality rate of those affected by smallpox was justification for vaccination.[148] However, vaccination was not in official and professional medical favor anymore. Polak did not receive permission to vaccinate newly arrived recruits, while he was told that in the case of death he would have to pay blood money, or worse, be judged according to the lex talionis (*qesas*).[149] Dr. Häntzsche who had re-introduced smallpox vaccination at the end of the 1850s in Gilan had to discontinue this activity due to religious opposition in Resht.[150] "Inoculation is the method pursued, *i.e.,*

---

[143] Government of Iran, *Vaqaye`-ye Ettefaqiyeh*, vol. 1, pp. 13-14 (nr. 3, 19 Rabi` II 1267/21 February, 1851).

[144] Binning, *A Journal*, vol. 2, p. 220.

[145] Polak, *Persien*, vol. 2, pp. 202-03.

[146] Government of Iran, *Vaqaye`-ye Ettefaqiyeh*, vol. 1, p. 83 (nr. 17, 27 Rajab 1267/May 13, 1851); vol. 1, p. 105 (nr. 22, 30 Ramazan 1267); vol. 1, p. 122 (nr. 25; 24 Ramazan 1267/July 23, 1851).

[147] Government of Iran, *Vaqaye`-ye Ettefaqiyeh*, p. 237 (nr. 45, 17 Safar 1268/12 December, 1851); Hajj Sayyah, *Khaterat*, p. 470; Hasanbeygi, *Tehran-e Qadim*, pp. 202-03 (for a romanticized and highly moralized version of the same events).

[148] Polak, *Persien*, vol. 2, pp. 292-93, 202.

[149] Polak, "Medicinische Briefe," p. 139.

[150] Häntzsche, "Physikalisch-medicinische Skizze," p. 569

the direct communication of the disorder by placing the patient in the same bed with one from suffering small-pox of the most virulent type."[151] This method seems to have been practiced nationwide, including among other nomadic groups than the Baluchis, and thus the disease was kept endemic.[152] According to Abbott, who traveled through the province of Fars in 1850, "I had heard before, and the information was here confirmed, that inoculation has been known amongst the tribes of Fars for centuries. The operation is performed on children at the wrist, and unless the pock makes it appearance in a general eruption over the body, it is not considered effective, and the operation is repeated. When thus induced, the disease is said to leave no mark. The cow-pock is, however, unknown amongst the tribes."[153] Under these circumstances, according to de Windt, "it is scarcely to be wondered at that the Shirazis die like sheep during an epidemic, and indeed at all times."[154]

Asaf al-Dowleh reported on April 20, 1870 that he had given instructions to start a vaccination campaign in Gilan, where he was governor at that time. To ensure its effective application he had given orders to punish the village chief (*kadkhoda*) if a child died of smallpox in his jurisdiction. There is no further mention on its actual implementation in Asaf al-Dowleh's published reports and letters, unfortunately.[155] By 1880, the mood started to change somewhat, for in that year, Naser al-Din Shah instructed E'tezad al-Saltaneh to begin compulsory vaccination, but nothing much came of it.[156] It did not mean that there was no more interest in the subject, for some vaccination took place. In 1894, `Eyn al-Saltaneh wrote in His Diary that at that time, "the barber (*dallak*) came to vaccinate (*abeleh kubidan*). They had made a strange discovery. In the past 90% of children died, and 10% survived; now 90% survive, and 10% die. People are really indebted to this English doctor; in Iran it is not yet widely used. Nothing is done at all in the villages for they are horrified to have their children vaccinated. In the days of `Abbas Mirza there was a lot of upheaval about this issue in Azerbaijan."[157]

However, during the first decade of the twentieth century there was still no vaccination campaign, and Persians continued to put their children with a person who had a mild case of smallpox, "or, oftener, inoculate him with it."[158] In Damghan, in the beginning of the twentieth century, when smallpox broke out some parents called for the services of an old woman from a village some five km from town. "She took the dried pocks of a child that

---

[151] Wills, *Persia*, p. 90.

[152] Collins, *In the Kingdom*, p. 168 ("Smallpox is kept endemic by the practice of inoculations, the fore-arm being selected as the seat of the operation.").

[153] Abbott, K.E. "Notes Taken on a Journey Eastwards from Shiraz to Fessa and Darab, Thence Westwards by Jehrum to Kazerun, in 1850." *JRGS* XXVII (1857), p. 171. In 1810, a British officer was assured that some pastoral tribes were exempt from small-pox. Malcolm, *The History*, vol. 2, p. 532, note *.

[154] De Windt, *A Ride*, p. 178.

[155] Asaf al-Dowleh, *Asnad*, vol. 2, p. 45.

[156] E`temad al-Saltaneh, *Montazam-e Naseri*, vol. 1, p. 242; vol. 2, 207; Greenfield, J. *Die Verfassung des persischen Staates* (Berlin: Franz Vahlen, 1904), p. 270.

[157] `Eyn al-Saltaneh, *Ruznameh*, vol. 1, p. 732.

[158] Malcolm, Mrs. Napier. *Children of Persia* (Edinburgh: Oliphant, Anderson & Ferrier, 1911), p. 85.

had had smallpox and put these on a stone, poured some water on it, ground it and made 'vaccine' and then put that substance on the back of my right hand. Another woman took my hand and the vaccination woman took a package of about 10 needles that were held together by a string in her hand and then, right on the spot where she had put the smallpox vaccine, stuck these needles till there came blood and then closed it." In the same village 22 children died of smallpox at that time.[159] The reluctance of parents to have their children vaccinated also existed in Bushire. Smallpox was endemic usually in early spring, but "people in general are not in favor of vaccination, even during an epidemic."[160] It was only as of 1909, that vaccination was happening on some significant scale, because Gilmour reported that it really had made a difference. For example, smallpox affected only nine persons in Bushire in 1914. This was ascribed to the fact that many children were vaccinated by the British Residency dispensary, where services were offered once a week to the public.[161] Nevertheless, it still fell far short of what was needed. For as late as 1934, Merritt-Hawkes commented: "It is hoped that smallpox vaccination will be compulsory in two years and also satisfactory, as vaccine is now prepared in Tehran. Arm to arm vaccination still spread syphilis. Twenty years ago it was thought that anyone who looked at a syphilitic patient would become infected and in some districts they were sent to remote villages where they had to look after one another."[162] There was no effort by the parents or family to isolate children who had an infectious disease such as smallpox or whooping cough.[163] In case of smallpox as well as of measles, the patients were kept warm and their hands tied to keep them from scratching.[164]

Measles or *sorkhcheh*, which, according to Baker had been introduced into Persia around the 1850s, could have devastating effects during winter. If left alone it would just run its course. However, the children were pestered with laxatives (physics) and enemas, which resulted in dysentery and diarrhea. Also, noma or lesion of the mouth (*akeleh*; *sartan-e juf-e dahan*) was seen.[165]

Scarlet fever (*makhmalek*) was unknown and there was not even a name for it, according to Polak. He had been informed that it occurred in Kerman under the name of *makhmalek*.[166] Baker believed that it had only been introduced into Persia around 1855.[167] However, according to Schlimmer the disease occurred in Persia well before that date, although Häntzsche had even denied its very existence in the entire Orient. The reason

---

[159] Keshavarz-Damghan, `Ali Asghar. *Sad Darvazeh. Mokhtasari as Tarikh va Joghrafiya-ye Damghan* (Tehran, 1352/1973), pp. 244-45.
[160] Government of Great Britain, *Trade Report 1920-21*, p. 1-2.
[161] Government of Great Britain, *Trade Report 1913-14*, pp. 6-7.
[162] Merritt-Hawkes, *Persia*, p. 148; Rice, *Persian Women*, p. 256.
[163] Rice, *Persian Women*, pp. 127.
[164] Sargis, Yacob Allahverdy. "Persia and Her Doctors," *Columbus Medical Journal* 25 (1901), pp. 586.
[165] Polak, *Persien*, vol. 2, pp. 293-94; Schlimmer, *Terminologie*, pp. 102, 493; Baker, "A few remarks," p. 323; Government of Iran, *Vaqaye`-ye Ettefaqiyeh*, vol. 2, pp. 842, 1175, vol. 3, p. 1561; Saad, *Sechzehn Jahre*, p. 134.
[166] Polak, *Persien*, vol. 2, p. 294; Saad, *Sechzehn Jahre*, p. 183.
[167] Baker, "A few remarks," p. 324.

that Polak and others denied its occurrence, Schlimmer ascribed to the fact that European physicians seldom saw this, or any other disease, in their early stage. Old women first treated the problem, and when that did not help or made it worse, recourse was first had to traditional Persian physicians. Only when everything else had failed European doctors were called in. He therefore maintained that in order to know the real health situation of the country you had to develop a good relationship with Persian physicians and from time to time attend to them in their clinics to learn their diagnostic terminology and healing methods. Only then, Schlimmer rightly argued, you would be able to form a solid opinion about the occurrence or not of this or any other disease. In this manner, Schlimmer was the first to diagnose the illness in Kerman in 1855, but he was not believed. In 1866-67, during his stay in Isfahan he was once again able to confirm the existence of the disease. The long-time existence of a group of Armenian women specializing in the treatment of this disease also led Schlimmer to believe that scarlet fever had existed already for a long time in Persia. Finally, with the outbreak of scarlet fever in Qazvin (1868-69) and in Tehran (1870), the Persian and European medical community was able to confirm Schlimmer's findings. In Khorasan, where scarlet fever sometimes acquired a serious nature, Persian physicians distinguished between benign scarlet fever (*makhmalek*) and lethal scarlet fever (*margijeh*). The latter could not be healed they found, and Schlimmer believed that it probably was gangrenous scarlet fever.[168]

Nettle rash (*ir*, *nabat al-leyl*, *kahir*, *anjoriyeh*) often broke out in the fall, in connection with severe intermittent fever. For those not acclimatized, *i.e.*, a recent arrival, the entire body was often covered.[169]

Pemphigus (*nefat*) quite often occurred among children. It was believed to be infectious, and indeed usually more than one child at the same time had it. It usually ran its course after two months, although babies often succumbed to the disease.[170]

Amoebic dysentery (*eshal-e khuni*, *eshal-e damavi*, *dhu santariya*) was endemic and sporadically lasted the entire year in cities. From August-mid November it was often dangerous and epidemic in nature. It occurred in all three known forms, which were described by Polak.[171] However, acute dysentery was relatively rare, according to Baker.[172]

Diphtheria or *khonaq* also occurred. Baker reported that it had been introduced into Persia in the 1850s. Later more cases certainly occurred and the disease is mentioned in private

---

[168] Schlimmer, *Terminologie*, pp. 501-03 (q.v. scarlatine); Moshtaq Kazemi, Morteza. *Ruzgar va Andisheha* 3 vols. (Tehran: Ebn Sina, 1350/1971), p. 12.
[169] Polak, *Persien*, vol. 2, p. 294; Schlimmer, *Terminologie*, p. 544.
[170] Polak, *Persien*, vol. 2, pp. 234, 295; Schlimmer, *Terminologie*, p. 429.
[171] Polak, *Persien*, vol. 2, pp. 311-14; Schlimmer, *Terminologie*, pp. 217, 283 (q.v. fièvre dysentérique or *nowbeh ba eshal-e damavi*), 191 (*eshal-e sadeh* or diarrhea). Persian doctors maintained that, "almonds are most excellent for dysentery. They scrub one out like soap. Pepper is also good," Stark, *The Valley*, p. 214 reported.
[172] Baker, "A few remarks," p. 324.

diaries of Persians. It also occurred much among Europeans.[173] However, according to another European physician diphtheria had only been introduced in Persia since 1874. It had then become so virulent that already two years later it had become endemic in a few towns, while in Tehran in 1876 it represented 20-30% of total deaths.[174] According to `Eyn al-Saltaneh, an American doctor, healed a patient in two weeks, where Persian doctors took three months. He therefore argued that all that was needed was an American-type hospital.[175] Amanollah Khan Ardalan's physician was Entezam al-Saltaneh. In 1896, they went to Tholozan for treatment of his diphtheria, who gave him a serum that just had been discovered in Paris.[176] One of the more normal methods of treatment was to "press the tonsils hard with index finger once every evening for three or four days and keep neck warm."[177]

As to non-communicable diseases little data is available. These concern dietary deficiencies, low calorific intake, and rickets. The first two were evidenced by the diet of most people in Qajar Persia, as discussed in the next section. Rickets was rather widespread among the young children working in the Kerman carpet industry.[178]

Generally speaking, Persians had good teeth.[179] According to Polak, caries (*kerm* or worm) did not occur often, and people kept their teeth till they reached old age. If people had caries, usually in the cities, chronic periostitis (*varam-e zariyeh, amas-e zariyeh*) occurred. As a result their teeth would drop out by themselves, or could be painlessly pulled out with one's fingers, due to atrophy of the root. Polak reported that Persians mistakenly believed that their gums receded, and every day he would hear the complaint, "*Gusht-e dandan raft*," (my gums have gone) for which they asked medicine to make the gums come back.[180] Later gum and other dental ailments apparently had become more widespread and loss of teeth was quite common in urban areas. Mostowfi wrote in his

---

[173] For example, Murdoch-Smith, the director of the Telegraph Department, lost three of his children within three days to the disease. Rubin, Micheal Allen. *The Formation of Modern Iran, 1858-1909: Communication, Telegraph and Society* (Yale University, unpublished thesis, 1999), p. 297; Ghaffari, Mohammad `Ali. *Khaterat va Asnad-e Mohammad `Ali Ghaffari, Na'eb-e Avval-e Pishkhedmat-bashi.* Eds. Mansureh Ettehadiyeh and Sirus Sa`dvandiyan (Tehran: Tarikh, 1361/1982), p. 329. In general, see Tholozan, J.D., *De la diphtérie en Orient et particulièrement en Perse* (Paris: Masson, 1878).
[174] G.D. "Sanitätsreformen in Iran. *Globus. Illustierte Zeitschrift für Länder- und Völkerkunde* 31 (1877), p. 300.
[175] `Eyn al-Saltaneh, *Ruznameh*, vol. 1, p. 871; Baker, "A few remarks," p. 323. In 1876, there was an epidemic of diphtheria in Tehran, according to Elgood, Cyril. *Medical history*, p. 519. Government of Iran, *Vaqaye`-ye Ettefaqiyeh*, p. 1198 (*khonaq*).
[176] `Eyn al-Saltaneh, *Ruznameh*, vol. 2, p. 1058; see also Sepehr, *Mer'at al-Vaqaye`*, p. 219; *Tarbiyat*, Index q.v. *Difteri*.
[177] Sargis, "Persia and Her Doctors," p. 586.
[178] Morton, *A Doctor's Holiday*, p. 217; Rice, *Persian Women*, p. 257. According to Polak, *Persien*, vol. 2, p. 328 rickets hardly occurred in Persia, and there was not even a word for the disease in Persian.
[179] Häntzsche, "Physikalisch-medicinische Skizze," p. 559.
[180] Polak, *Persien*, vol. 2, p. 310; Schlimmer, *Terminologie*, pp. 431-32.

autobiography, "Like most victims of this disease, I lost my teeth one at a time."[181] The increase in caries may have been occasioned by the increased consumption of sugar, after 1870.[182] According to Schlimmer, although the 'real' cause of caries of the teeth (*dandan-e kerm khordeh*) had been explained to the new generation of doctors, the old practitioners persisted in their old ways. Rather than adopting new knowledge, the nature of which Schlimmer did not describe, they continued to make an effort and show that the real cause of caries was worms. To that end they put the open mouth of the sufferer over a small stove with burning charcoal on which they threw henbane. The anodyne smoke that resulted from the slow torrefaction of the seeds usually immediately took away the pain. Once the running of saliva had stopped the Persian healer told the patient and his assistants that the worms that had been in the patient's mouth and had caused the caries now had been burnt and were part of the charcoal ashes. However, these so-called worms were but the rudimentary embryonics of the henbane, which, if not touched, maintained their form.[183]

Although <u>drug addition</u> such as alcoholism was marginal, when compared with the Western world, there was nevertheless heavy drinking by certain groups, resulting in public disorder. Opium addiction was a worse problem, for it was widespread and in certain towns reached a level of 50%.[184]

<u>Hemorrhoids</u> (*bavasir*) were a chronic disorder. A snake doctor's family in Tabriz fumigated (probably imbued with arsenic) the tubercles to get rid of them. But the patients died.[185]

<u>Urinary problems</u> were very widespread, in particular in Azerbaijan, Hamadan, Qazvin, Tehran, Qom, Caspian littoral, and Shahrud-Bestam. South of Qom it occurred much

---

[181] Mostowfi, `Abdollah. *Sharh-e Zendegani-ye Man* 3 vols. (Tehran: Zavvar, n.d.), vol. 1, p. 529. Landor, *Across*, vol. 1, p. 208, however wrote that "young men and women have good teeth, and frequently so firmly set in their sockets as to allow their possessors to lift heavy weight with them, pulling ropes right, etc."

[182] On the consumption of sugar see Floor, Willem. *The Traditional Crafts of Qajar Iran* (Costa Mesa: Mazda, 2002), pp. 332-44.

[183] Schlimmer, *Terminologie*, p. 185 (q.v. dent).

[184] Neligan, "Public Health," part III, pp. 742-44; Rice, *Persian Women*, p. 258. The women of the royal harem and of those of male members of the elite drank themselves into a stupor, according to De Gobineau, A. *Les Réligions et les Philosophies dans l'Asie Centrale* 2 vols. (Paris: G. Crès et Cie., 1923), vol. 1, p. 78. Alcohol use was not limited to the political elite; it also occurred among the olama and the public in general. See, for example, Sirjani, Sa`idi. *Vaqaye`-ye Ettefaqiyeh. Gozareshha-ye khofyeh-nevisan-e englis* (Tehran: Now, 1361/1982), Index q.v. *neza` va masti*; Sheykh-Reza'i, Ensiyeh and Azari, Shahla ed. *Gozareshha-ye Nazmiyeh az Mahallat-e Tehran* (Tehran: Sazman-e Asnad-e Melli, 1377/1998), Index, q.v. *shorb*; Floor, *Agriculture in Qajar Iran*, pp. 457-60.

[185] Polak, *Persien*, vol. 2, p. 315; Schlimmer, *Terminologie*, pp. 467 (q.v. polype), 312 (q.v. hemorrhoides); Saad, *Sechzehn Jahre*, p. 184; Jozani, *La beauté*, pp. 204-09. The "tareh, a small plant resembling garlic and with a similar smell, said to be good for haemorrhoids." Browne, *A Year*, p. 424. In Ardabil a plant called cat's nail or *pishik jirnakhi* was believed to be effective as well against hermorrhoids. Safari, *Ardabil*, vol. 3, p. 497.

less, in fact, it was rather rare. People generally thought that they had gonorrhea, because they often stated: *suzanak daram*. It allegedly occurred more in the south than in the north. According Polak, who often performed lithotomy, as did his students after him, opined that traditional doctors rarely performed the operation (*estekhraj-e sang-e methaneh az shekaf-e `ojan*). Normally, Persian doctors stuck to the belief in the efficacy of their drugs that dissolved the stones and thus the disorder.[186]

WOMEN'S 'DISEASES'
One of a woman's functions in Qajar Persia was to get pregnant. That sometimes did not happen, for whatever reason. The absence of pregnancy was the woman's failure, if not fault, and women therefore, whether their husband was fertile or not, went out of their way to invoke the powers that be to grant them pregnancy. For barrenness "was considered the greatest curse."[187] Yate observed that near the Surab gate at Mashad "stands an old and broken figure of a tiger, carved out of a block of stone." There was always a group of women "around this tiger, and one woman in the center astride of it. ... The woman is seated on the stone tiger, and various incantations are gone through, such as the cutting of a string with forty knots, and other things, and the ceremony is over."[188] Near Kerman there is a spring gushing forth from the hard rock due to a blow by the Imam `Ali. On the steep mountain the words Ya `Ali are painted, and below them the merest trickle of water exudes. "All day long women climb up to this spot to collect the slowly-dripping water from the sacred stream, and to hang tallow-dips from the branches of the one small tree growing by it, which votive offerings will ensure to them the joys of motherhood. Sick women, on the other hand, made their pilgrimage to a spur of the hills on which are the old fortresses, and deposit bread, meat, sugar, and fruit in a small mud room. If on their return their offering are eaten, they believe that the Queen of the Fairies has taken pity on them, and will cure them of their complaints."[189] Persian doctors also prescribed camel-rennet (*mayeh-ye panir-e shotor*) to ensure conception, but the conditio

---

[186] Polak, *Persien*, vol. 2, p. 317-22; Schlimmer, *Terminologie*, p. 527 (q.v. taille); Baker, "A few remarks," p. 325. Savage-Smith, "The Practice," p. 317 suggests that Islamic doctors performed minor surgery of a non-invasive character only. Among the kinds of operations performed she mentioned tonsillectomy. I have not yet come across anyone recording this being done in Qajar Persia. Even lithotomy, as when the stones were in the neck of the bladder, seems to have been an operation of limited occurrence. Wishard, *Twenty Years*, p. 210 mentioned that a Persian doctor did not even recognize the nature of the rather large stones that he had extracted when he showed it to his colleague, and he asked whether they contained diamonds.
[187] Wilson, *Persian Life*, p. 261.
[188] Yate, C.E. *Khurasan and Sistan* (London: William Blackwood & Sons, 1900), p. 337.
[189] Sykes, Ella. *Through Persia on a Side-Saddle* (Philadelphia: John MacQueen, 1898), p. 96; Landor, *Across*, vol. 1, p. 458 for a picture of "wives returning from the pilgrimage for sterile women." Reitlinger, *A Tower*, p. 109 related the rather amusing story of two villages that shared one imamzadeh, where women hang their offerings on the tomb to ensure fertility. When denied access to the imazadeh by the village in which the imamzadeh was located, the people of the other village acquired a mollah to take care of their spiritual needs. When, one year later, the birth rate had not increased the villagers found the mollah wanting. They killed him and built a shrine over his corpse, where the women of the village could hang their votive offerings to ensure pregnancy and other beneficial things. If true, it shows how serious people took their needs and beliefs and how practical they were to ensure that they could practice their faith.

sine qua non for its success was that the woman had to swallow it without knowing that she did![190] Praying in an Imamzadeh also was considered to be helpful.[191] In Urumiyeh, in the Catholic church built in the Mart Mariam quarter, the local women, whether Christian or Moslem, came to light wax candles and incense to beseech the blessing of the Virgin Mary to make them pregnant.[192] Similarly, the Pearl Cannon (*Tup-e Marvarid*) in Artillery Square in Tehran was allegedly endowed "with miraculous powers, even with the gift of granting children to barren women who touch its brass mouth."[193]

> In case of sterility women also apply to the magicians who in such cases fill a copper bowl with water and build a small fire. The magician then requires the lady to sit close to this while he takes a large sheet and covers himself and her while the smoke fills the space. He now utters some incantation in the Arabic language which means that he is calling out the devils. The lady now looks upon the water which by some extraordinary spell he makes to move in the bowl. This the lady sees and at that time he rubs together some needles that he has with him or some thing else that produces a chirping sound like a bird. This the lady hears and verily believes that devils are now present. After this he writes a prescription and instructs her what to do with it and tells her that some time in the future she will dream that she sees a man coming to her and giving her a red apple. That is to presage the birth of a child. In order to make her doubly sure that this is to take place he tells her that she will find a birthmark upon the face or some other part of its body. She returns home expecting that year and next and the next and so on to become the mother of a child, but of course never does.[194]

Not only Moslems and Christians tried to bring about pregnancy by magical means, adherents of other religions did the same. Among the Jews, for example, a great rabbi would recite a blessing over barren women and then write amulets for them to become pregnant.[195]

Other related remedies included love charms. For example, when a hyena was killed, "its stomach was cut out ... as being an infallible love-charm."[196] Or, a diamond worn at the neck would let drop painful teeth without pain and made women desirable.[197] There were old brass bowls on which the signs of the zodiac were inscribed all round the outside, and on the inside were engraved descriptions of the different diseases, combined with prayers

---

[190] Schlimmer, *Terminologie*, p. 97 (q.v. caillette).

[191] Homayun, *Molk-e 'Anbir-amiz*, p. 118.

[192] Wilson, *Persian Life*, p. 95; de Gobineau, A. *Les Réligions et les Philosophies dans l'Asie Centrale* 2 vols. (Paris: G. Crès et Cie., 1923), vol. 1, p. 9.

[193] Jackson, A.V. Williams. *Persia Past and Present, a book of travel and research* (London: MacMillan, 1909), p. 422.

[194] Knanishu, J. *About Persia and its People* (Rock Island, Ill., 1899), p. 82.

[195] Sabar, Yona. *The Folk Literature Of The Kurdistani Jews: An Anthology* (New Haven: Yale UP, 1982), pp. 172-73.

[196] Goldsmid, Sir Frederic J. *Eastern Persia, An Account of the Journeys of the Persian Boundary Commission 1870-71-72*, 2 vols. (London: MacMillan & Co, 1876), vol. 1, p. 274; see also Polak, *Persien*, vol. 1, p. 222 about how to get a man.

[197] Serena, C. *Hommes et Choses en Perse* (Paris: G. Charpentier, 1883), p. 135.

to Allah. "Women wishing to gain the love of their husbands, use these bowls, repeating an invocation to the Prophet as they pour the water over their heads."[198]

Men, from their point of view, also tried to be helpful by trying to overcome impotency to which end Indian liquorice (*chashm-e khorus*) was used in a dosage of five grams mixed with oxymel (*taranjabin*).[199] E`tesam al-Molk, when consulting a physician in Mashad, received two prescriptions, one for hemorrhoids (*bavasir*), the other for *qovveh-ye bah* (potency).[200]

Women also used remedies to prevent conception. For example, a piece of wolf worn by a woman prevents conception and allows her to indulge in her caprices without fearing any consequence.[201] Malijak, Naser al-Din's mignon, said during a social gathering, that the shah's wives had the intention to give the shah bear's liver so that he would not have any more children.[202] Women in childbirth pain had to pass a thread through the root of doronic (Roman's leopard's bane) and to hang it over the uterine region, provided that the woman did that herself while giving birth.[203]

Because children were in great demand, *abortus provocatus* was relatively rare. Landor even went so far as to state that "Abortion seldom occurs naturally, and is never artificially produced." However, in the first volume of his travelogue he stated the contrary, writing that, artificial abortion "has become frequent for the prevention of large families that cannot be supported."[204] There were indeed a few physicians and midwives who also dealt in abortion, but they were not aware of the drugs and techniques used in Europe to bring about an *abortus provocatus*. As ecbolics (*adviyeh-ye mosqateh-ye janin*) they used several herbs such as the small, fresh leaves of the date palm (*Phoenix dactilifera*), which they cultivated in pots in their own yard. They were cut whenever there was a need for them and made into a suppository. Women with a bad reputation, who conceived, swallowed strong dosages of asafetida (*stercus diaboli*), which, allegedly, never failed to bring about delayed courses and made them sterile after they swallowed the same dosage at each subsequent menstrual period. The same effect, according to Schlimmer, might be also achieved by vaginal injection of Sprititus vini, which had been obtained by fermentation of *Uvae passulae minores*.[205] In fact, Neligan reported in 1926, midwives introduced substances that "provoke abortion. The latter practice has become regrettably common in the capital, and is not always the work of uneducated women."[206]

---

[198] Sykes, *Through Persia*, p. 46.
[199] Schlimmer, *Terminologie*, pp. 8-9; Saad, *Sechzehn Jahre*, p. 184.
[200] E`tesam al-Molk, *Safarnameh-ye Mirza Khanlar Khan E`tesam al-Molk*. ed. Manuchehr Mahmudi (Tehran, 1351/1972), p. 104.
[201] Serena, *Hommes*, p. 135.
[202] E`temad al-Saltaneh, Mirza Hasan Khan, *Ruznameh-ye Khaterat*. ed. Iraj Afshar (Tehran: Amir Kabir, 1345/1966), p. 192.
[203] Serena, *Hommes*, p. 135-36.
[204] Landor, *Across*, vol. 2, p. 182, vol. 1, p. 208; .
[205] Schlimmer, *Terminologie*, p. 8. (q.v. abortifs; also *althea officinalis*); Polak, *Persien*, vol. 1, pp. 217-18. As to asafetida see Floor, *Agriculture*, pp. 485-90.
[206] Neligan, "Public Health," part III, p. 742.

Barrenness was not women's only problem. Skinniness (*hezal* or *lagheri*) was also a disaster for Persian women and it was a cause for divorce. Men desired round, fat women. Merrit-Hawkes remarked, "whilst the European and Persian ideas about men are the same, they differ with regard to women, for the Persians haven't any more admiration for the slim women than we have for the fat. Legs which we consider elephantine some Persians consider worthy of a poem."[207] Skinny women, therefore, went to doctors to be helped. Persian physicians were greatly interested in this issue. Modern Persian medical treatises proposed untenable theories and preposterous remedies, according to Schlimmer. Many drugs were prescribed, the most popular one for idiopathic skinniness was the fat of a camel's hump, taken every day, at fixed times and at fixed quantities (2 to 3 grains/day). Local physicians assured Schlimmer that they had success with this treatment. Sarcocolla also was used. Schlimmer had seen thin women grow fatter by long-term use of cod-liver oil or of pulverized stearine, which he had prescribed, with success, for a long time in case of scrophula and beginning tuberculosis.[208]

Because most mothers were still children there arose a myriad of problems, both psychological and medical. Dr. Morton opined that, "Child marriages have been responsible for an untold amount of suffering, often bringing lifelong misery to women from the resulting complications."[209]

Many women, as well as men, also suffered from hysteria or neurasthenia due to their cloistered life in urban areas. Persian doctors prescribed rennet (*mayeh-ye panir*), preferably from a rabbit.[210] How bad this situation could be is clear from a report by Lady Sheil. "This reminds me of a curious circumstance which I heard relative to the women of the upper classes of Tabreez. Instead of being stricken with fear at the rumour of these scourges, these capricious ladies hail with glee the approach of cholera or plague, which to them brings freedom and release from monotony. Wearied with every-day life, they joyfully prepare to quit the city and seek refuge in the yeïlâks (the high summer mountain lands), in which and in tent-life all Persians delight."[211] For the same reason many women developed imaginary diseases just to get a visit from a doctor and see a new face, or even better, to have a discussion with a new person, as will be discussed in what follows. There

---

[207] Merritt-Hawkes, *Persia*, p. 59. Mirza Abu'l-Hasan Khan told the Prince of Wales, "I like women as plump and as tall as a cypress tree.... Thin women do not atttract me at all." Mirza Abu'l-Hasan Khan. *A Persian at the Court of King George 1809-10. The Journal of Mirza Abul Hassan Khan.* translated and edited by Margaret Morris Cloake (London: Barrie & Jenkins, 1988), p. 131

[208] Schlimmer, *Terminologie*, pp. 32 (*ferbeh shodan* or to fatten up), 305 (q.v. graisse de la bosse); Serena, *Hommes et Choses*, p. 136; Yonan, *Persian Women*, p. 86; Shahri, *Tarikh*, vol. 4, p. 327. On the various aspects of the body and their appreciation see Jozani, *La beauté*, pp. 74-76, and skinniness as seen by popular Persian culture and the remedies to cure this problem, Ibid. pp. 93-97.

[209] Morton, *A Doctor's Holiday*, pp. 216, 235; Polak, *Persien*, vol. 1, p. 217f.

[210] Hume-Griffith, *Behind the Veil*, pp. 161-62; Rice, *Persian Women*, p. 256; Schlimmer, *Terminologie*, p. 97 (q.v. caillette); Morton, *A Doctor's Holiday*, p. 216; Drouville, *Voyage*, vol. 2, p. 167. Wilson, S.G. *Persian Life and Customs* (New York: Fleming. H. Revell, 1895), p. 262 related the story of a young girl who feigned madness because she had been married against her will.

[211] Sheil, *Glimpses*, p. 93.

also were real reasons to see a doctor, for "many people, often women, are injured in fighting with each other, generally over very small matters."[212] In Tehran, in the 1920s, hysteria was one of the diseases listed as a cause of death among its population.[213] The newspaper *Tarbiyat* published several article about the disorder to acquaint its readers with its cause, the symptoms, and treatment and how particular behavior could make it worse.[214]

Finally, diarrhea was quite common, among both adults and children. It occurred mainly during the summer due to excessive consumption of fruit, and when it became chronic it was difficult to treat. It was a main cause of infant death.[215]

DARD-E DEL

There was also "that universal, but somewhat vague complaint entitled *dard-i-dil* (heartache)."[216] Indeed, in Memoirs of contemporaries you read about authors or other personalities being indisposed for unclear reasons. For example, E`tesam al-Molk, noted that he did not feel well and had *dard-e del*; it was a severe case. "I drank some oxymel (*sekanjebin*), warm water and salt, and then vomited, and felt better."[217] Similarly, headache was treated in the same way. `Eyn al-Saltaneh wrote in his Diary that the weather was cold and that he had a severe headache. "However much snuff I took I did not sneeze. Smelling some essence of vinegar (*sarkeh*) did not help. Later I sneezed and I felt better. The next day I still had a headache. I took a purgative (*moshel*; *i.e.*, a medicine that carries off the phlegm) known as *sadliz* (Seidlitz salt), which is a hot (*jush*) medicine; I took three *khorak*s [*i.e.*, an unspeficied dosage]. Later the pain became less."[218] E`temad al-Saltaneh

---

[212] Rice, *Persian Women*, p. 259; Ibid., *Mary Bird*, p. 118.
[213] Gilmour, *Rapport*, pp. 65-66.
[214] *Tarbiyat*, Index q.v. *Saksakeh*, *Histeri*.
[215] Baker, "A few remarks," p. 324. On the treatment of baby disorders see Jozani, *La beauté*, pp. 99-104.
[216] Sykes, *Through Persia*, pp. 142, 146; see also Safari, *Ardabil*, vol. 3, p. 483, who writes that in Ardabil this disorder was called *sanji* and classed as a stomach disorder (see Ibid., vol. 3, p. 490 with a sample of a prescription against this disorder)
[217] E`tesam al-Molk, *Safarnameh*, p. 166.
[218] `Eyn al-Saltaneh, *Ruznameh*, vol. 1, p. 332. "A Seidlitz powder was, in fact, two powders — one wrapped in blue paper and one in white paper. The powder in the blue paper, containing sodium potassium tartrate and sodium bicarbonate, was thoroughly dissolved in half a pint (275ml) of water and the contents of the white paper, tartaric acid, added. The resulting solution was drunk while it effervesced. Hooper's Medical Dictionary (1839) stated: The diseases for which this water is recommended are crudities of the stomach, hypochondriasis, amenorrhoea, and the anomalous complaints succeeding the cessation of the catamenia (menstruation), oedematous tumours of the legs in literary men, haemorrhoidal affections, and scorbutic eruptions. Synonyms for magnesium sulphate have included Seidlitz salt as well as Epsom salt." See for further details, the following website, http://www.pharmj.com/Editorial/20011222/christmas/seidlitz.html. A sneeze is a bad omen; however, "a second sneeze immediately following counteracts the evil nature of a single sneeze, and is often, at all events by foreigners, simulated." Rice, *Persian Women*, p. 248 and in particular Donaldson, Bess Allen. *The Wild Rue. A Study of Muhammadan Magic and Folklore in Iran* (London: Luzac & Co, 1938), pp. 182-83. When Mozaffar al-Din Shah en route to a racing event, to which the entire diplomatic community had been invited, sneezed and could not sneeze a second time he postponed the event till after his second sneeze, according to De Lorey, Eustace & Sladen, Douglas. *Queer Things About Persia* (Philadelphia-London: J.B. Lippincot Co, 1907), p.

had a similar experience. He wrote, "I suffered from distemper (*mazaj*) due to the taking of a purgative. I took 12 *methqal*s (55.2 grams) of sugar. It did not help. Then I took 20 *methqal*s (92 grams) of *shirkhesht*. I took it seven times, and it helped."[219] E`tesam al-Molk took a similar medicine. "I drank oxymel (*sekanjebin*) because I had a head-ache (*soda`*)."[220] Basir al-Molk, when he felt down, took ginger (*zanjabil*).[221] When the British diplomat Eastwick felt a bit parched after a day's outing, and possibly somewhat feverish as he stated later, he asked for some rice congee to quench his thirst. "Then I discovered that the cook had half filled the glass with salt! Such is the nursing that sick men find in Persia."[222] What Eastwick did not know was that the cook just had given him a standard restorative or pick-me-upper. For example, E`temad al-Saltaneh reported in his Diary that "To-day I took 14 *methqal*s [64.4 grams] of salt and two *methqal*s [9.4 grams] of *shirkhesht*." He also ate watermelon, and then had the runs. As a result, E`temad al-Saltaneh "became so weak that if I had not taken an egg and wine I would have fainted."[223]

PSYCHIC DISORDERS

Insanity (*jonun* or *divanegi*) was not common in Qajar Persia. In fact, according to Schlimmer, there were fewer mentally ill people in Persia than in Europe, relatively speaking. He had only seen a handful.[224] However, according to Dr. Emmeline Stuart, the insane were numerous in the early twentieth century.[225] There was no lunatic asylum in Persia until 1918, or thereabouts. Psychic disorders were thought to be due to supernatural interference, *i.e.*, demon possession or other spiritual intervention. In Astarabad, for example, centennial lime trees were supposed to bewitch people who would stand under their spreading boughs after sunset. "Half-witted people are pointed out among the population, and the Astarabadi will tell you, with a grave shake of the head, that 'that is what comes of standing under such-and-such a tree after night-fall.'"[226] The demonic nature of psychic affliction determined the manner of treatment that psychic persons received. "Idiots and harmless, being looked upon as persons of particular sanctity, are allowed to wander about unmolested; while the unfortunates suffering from acute mania are confined in dark cellars, manacled, starved, and beaten, till death soon terminates their sufferings."[227] Idiots remained in their homes with their family, because they were not considered dangerous. In fact, they were considered to be the innocents of God, and when they spoke gibberish it might be a message from God, and therefore

---

326; Powell, E.A. *By camel and car to the peacock throne* (New York: The Century Company, 1923), pp. 320-21; Stark, *The Valley*, p. 283; Linton, *Persian Sketches*, p. 12.

[219] E`temad al-Saltaneh, *Ruznameh*, p. 383.

[220] E`tesam al-Molk, *Safarnameh*, p. 178.

[221] Basir al-Molk Sheybani. *Ruznameh-ye Khaterat*. eds. Iraj Afshar and Mohammad Rasul Daryagasht (Tehran: Donya-ye Ketab, 1374/1995), p. 420.

[222] Eastwick, *Journal*, vol. 2, p. 175.

[223] E`temad al-Saltaneh, *Ruznameh*, p. 521.

[224] Schlimmer, *Terminologie*, p. 26

[225] Stuart, Emmeline M. *Doctors in Persia* (London: CMS, n.d.) p. 23

[226] O'Donovan, *The Merv Oasis*, vol. 1, pp. 186-87.

[227] Wills, *Persia*, pp. 80-91; Schlimmer, *Terminologie*, p. 26 (q.v. alienation); Polak, *Persien*, vol. 2, p. 326.

worth listening to.²²⁸ When visiting Key Khosrow Beg, the local Jaf chief in his camp at Lake Zeribar (Kurdistan), Rich was exposed to

> some Persian singing by two Mullas. Some Indian Fakeers were present; and an elderly woman perfectly naked, but very quiet and well behaved. It was a disgusting sight. She is subject to the epilepsy, and was once mad, when she threw off her clothes and took to the mountains, where she lived for some years in a perfect state of wilderness. She was at last reclaimed, and is now quiet, but cannot be persuaded to put on clothes. She sometimes visits Sulimania, where she walks about the streets in a state of perfect nudity.²²⁹

Frey Stark met a half-wit among the Lurs, who had a better life than in an asylum. She remarked that, "such people are treated with tenderness by the tribesmen. This specimen had just had a wife found for him, the young man told me with a delighted amusement."²³⁰

However, mad persons usually were dealt with in a harsh manner. Ella Sykes was quite explicit about their treatment and lot. "Lunatics meet with no mercy in Persia. These unfortunates are put in the stocks, and their hands fastened with chains to the wall above their heads; they are alternatively beaten and starved, with the laudable intention of driving the devil out of them; they are dowsed with a decoction of herbs poured over them when violently roused from their slumbers by the yells of their misguided friends; and they are confined in horrible dungeons."²³¹ The idea was that illnesses such as epilepsy were caused by jinns and devils, and the aim of the treatment was to break their influence over the afflicted person, so that the patient could recover.²³²

> For the insane, and all suffering from striking nervous symptoms, medicine is considered of but little value. Here spirits or devils are manifestly present, and to treat these genii something more spiritual than ordinary medicae must be used. For those possessed of a devil (any form of insanity, epilepsy, chorea, etc.) one of the first things to try is to get from a prayer doctor the first chapter of the Koran, written seven times, with musk and saffron on the inside of some vessel, after which it is washed off with pure water, and this is given to the patient to drink. If this fails, a little yarn that has been spun by a young girl is taken and a seven-fold cord is made with it. The ninety-eighth chapter of the Koran must be read seven times and then this cord is knotted and fastened to the arm of the patients. There are many Nestorian Christian churches whose departed saints after whom the churches are named, enjoy the reputation of curing these

---

²²⁸ Cochran, "Treatment," p. 105.
²²⁹ Rich, Claude James. *Narrative of a Residence in Koordistan ... and of a visit to Shirauz and Persepolis*. 2 vols. (London: James Duncan, 1836), vol. 1, p. 190; for naked deranged man in Kazerun, see Pirzadeh, *Safarnameh*, vol. 2, p. 421. For what seems to be a similar case of a deranged naked woman see Alexander, *Travels*, p. 196. For a deranged European, who even got away with lifting women's veils in the street see de Gobineau, *Trois Ans*, vol. 1, pp. 241-44.
²³⁰ Stark, *The Valley*, p. 82.
²³¹ Sykes, *Persia and its People*, p. 340.
²³² Rice, *Persian Women*, p. 260; Ibid., *Mary Bird*, pp. 131-33. According to Polak, *Persien*, vol. 2, p. 327 epilepsy (*sar`*) frequently occurred.

[psychic] diseases. Even the Muhamadans frequently take their sick to these churches, carrying as an offering a lamb or a sheep, which is sacrificed to the saint, and the patient is locked up for a night in an underground dungeon built for the purpose. It is a fortunate thing that insanity, relatively, is much less frequent than in America, for after the friends have used such means as these described, or others of like value, the patients is allowed to wander where his genii lead, sometimes violent, and again perfectly harmless, sometimes clothed and often entirely nude, followed and taunted by the boys and girls of the towns. Where these patients are known to be very dangerous, they are usually chained to some pillar or post in the house or stable, and remain there till ends their misery.[233]

Dr. Sargis confirms this and described the arrangement at the church of Mar-Sargis, 15 miles west of Urumiyeh. "A narrow door leads downstairs. In a crouching position you may be able to enter here; the room is dark; there are no windows, and no light is brought into this room. The highest point is six feet, the widest about six and half feet. It may be a comfortable grave for the dead, but a poor hospital for the living. Here are brought insane people from all over the country, and after leaving the insane in this place they roll a large stone against the door so there is no way of escape. He will be left there entirely alone two or three days, at the end of which time they either become cured or die. They imagine while the insane are confined in this place, the saint comes and touches them, curing them. In case they die (as about 98 per cent. do), they say the saint must have been out visiting some of his other shrines."[234]

In Tehran, there was a famous panegyricist (*rowzeh-khvan*), Sayyed Abu Taleb Sadr al-Dhakerin, who was very respected, especially among women, and who was also a famous jinn catcher. Hedayat related a case where the sayyed concentrated totally on driving out the jinn from the body of a woman. Finally, after having made movements as if he put his hand a few times in the woman's bosom, he had caught the attention of the jinn, and said, "You are a real villain, you better come out now." He then took the jinn from the woman's breast, and put it in a bottle, which he sealed securely. The woman, who had been standing below the doorway, put an *ashrafi* on the doorstep and left.[235]

Although there is no contemporary description of the procedure, among the Bakhtiyaris, and may be among society at large as well, trephining was still practiced as "treatment of head injuries, mental illness or 'possession.'" in the 1950s. The procedure consisted of

---

[233] Cochran, "Treatment," pp. 106-07; Sykes, *Through Persia*, p. 111-112 ("a Persian afflicted with an epileptic fit is said to be undergoing a beating at the hands of devils."); Safari, *Ardabil*, vol. 3, p. 497. See also Speer, Robert E. *Hakim Sahib, the foreign doctor; a biography of Joseph Plumb Cochran* (New York: Revell, 1911), p. 324. Christians also consulted dervishes with much respect, see de Gobineau, *Les Réligions*, vol. 1, p. 9.
[234] Sargis, "Persia and Her Doctors," pp. 587-88. See also Wigram, *The Cradle*, p. 206 ("inscriptions in the church indicate that under certain circumstances it is allowable to sleep in the *bait shidâni* by proxy.").
[235] Hedayat, *Khaterat*, p. 88.

exposing the cranium, cut the bone, drill or scrape with an instrument to make an opening into the skull. The operation was only done when the patient was conscious.[236]

Not only mental illnesses and epilepsy, but also physical deformities and abnormalities were considered to be a sign of demonic possession or of having been tainted by contact with evil. For example, Hume-Griffith related that the parents of a twelve-year old boy from an outlying village with a harelip came to see him for treatment. Because Persians believed a harelip to be the mark left by the foot of the devil, the boy was known in his village as the little devil. He was successfully operated upon, and the boy happily cried, "I am no longer a little devil."[237] Another case was that of a child with an abnormally big head was believed to be possessed by a demon. "The cure recommended by the native doctor had unfortunately failed in its effect. The prescription had been to leave the child for some hours in an open grave, during which time the malignant spirit would either kill or quit its little victim. The parents fed the child well, and it soon feel asleep in its novel cradle." It awoke feeling not a whit worse or the better, Ella Sykes commented.[238] Among the Nestorian Tiyari tribe in Kurdistan, "when all visits to church of Name fail, the patient is absolutely buried alive. He is prepared for burial exactly as if he were a corpse, borne to the graveyard on a bier, and interred with the full church service. A small opening is left for him to breathe through; and at the end of twenty-four hours, he is carefully resurrected. The nervous shock has often beneficial results; but naturally not always."[239]

Cemeteries seem to have been a cure of choice to treat people believed to be possessed by demons. Among the Bakhtiyaris, "Possession by bad spirits is believed in, and cowardice is attributed to possession. In the latter case medicine is not resorted to, but a *mollah* writes a text from the Koran and binds the paper on the coward's arm. If this does not cure him he must visit a graveyard on the night of the full moon, and pass seven times under the body of one of the sculptured lions on the graves, repeating an Arabic prayer."[240] Among the Jews of Kurdistan and Shiraz, and most likely elsewhere, there was a strong belief in the curative power of amulets, because they believed that illness, somatic and psychological, was caused by a touch of a demon. The disorder could be cured by a charm written or made by a rabbi.[241]

A totally different approach to spirit possession of human beings existed throughout the southern part of Persia from Khuzistan to Baluchistan, where people strongly believed in

---

[236] Roney Jr., James G. "The Occurrence of Trephining Among The Bakhtiari," *Bulletin of the History of Medicine* 28 (1954), pp. 489-91.
[237] Hume-Griffith, *Behind the Veil*, p.141.
[238] Sykes, *Through Persia*, p. 111-112.
[239] Wigram, *The Cradle*, p. 308.
[240] Bird, *Journeys*, vol. 2, p. 75. For the same reason *piyaz* (onion), `onsul` (wild onion), or *piyaz-e Gurestan* (cemetery onion), was part of the Persian medical arsenal. It was thus called, because "it sometimes grows among the tombs. This plant is known to the Persian apothecaries, and used, if I recollect right, as an astringent." De Bode, C.A. *Travels in Luristan and Arabistan*. 2 vols. (London: J. Madden & Co, 1845), vol. 1, p. 377.
[241] Sabar, *The Folk Literature*, pp. 189-90; Loeb, *Outcaste*, pp. 220-21.

metaphysical forces (*zar*; *gowat* in Baluchistan). These spirits were like invisible winds (*bad* in Persian) with the ability to speak a human language. The groups of people most affected by the *zar* spirits were male and female descendants of African slaves, usually lower class people working in palm groves or as sailors. Those who were possessed by one of these winds were called *Ahl-e Hava* (people of the air). To drive out the spirits the adherents of the *zar* belief performed a ceremony during which they sang special songs and beat the drum (*dohol*), while supporting this with rhythmic movements of head and body to ward off evil spirits from the body.[242]

The *zar* approach was a form of less violent demonic exorcism, which was also practiced in Persia. Ella Sykes reported about the case of a Persian woman who was indisposed, due to a demon, it was believed. A general (*sartip*), who was a reputed exorcist, did the following. "The procedure adopted was to light dozens of little lamps and place them all around the divan on which the patient lay, and the *sartip* then asked her again and again what she saw, but the answer was always the same, 'Nothing, but lamps.'" The general was desperate and thus called an old woman whom he had cured from a similar affliction to assist him. He asked her what she saw. She said that she saw the devil. He had flown past the house and had been beguiled by the lady's beauty. The general told the old woman that she should tell the devil that he had to release the lady. The old woman told the general that the devil refused. The general then became very angry and told the woman to tell the devil that if he did not leave immediately he would turn him into a Moslem. The devil departed immediately. Unfortunately, the lady's situation did not improve. Finally an English doctor cured her.[243]

It also could happen that someone with the evil eye wanted to be cured. Such a request was made to British missionaries in Kurdistan. The men of the afflicted person's village told that, "if he looked at a crock of milk, it upset; if at a sheep, the wolf got it; if at a child, it was likely enough to tumble into the fire. They were quite fair about the matter, fully recognizing that it was the poor fellow's misfortune, not his fault." Although they had Nestorian charms against the evil eye the missionaries felt it was not proper to use them and sent the villagers on their way. Among the Nestorians there were so-called 'books of remedies' and collections of charms, whose texts were almost identical to those found on Babylonian tablets. One of the charms the missionaries possessed had an invocation of the Archangel Gabriel against 'that light and vile daughter of perdition' with power to send it away 'into the desolate land, where cocks crow not and foot of

---

[242] For more more information on the *zar* phenomenon see Riyahi, `Ali. *Zar va Bad va Baluch*, (Tehran: Tahhuri, 1356/1977); Hamidi, Hoseyn. *Hasht Behesht*, (Tehran: Mahur, 1996); During, Jean. "African Winds and Muslim Djinns. Trance, Healing and Devotion in Baluchistan" in *1997 Yearbook for Traditional Music*, Dieter Christensen, ed. (UNESCO, International Council for Traditional Music, 1997); Darvishi, Mohammad Reza *Baluchistân* (Tehran: Mo'asseseh-ye Farhangi va Honari-ye Mahur, 1378); Sa`edi, Gholam Hoseyn. *Ahl-e Hava* (Tehran: Daneshgah, 1342/1963); Littman, Enno. *Arabische Geitsterbeschwörungen aus Ägypten* (Leipzig, Harrassowitz, 1950), and Bolukbashi, `Ali, "Ahl-e Hava," *Dar al-Ma`aref-e Bozorg-e Eslami*, vol. 10, pp. 478-81.
[243] Sykes, *Persia and its People*, p. 338.

beasts tread not, there to walk up and down in dry places, seeking rest and finding none.'"[244]

From the above it is clear that Qajar Persia was an unhealthy place to live in, but not more so than many other countries at that time, including European ones. Ebrahimnejad has suggested that there was nevertheless an increased prevalence of cholera epidemics, which triggered political consciousness and stimulated medical science in Persia. The problem with this statement is that we do not know whether the nineteenth century had more epidemics than the preceding centuries.[245] It therefore may also have been the presence of European physicians at the royal court that gave rise to this higher awareness of the need to take action about the public health situation in Persia.

---

[244] Wigram, *The Cradle*, pp. 328-29.
[245] We are better informed as to the situation in the Ottoman Empire, see Panzac, D. *La peste dans l'empire Ottoman 1700-1850* (Louvain, 1985). There is no similar book or article describing the situation in pre-Qajar Persia.

PUBLIC HYGIENE

The spread of the various endemic and other diseases that prevailed in Qajar Persia was facilitated by the presence of many insect vectors of disease as well as by unsanitary food and water supplies. Flies, fleas, lice, bugs, mites, and mosquitoes were omnipresent and no measures were taken to prevent their occurrence and their contact with human beings. Though many houses had latrines, refuse and excreta disposal was done in an unhygienic manner and, as a result, the towns and villages were often like open cesspools. Also, the latrines were not dry thus offering a source of fly breeding. In the rural areas there were no latrines. As a result, the excreta and other contaminants came into contact with drinking and washing water, which became a carrier of infectious diseases.

The problem was made worse by the lack of personal hygiene that also contributed to the spread of disease. The structural problem underlying the spread of disease was the lack of understanding what caused disease resulting in an almost total absence of personal hygiene. Forbes-Leith, who for years had intimate contact with the rural population as their only source of modern medical assistance, wrote, "people were entirely ignorant of the elementary principles of hygiene, and most of them lived their whole lives in surroundings of indescribable filth. Their deeply ingrained and totally false ideas on all matters relating to health and sickness were extremely difficult to dispel, and an endeavour to improve their conditions proved a difficult job."[1] Moreover, many peasants had "only one suit of clothes, which consisted of the one they wore as children."[2] Furthermore, "among the common people the clothes are only washed once a year, and then in cold water, with the root of a very sticky soap wort."[3] Also, soap was not always available, and of varying quality. In the rural areas, where soap was not always available, peasants made use of a variety of products.[4] Even in major towns such as Tehran in 1920, the sale of soap was limited to a few fixed locations. Of the total of 21 shops there were 16 in the Bazaar quarter, three in 'Owdlajan and one in Sangalaj and one in the Hasanabad quarter.[5] There were, of course, itinerant traders who also sold soap, but this configuration shows that soap was not a very accessible product. Clothes' washing was further limited by the scarcity of water. People's clothes were therefore crawling with vermin. The Prussian ambassador von Minutoli was an avid collector of insects. When in Miyaneh, he asked one

---

[1] Forbes-Leith, *Checkmate*, p. 88; Lichtwadt, "Western Medicine," p. 237 ("Sanitation was primitive (to put it mildly) and knowledge of hygiene was nil.").
[2] Forbes-Leith, *Checkmate*, p. 90.
[3] Bird, *Journeys*, vol. 2, p. 75.
[4] Floor, Willem. *The Traditional Crafts of Qajar Iran* (Costa Mesa: Mazda, 2003), pp. 313-21; Stark, *The Valley*, pp. 22 (the Lurs had no soap), 208 (even soap was an unknown luxury in the Shah Rud valley), 216 (the usual absence of soap in the village).
[5] Baladiyeh, *Dovommin Salnameh*, pp. 78-79. The situation was similar in Qazvin, where in the Meydan-e Gosfand quarter there were two soap sellers (*sabuni*) for a total of its seven neighborhoods. Sadvandian, Cyrus. "The Inhabitants of Meydan-Gusfand", *The Journal of the Middle East Studies Society at Columbia University* 1 (1987), p. 53.

of its inhabitants to find him the dreaded Miyaneh bug. The man opened his girdle sash and immediately took out a dozen from its folds.[6]

The water that Persians used for drinking, food processing, and clothes washing purposes was often heavily polluted and a carrier of infectious diseases. Most houses had a water basin that teemed with mosquitoes, but health officials found that "householders are reluctant to permit any preventive measures."[7] Moreover, because of Islamic precepts, "These primitive people have it firmly ingrained in their minds that any water that is running is pure and fit to drink." For example, a corpse [that had died of enteric fever] was washed in a stream and a few yards downstream "women filled their brass storage pots with water for domestic use."[8] Vambery described that the following scene shocked him:

> In the center of the yard of the caravansary is placed a basin full of water, originally intended for the performance of ritual lavations, but, I saw that whilst at one side of the reservoir some were washing their dirty things, others placed half-tanned skins into the same water for soaking, and a third was cleansing his baby, there were standing men on the opposite side of the basin, gravely performing their religious washings with the identical water, and one of them, who must have been thirsty indeed, crouched down and eagerly drank of the dark green fluid I could not repress at the sight a manifestation of loathing. A Persian, standing near, immediately confronted me and reproved me for my ignorance. He asked me if I did not know that according to the *Sheriat* (the holy law) a quantity of water, in excess of a hundred twenty pints, turns blind, that is, it cannot become soiled or unclean.[9]

What the European observers failed to understand was that Moslem law does not refer to biological or chemical purity or cleanliness of water, but rather its ritualistic aspect of purification. The washing of the body had nothing to do with hygiene; it was a religious act, done for a religious purpose. The fact that the water was contaminated was unfortunate, but did not negate the religious import of the rite. Nowadays that Moslems can make sure that the water they use is really clean they can have both the religious and health benefits by practicing their purification rite.[10]

---

[6] Brugsch, H. *Die Reise der K.K. Gesandtschaft nach Persien 1861-1862*, 2 vols. (Berlin: J.C. Hinrichs, 1863), vol. 1, p. 182.
[7] Government of Great Britain, *Trade Report 1920-21*, p. 1-2.
[8] Forbes-Leith, *Checkmate*, p. 91; Wigram, W.A. and Wigram, T.A. *The Cradle of Mankind. Life in Eastern Kurdistan* (London: A&C Black, 1936), p. 207. For caricatures of this situation see, for example, *Shekufeh*, p. 44 (year 1, nr. 11, 12 Rajab 1331/June 17, 1913).
[9] Vambéry, Arminius. *His Life and Adventures* (London: Fisher Unwin, 1884), p. 57; see also Powell, E.A. *By Camel and Car to the Peacock Throne* (New York: The Century Company, 1923), pp. 237-38 (a brook with pillowogs, a discarded shoe, and a dead cat served as the source of watersupply for a rural tea-house); Benn, *An Overland*, p. 156 ("a huge green pond of stagnant water, which is, at one and the same time, the drinking supply, the wash-tub, and the refuse pool of the inhabitants.").
[10] Heiler, *Erscheinungsformen*, pp. 177-78

Given the lack of knowledge about public health conditions and requirements among the Persian administrative, medical, and religious authorities as well as the traditional notions about the cause of disease among the professional medical class and the population in general, one could not expect otherwise. Persians also had no idea about the danger of contagious diseases. They did not isolate persons affected and small children "covered with the scales of confluent small-pox are allowed to play with others."[11] Cemeteries were found right in the middle of the towns, and the corpses were not buried deep enough, because of religious law. It happened that corpses became partially uncovered and the air was polluted with their putrefaction. The situation was worse with the space set aside for the storage (*emanat*) of corpses that were to be transported to one of the holy sites. The practice to transport dead bodies to the Holy Cities (Karbala, Mashad, Qom) was a public health disaster. The storage space was not properly closed off, and corpses were not embalmed or otherwise treated. They were just packed in felt and put on the back of mules.[12] The situation was even worse en route and when the corpses arrived at the shrine for burial. Taj al-Saltaneh described the sight she saw during her visit of Qom. "By the time they reached the shrine of Ma`suma, the coffins were in pieces, the shrouds ripped to shreds, and the corpses' heads and limbs broken. ... There were so many corpses piled atop one another in the graves that there was no room for others. So they had to open the graves and lay the new corpse on the others and cover them all with a little dirt."[13]

Regular cleaning of the body would have gone a long way to improve personal hygiene. Although Islamic law prescribed the washing after sexual intercourse this was only possible in those locations where a public bath was available. In many parts of the rural areas there were not such facilities, and people therefore did not wash themselves completely.[14]

A positive development was that the number of houses per unit of bath had decreased in Tehran, thus potentially improving the problem. In 1852, there was only one bath for 148 houses in Tehran, while this was one bath for 89 houses in 1902, thus, an increase of 40% in fifty years. At the same time, buildings that served the needs of the soul fell significantly during the same period. The number of shops serving the population also seem to have increased although the figure given (1.72) in Table 4 cannot be right, because it would mean that every third dwelling was a shop.[15]

---

[11] Baker, "A few remarks," p. 323.
[12] Baker, "A few remarks," p. 326; Greenfield, *Verfassung*, p. 272; Benn, Edith Fraser. *An Overland Trek From India* (London: Longmans & Co, 1909), p. 218 (graveyard, as usual, occupied a site at the head of the water).
[13] Taj al-Saltaneh. *Crowning Anguish*, p. 296.
[14] If there was no public bathhouse "the women find a warm place in the stables, where they take jars of hot water and spend a few hours bathing and chatting." Yonan, *Persian Women*, p. 104; see also Stark, *The Valley*, p. 77.
[15] Ettehadieh, Mansureh."Patterns in urban development; the growth of Tehran (1852-1903), in Bosworth, Edmund and Hillenbrand, Carole eds. *Qajar Iran. Political, Social and Cultural Change 180-1925* (Edinburgh, Edinburgh UP, 1983), p. 208.

Table 4: The number of houses per unit of bath, shop, *masajed va madares* and *takaya* in Tehran 1852-1902

Building type	1269/1852-53	1286/1869-70	1320/1902-03
One bath per	148 houses	105 houses	89 houses
One shop per	21 houses	-	1.72 houses
One *masjed va madresh* per	65 houses	116 houses	203 houses
One *takiyeh* per	140 houses	280 houses	378 houses

Source: Ettehadieh, "Patterns in urban development," p. 208.

There were, of course, differences per city quarter as shown in Table 5. The Dowlat quarter was a new one and therefore shows the highest change, and it was also a very large quarter, bigger than the other ones.

Table 5: Changes in the number of baths in Tehran between 1269-1320/1852-1903

Quarter	1269	1320	Change	% of change
`Owdlajan	30	53	+23	+76%
Chalmeydan	28	16	- 12	- 42%
Dowlat	-	38	+38	+100%
Sangalaj	59	33	- 26	- 44%
Bazar	27	30	+ 3	+11%
Ark	14	-	-	-

Source: Ettehadieh, "Patterns in urban development," p. 205.

However, having enough bathhouses was not necessarily a condition for better public health. According to Dr. Edward Dodson of the CMS in Kerman, "As poorer people seldom bathe their entire bodies, sweat accumulates, both in the torrid summer and, as clothes are seldom changed, also during the freezing winter weather. Clothes are changed when the *hammam*, or public bath, is visited; then everything is put on fresh. But many, having no clean clothes, do not go to the public baths for months. Unfortunately, it is quite a usual thing to go after acquiring an infectious disease. Some of the germs may be destroyed but many are still active, and thus the disease is transmitted. Ignorance makes illness an inescapable hazard."[16]

Thus, the public baths that people used once in every two or three weeks, when accessible, were not the ideal of public health either. For public baths constituted the ideal method for spreading diseases such as fungus, trachoma, skin and respiratory diseases and intestinal disorders. In fact, it was one of the major sources of infection, for "the water was only changed about three times a year, so the rapid way in which disease spread was hardly to be wondered at."[17] Also, the mistaken belief that running water was safe and not polluted according to Islamic law contributed to the spread of disease. Often running water was

---

[16] Morton, *A Doctor's Holiday*, p. 217-18.
[17] Forbes-Leith, *Checkmate*, p. 89.

already polluted before if reached a village.[18] Also, doctors usually prescribed an enema with water from the bathhouse.[19]

Concomitant with a general ignorance of, and thus disregard for, personal hygiene, housing, whether in towns or villages, generally also was unhygienic. From a public health point of view the hovels, huts, dwellings, homes, houses or whatever label one wants to attach to these constructions that gave shelter to most Persian families and its animals were a disaster. They were all filthy and full of vermin. There was no sanitation whatsoever. In rural areas, in many cases the 'latrine' was referred to as *kenar-e ab*, or 'at the water', thus ensuring the pollution of the water source. Inside the dwelling, in wintertime, man and animals lived together, and the soil was saturated with urine. Finally, there was the inevitable vermin-breeding cover over the open fireplace (*korsi*) in the middle of the dwelling.[20]

Outside the dwelling the situation was also very unhealthy. Dead animals were thrown at 30 paces from the village for the dogs, jackals, and the crows. Entrails and other slaughter were left rotting in front of the houses. People seldom had outhouses, and usually relieved themselves in the open. Villages that had a public bath were not necessarily better off from a hygienic point of view, for the bath was a breeding ground for all kinds of diseases. The water was only occasionally refreshed and was used by everybody. Also, village women came into regular contact with dung, when making the store of winter fuel, which consisted of a combination of animal dung and straw and constituted a health risk.[21] The situation in pastoral areas may have been slightly better, because the nomadic groups moved most of the year. Nevertheless, among the Bakhtiyaris, "The skin maladies and some of the eye maladies come from dirt, and the parasites which are its offspring," according to Isabella Bird.[22]

The situation in the urban areas was not different. Most houses resembled those of the rural areas. Only the houses of the rich and the middle class were better built and more spacious. But, more importantly, the very organization of urban life was a public health disaster.

> There was no organization whatsoever to deal with public health, which was left to look after itself. The towns were crowded, badly built, and devoid of roads other than gaps between the houses. Inside the towns there was no water supply

---

[18] Watelin, *La Perse*, p. 80.

[19] Greenfield, *Verfassung*, p. 273.

[20] Floyer, *Unexplored Baluchistan*, p. 421; Binder, *Au Kurdistan*, p. 351, Johnson, Lieut. Col. *A Journey from India to England through Persia, Georgia, Russia, Poland and Prussia in the Year 1817* (London: Longman, Hurst, Rees, Orme, and Brown, 1818), p. 86; Harris, *From Batum*, pp. 157-158; Polak, J.E. "Beitrag zu den agrarischen Verhältnissen in Persien", *Mittheilungen der K.-K. Geogr. Gesellschaft* VI (1862), p. 121; De Morgan, J. *Mission Scientifique en Perse. Etudes Géographiques* 5 vols. (Paris, 1894), vol. 1, pp. 253, 255; Heinrich, *Auf Panthersuche*, pp. 69, 76.

[21] Binder, *Au Kurdistan*, pp. 352-353; see also Anonymous, *Woman and Her Saviour in Persia by a Returned Missionary* (Boston: Gould and Lincoln, 1865), p. 96; Wilson, *Persian Life*, p. 167; Moore, Benjamin Burges. *From Moscow to the Persian Gulf* (New York: G.P. Putnam's Sons, 1915), p. 333.

[22] Bird, *Journeys*, vol. 2, p. 75.

other than the rainwater tanks in the houses, and arrangements for conservancy would be complimented when described by the adjective primitive. Refuse, excreta, human and animal, were deposited or thrown indiscriminately into the mud lanes that separated the houses from each other and are generously distributed over the town by the traffic that passes through these lanes. Many of the houses had their drains opening up to the lanes; in other pits in the houses were used for this purpose and the putrifying contents of these pits, often the accumulated filth of years, drained into such wells as exist and sent their stench to the air of the houses and the town. No records of births and deaths appear to be kept.[23]

Although the above situation referred to the town of Bushire, the situation was not different in any other Persian town.[24] Some towns, such as Shushtar, even Persians considered to be filthy.[25] "As in practically every other town of the Persian Caspian provinces, sewers are unknown at Barfrush" as a result there was much typhoid and smallpox, and also outbreaks of cholera.[26] The situation inside the houses also contributed to this unhygienic situation. A typical situation was where "The latrine was a hole in the ground, which lead, by a sloping shoot, to a pit about 12 to 20 feet deep. When the pit was full it was either dug out and carried away to be used as manure or emptied by rope and bucket and dumped in the street or some open space. In poor people's houses the pits often were not emptied for a long time and were allowed to overflow. The sewage then polluted the ground water, from which people drew their water supply through nearby wells."[27]

---

[23] Government of Great Britain, *Trade Report 1921-22*, pp. 1-2; Ibid., *Trade Report 1920-21*, pp. 1-2 ("Sanitation is practically non-existent. Fitful efforts at cleaning the streets occur from time to time with little result. Drainage is non-existent and during the rains each street is a conduit unto itself."); Ibid., *Trade Report 1913-14*, p. 1 ("The practice of throwing the foulest garbage into these thoroughfares.")

[24] Smith, Major. "Report on the condition of the working classes in Bushire," November 11, 1870, in Government of Great Britain, *Accounts &Papers*, vol. 68 (1871), p. 407; "Report by consul-general Jones on the condition of the industrial classes in Tabrees", Tabriz October 15, 1870, in Government of Great Britain, *Acounts &Papers*, vol. 68 (1871), p. 419; "Report by Mr. Jenner on the condition of the working classes in Persia," Tehran, 2 November 1870, in Government of Great Britian, *Accounts and Papers* [A & P], vol. 68 (1871), p. 398; De Penisse, Comte. *La Russie, la Perse, l'Inde – souvenirs de voyage 1865-1866* (Paris, 1867), p. 110. For the situation in Tehran see Willem Floor, "Sécurité, Circulation et Hygiene dans les rues de Teheran a l'époque Qajar," in: in Adle, Charyar et Hourcade, Bernard eds. *Téhéran Capitale bicentenaire*, Institut Francais de Recherche en Iran, 1992 (Bibliotheque iranienne, vol. 37), pp. 173-198; for Abadan see Neligan, "Public Health," part II, p. 690.

[25] E`temad al-Saltaneh, Mirza Hasan Khan. *Mer'at al-Boldan* 4 vols in 3. ed. `Abdol-Hoseyn Nava'i and Mir Hashem Mohaddeth (Tehran: Daneshgah, 1368/1989), vol. 1, p. 692; Nezam al-Saltaneh Mafi, *Khaterat va Asnad*, vol. 2, p. 58; `Eyn al-Saltaneh, *Ruznameh*, vol. 1, pp. 381 (Hamadan), 651-52 (Tehran); vol. 2, p. 1183 (Qazvin); Najm ol-Molk, `Abdol-Ghaffar. *Safarnameh-ye Khuzestan*. ed. Mohammad Dabir-Siyaqi (Tehran: Elmi, 1342/1963), pp. 13-14 (Borujerd), 21, 133 (Dezful), 27, 133 (Shushtar), 90-91 (Mohammarah, where people used the streets as a public toilet); Asaf al-Dowleh, *Asnad*, vol. 2, p. 124 (general), 174 (once the streets are clean, people gradually would also want to keep streets clean).

[26] *DCR* 4812 (1910-11, p. 4.

[27] Adamec, L. *Historical Gazetteer of Iran*, 4 vols. (Graz: Akademische Verlag, 1981), vol. 2, p. 483.

The streets were stinking and wafting with the odors of decomposing animals and excreta. The uncovered water mains (*jub*s) transported the water with all kinds of pollution, including industrial such as from tanning etc., throughout the city. In 1880, or thereabouts, Naser al-Din Shah had ordered that the streets and squares had to be cleaned and to get the dangerous stuff out of the uncovered water mains,[28] but this royal order did not yield any result, because its execution lapsed after some time. The most effective street cleaners were the street dogs.[29] In other towns, occasional clean up operations were initiated, but these were haphazard and intermittent occurrences.[30]

The removal of refuse of householders, including private and public toilets, was the responsibility of the homeowners. It was, *inter alia*, the task of the *tanzif* department to see to it that homeowners took care of the removal of their refuse. A special group of people, known as *kannas*, made a living of this. They transported the city's waste matter towards the surrounding villages where they sold it as fertilizer. Of course, the government taxed even this despised activity, for sewage removal was a lucrative investment. The right to clean out the public toilets commanded a high price. For example, those of the Shah Mosque in Tehran with 40 toilets had a *sar-qofli* of at least 30,000 tomans per year. It is clear that it was not the sewage men who made a lot of money, but rather those who employed them. In Isfahan there were some 150 *kannas* in the 1870s.[31]

The cause of much illness was attributable to the existing water supply, which in rural areas water was from wells, springs, *qanat*s and/or rivers. All of them were polluted. In the town water was obtained from uncovered water mains (*jub*), wells, *ab-anbar*s (i.e., small rain-water reservoirs) in the courtyards of the houses. The gutters were polluted with refuse and other dross, while the wells and cisterns teemed with mosquitoes. Householders were reluctant to permit any preventive measures, however. They were bolstered in their belief by the mistaken Islamic tenet of faith that running water, or stagnant water of a certain size, will not be polluted by unclean elements. However, this may be true from a religious point of view, but certainly not from a medical scientific one. The basic problem, of course, was that the religious law is concerned with ritual purity, not with medical hygiene. Thus, the washers of the dead, for example, used the same water that other people used for all their daily needs. In 1869, in Tabriz, there were 100 *mordeh-shur*. They were lower-class men and women, who had no idea of hygiene.[32]

---

[28] E'temad al-Saltaneh, *Montazam-e Naseri*, vol. 1, p. 243; Ussher, John. *A Journey from London to Persepolis* (London: Hurst and Blackett, 1865), p. 614.
[29] Greenfield, *Verfassung*, p. 273.
[30] Farmanfarma, Firuz Mirza. *Namehha-ye Hokumati* ed. Fathollah Keshavarzi (Tehran: Sazman-e Asnad-e melli, 1377/1998), p. 93 (Hamadan); Asaf al-Dowleh, *Asnad*, vol. 2, p. 114 (Enzeli at the occasion of the expected visit of a Russian arch-duke in 1870).
[31] Tahvildar, Mirza Hosein Khan. *Joghrafiya-ye Isfahan*, ed. M. Setudeh. (Tehran: Daneshgah, 1342/1963), p. 121, 125; Höltzer, Ernst. *Persien vor 113 Jahren* ed. Mohammad Assemi (Tehran: Vezarat-e Farhang va Honar, 2535/1976), p. 23; Shahri, Ja'far. *Tehran-e Qadim*. 5 vols. (Tehran: Mo'in, 1377/1999), vol. 1, p. 60.
[32] Javadi, Shafi'. *Tabriz va Peyramun* (Tabriz: Bonyad-e Farhang-e Reza Pahlavi, 1350/1971), p. 228; Morton, *A Doctor's Holiday*, p. 221; Alexander, *Travels*, p. 165 (rural house for washing the dead), also Homayun, *Molk-e 'Anbir-amiz*, p. 118 and Keshavarz-Damghan, *Sad Darvazeh*, p. 245.

Food poisoning (salmonellosis, botulism and staphylococcus infection) also occurred due to the absence of hygiene and food preservation as well as the omni-presence of the housefly as a vector. Persians ate many dairy products such as cheese and yogurt (*mast*). Because these were made from boiled milk disease vectors were killed. The problem occurred where yogurt was diluted with polluted water and drunk as sour milk (*dugh*). Furthermore, the consumption of cheese and butter, which products were made from raw milk produced by often sick (t.b.) animals also could cause food poisoning. Vegetables eaten, if not boiled or well washed, were polluted, because of the use of night soil as fertilizer and polluted water for irrigation. Fruit, one of the population's staple foods, was dried on the roof and the dirt ground. Many unwashed hands handled it, because they had to be turned around, and they were not washed, while flies and dust left deposits on them. Also, due to lack of preservation means as well as open-air display (often covered with flies) raw and prepared food also was infected.[33] Whenever the population suffered from undernourishment due to famine or other reasons sickness and epidemics struck the unfortunate affected population, as was the case during the 1917/18 famine.[34]

The diet of the urban poor was very simple; "fruit, and cheese form their usual repast."[35] There was, of course, variety in diet among the various regions of Persia. For example, dates were eaten where they abounded, in the south, but not in the north. "All classes of labourers live very much alike, in the most frugal manner, and a man who earns his 0.5 kran may be taken as an average specimen. His food will be a lump of dates before going to work, some bread (unleavened) and salt fish for dinner, and some boiled rice for supper."[36] The poor seldom ate meat, eggs and milk, because they could not afford it. When the poor could afford to buy meat, they ate "beef, not lamb, usually obtained from slaughtered carcasses of diseased cattle or camels, which is hardly fit for consumption." The butchers only offered beef by special arrangement.[37]

By confining themselves to the above diet, the workmen in this country can just manage to keep body and soul together.[38] The very poor, those without a regular income, lived a hard and desperate life. According to Hajj Sayyah, when describing the situation in Kerman in the 1880s, "Of 100 houses not one has the means to light a night lamp, some even go for some days without bread, and make do with turnip and beets, if they can find them."[39] The very poor only had occasionally had the chance to get a good meal, usually at the occasion of some public or religious holiday. "Further aid is provided through alms. Once a year,

---

[33] Morton, *A Doctor's Holiday*, p. 218; Baker, "A few remarks," p. 324. On fruit preparation and handling see also Willem Floor, *Agriculture in Qajar Iran* (Washington, DC: Mage, 2003), pp. 288, 327.

[34] Barton, James L. *Story of Near East Relief 1915-1930 An Interpretation* (New York: MacMillan, 1930), pp. 95-100, 192-93.

[35] "Report by consul-general Jones," p. 419; Smith, "Report on the condition," p. 402.

[36] Government of Great Britain, "Report …working classes in Bushire," p. 402, see also p. 405.

[37] Adamec, *Historical Gazetteer*, vol. 2, p. 484. There was also much opium addiction in Mashad. Ibid., vol. 2, p. 486.

[38] Great Britain, "Report by Mr. Jenner," p. 397.

[39] Hajj Sayyah, *Khaterat-e Hajj Sayyah,* ed. Hamid Sayyah (Tehran, 1346/1967)p. 164.

during a period of three days the poorest man may sit down to a comfortable dinner, which is furnished to him by the devotees of Hassan and Hossein, which is equivalent in Persia to saying all those who can afford it."[40] Clothing and footwear also were inadequate given temperatures during the winter.[41]

Despite these living conditions and the plethora of diseases that Persians were exposed to many survived their onslaught, and there was even an increase in population, which was mainly due to "the extraordinary power of resistance possessed by the peasants [that] was remarkable."[42] Isabella Bird noticed the same resistance among the nomadic Bakhtiyaris, who "are rigid 'abstainers,' and *arak* is not to be procured in the Bakhtiyari country. This partly accounts for the extreme and almost startling rapidity of the healing of surgical wounds."[43] John Malcolm also noted "the abstemious habits, and consequently healthy state of the body of the patient, often obtain extraordinary credit to the untutored practitioner."[44] Finally, the quick healing of wounds also astonished Polak and other European physicians.[45]

---

[40] Great Britain, 'Report by Jenner," p. 398.
[41] Great Britain, *Trade Report 1915-16*, p. 5. Also, many did not wear shoes Sani` al-Dowleh, Mohammad Hasan Khan (E`temad al-Saltaneh) *Mer'at al-Boldan* 4 vols. (Tehran, 1294-97/1877-80), vol. 1, p. 480. In general, see Polak, *Persien*, vol. 2, pp. 290-348.
[42] Forbes-Leith, *Checkmate*, p. 88.
[43] Bird, *Journeys*, vol. 2, pp. 74-75.
[44] Malcolm, *The History*, vol. 2, p. 534.
[45] Polak, *Persien*, vol. 2, pp. 347-48; Ibid., "Medicinische Briefe," p. 175; Dequevaullier, "Notice," pp. 5, 21; Häntzsche, "Physikalisch-medicinische Skizze," pp. 568-69.

MEDICAL KNOWLEDGE

The kind of traditional medicine practiced in Qajar Persia drew upon three different sources of knowledge. First, there was the Greek, so-called Galenic system (*tebb-e yunani*). It is the one that is invariably presented as the mainstream medical system, although in actual fact it was the least important one of the three systems. However, since it was the system that was practiced by the elite, some of whom wrote theoretical treatises about it, the Galenic system also has drawn most attention of scholarly activity so far.[1] Second, there is the theurgic, magical, or folk medicine (*tebb-e sonnati*). It was the oldest and most important medical system, because everybody practiced it; it was deeply ingrained in popular culture, and it retained many of its pre-Islamic characteristics. It also has received the least attention from the scholarly community, partly because its practitioners left very few written accounts. Third, there was Prophetic medicine (*tebb al-nabi*), which was an attempt to domesticate Galenic and folk medicine by giving it a Moslem veneer, while, at the same time, legitimizing questionable practices, *i.e.*, from an Islamic religious point of view, of folk and Galenic medicine. In the case of Persia, the medical counsel attributed to the Shi`ite Imams, *tebb al-a'emmeh*, was added to the framework of Prophetic medicine. The latter has been better studied than folk medicine. Its importance does not so much lie in its medical message as in providing religious justification for the practice of both Galenic and folk medicine.[2]

Greek medicine (*tebb-e yunani*) had been developed in Greece and had spread throughout the Hellenistic world. Galenic medicine, developed in the second century CE, also reached Persia and beyond. Its heir was Islamic medicine that became the main medical system of knowledge in the Islamic world as well as in Western Europe. In Western Europe this system was replaced by a system of modern medicine based on verifiable scientific principles. However, in the *Dar al-Islam*, and in the case of Qajar Persia (1787-1925), the Islamic-Galenic system continued to be the guiding principle for the formal practitioners of medicine.

The system was characterized by the belief that there are "four elementary constituents of the body. The excess of any one of these elements: blood, bile, phlegm and black bile (the element which produces all skin affections) is in preponderance, the physician's aims is to diminish it by direct means as well as by restricting the food to those articles which are believed to produce that particular element."[3] For the aim is to keep these elements in balance and to seek symmetry; if one element was bringing the system out of balance, its natural opposite element had to be increased as a counter-balance. This meant that

---

[1] See, for example, Elgood, *Medical History*; Browne, E.G. *Arabian Medicine* (Cambridge, Cambridge UP, 1921); Ghani, Qasem. "Tarikh-e Mokhtasar-e Tebb-e Eslam," in *Yaddashtha-ye Doktor Qasem Ghani* 9 vols. ed. Sirus Ghani (Tehran: Zavvar, 1367/89), vol. 7, pp. 10-71; Najmabadi, Mahmud. *Tarikh-e Tebb dar Iran pas az Eslam* (Tehran: Daneshgah, 1353/1974).
[2] In this context it is of interest to note that the entry on "Medical Science" under the lemma "Iran" in the *Dar al-Ma`aref-e Bozorg-e Eslami*, vol. 10, pp. 669-71 only concerns Galenic medicine.
[3] Cochran, James P. "Treatment of the Sick and Insane in Persia," *The American Journal of Insanity* 56 (1899), p. 105.

doctors had to establish whether the illness was hot or cold, and in which degree, and whether the disease proceeded from too much heat or too much cold. Consequently, Persian medicine rested on the axiom that opposites repel each other, *i.e.*, heat must be repelled by cold, and cold by heat.[4] "Besides the hot and cold classes of disease, an additional distinction is made into those of hararet (heat and inflammation) and rutubut (humidity). Bleeding and purging are the remedies of the former, but carried to such excess that they generally terminate the case; while large doses of quinine and powerful aromatics administered in wine, with warm infusions are given for the latter."[5] Finally, Persian physicians had no practical knowledge at all of anatomy, and surgery was hardly practiced and was restricted to bone setting, teeth pulling and cautery. The Galenic doctors or *hakim*s referred these cases to popular healers such as the barber.[6]

The nature of the development and acquirement of knowledge of the Galenic system is also important in this context. Traditionally there had been a difference between theoretical (*nazari*) and practical medicine (`*amali*). The former had, or even developed new, knowledge of the humors, temperaments, and qualities as well as of theoretical anatomy and the like. The latter actually tried to heal patients through diets and medications. This meant that there was no effective linkage between theory and practice, and thus little development of new ideas and insights. The available medical texts were written for anybody who could read and grasp the concepts developed in them. One might therefore argue that the term layman had no meaning in this context, for the difference between someone who devoted all his or her time to the practice of medicine and somebody who did so occasionally was irrelevant.[7]

It was a system based on trial-and-error, of the kind, which Dr. Grant so amusingly characterized with the following story:

> A Persian physician "called on a tailor who was ill with intermittent fever. After feeling his pulse, looking wise and mentally invoking the aid of Allah, he left his directions and went his way. He returned next day and found the tailor well enough to be up and around. 'Alhamdulillah,' he exclaimed, 'I see you followed my directions!' 'No,' rejoined the tailor, 'I did not.' 'Then what did you do?' 'Why, nothing in particular, except that I drank a bowl of cabbage soup.' The physician at once reached the conclusion as to the proper method of treating low fevers. Exit physician, jotting down as an important item, 'Cabbage soup will cure low fever.' Next day he was summoned to the house of an upholsterer and found him very ill with apparently the same symptoms. At once he prescribed

---

[4] Kotzebue, Moritz von. *Narrative of a Journey into Persia in the suite of the Imperial Russian Embassy in the year 1817* (Philadelphia: Carey & Sons, 1820), p. 148; Waring, Edward Scott. *A Tour to Sheeraz* (London, 1807 [New York: Arno, 1973]), pp. 48-49; Hume-Griffith, *Behind the Veil*, p. 160; Collins, *In the Kingdom*, p. 168.
[5] Wills, C. J. *Persia As It Is* (London, 1886), p. 87; Olivier, *Voyage*, vol. 5, pp. 110-11.
[6] Waring, *A Tour*, pp. 48-49; Malcolm, *The History*, vol. 2, p. 531; Fowler, *Three Years*, vol. 1, p. 59 ("As to surgery in Persia I should say there is no such thing."). According to Lichtwadt, "Western Medicine," p. 237 "his surgical instruction was very elementary, and consisted in demonstrations of the opening of the boil."
[7] Ebrahimnejad, "Theory and Practice," p. 173.

'plenty of cabbage soup.' On returning next day to see how rapidly his patient was recovering, he was astonished to learn that the man was dead. 'Allah akbar!' he exclaimed, ''twas the will of Allah!' The he departed. Jotting down in his memorandum book this astonishing medical discovery. 'Cabbage soup will cure low fever in a tailor, but will kill an upholsterer.'"[8]

Because the hot-cold dichotomy also applied to plants Persian doctors general had a good knowledge of the nature and characteristics of herbs and plants. In 1828, Dr. Stirling noted that "the [medical] art is said to be better known and the [practitioners] more learned [in Shiraz] than many other places in Persia. Of their knowledge I am inclined to have a good opinion, but from an ignorance of their practice and the books they consult, generally it seems certain that they are well acquainted with the virtues of [a] number of vegetables, which they are in the habit of using and applying as remedies, and it must be granted that they are completely masters of the art as handed down by their fore-fathers the Arabians and the Greeks. I do not know that they have made any additions to the knowledge of the ancients."[9] The latter, and not without merit, had indeed occurred. For John Malcolm reported that the most learned Persian doctors boasted of "the discovery of many new remedies. Salvation is quickly produced, by inhaling, through the common pipe of the country, a lozenge made of cinnabar and flour: and this speedy mode of affecting the system is universally practiced, where the case is deemed of a nature to require it."[10]

The second system of medical practice was that of folk medicine. Persians lived in two worlds. One, the physical world that everybody could see, feel and smell and that was peopled with human beings. The other was a spiritual world that was populated with ghouls, goblins, *div*s (demons), jinns, afrits, and *pari*s (elves, fairies), which apparently only could be seen or experienced by Persians. The fact that the Koran and the Traditions (*hadith*) acknowledge the existence of jinns or demons meant that demonology is a legitimate concern for Moslems. It also made it a seamless effort to adopt the pre-Islamic Persian demonic world into the Islamic world. Many Europeans reported that, "The ordinary Persian has a profound belief in ghouls, divs (demons) jinns, and afrit."[11] This array of sprits, most of which were malevolent, was found everywhere. Jinns were "in keyholes, *jins* in the *qan'ats*, *divs* in the mountains, *divs* in the rocks, anywhere, everywhere, a vast population filling up the huge interstices left by Nature."[12] In

---

[8] Yonan, *Persian Women*, pp. 121-22. For the same story see also Sargis, "Persia and Her Doctors," p. 585. For a similar comparison see Olivier, *Voyage*, vol. 5, p. 112.
[9] Stirling, *The Journals*, p. 66.
[10] Malcolm, *The History*, vol. 2, p. 534.
[11] Sykes, Ella. *Persia and its People* (London: MacMillan, 1910), p. 325; Landor, *Across*, vol. 2, p. 365; Brugsch, Heinrich. *Im Lande der Sonne. Wanderungen in Persien* (Berlin: Algemeine Verein f. Deutsche Literatur, 1886), pp. 204-07; Polak, *Persien*, vol. 1, p. 346; Ussher, *A Journey*, pp. 610-11 (ghouls). In general see Donaldson, *The Wild Rue*, pp. 34-47. Jews also believed in jinns and demons, see Sabar, Yona. *The Folk Literature Of The Kurdistani Jews: An Anthology* (New Haven: Yale UP, 1982), pp. xv, 59, 65-66, 77, 87, 187, 189, 190-93; Loeb, Laurence D. *Outcaste. Jewish Life in Southern Iran* (New York: Gordon and Breach, 1977), pp. 216-19. For a drawing of the Spirit of the Mountains, see Feilberg, *Les Papis*, p. 152.
[12] Malcolm, *Five Years*, p. 121-22. For references to jinns and their deeds see Stewart, C.E.

Kurdistan, people believed in fairies, jinns, *pir*s (saints to whom votive offerings of rags were made), and *shait*s, "a curious class of supernatural beings, for among them are classed all the martyrs of Islam and many Kurds who have fallen in defence of their tribe, ... and desirous of helping the mortal Kurd to his desires."[13] Jinns could assume any form. For example, in the north-west of Persia lizards were "classed as believers and infidels; it is lawful to kill the latter."[14] To Persians these spirits, demons, goblins, and fairies were as real as human beings and they could not understand why Europeans did not see them, when it was clear to them that they were out there, you heard them, you saw them, you felt them, you lived with them, and they might cause you problems or illness. Consequently, there was a strong belief in the power of ghouls etc. against which European drugs were useless.[15] This belief in demonic possession and demonic interference in human life in general also prevailed among well-educated Persians. Hume-Griffith had one of them among his patients, who suffered from an attack of chorea (St. Vitus' dance). According to the patient, his illness had been caused because he had chanced upon a group of goblins, who had pelted him with stones.[16] Traditional faith healers, therefore, would look into the Koran or other books to determine which particular demon was afflicting the patient, and then gave the patient an appropriate charm to be drunk and/or to be attached to his arm.[17]

So widespread was this belief that fairies and demons had almost as large a place in people's life as did God and the Imams. This was quite understandable, because, according to Moslem creed, jinns are everywhere. They may assume the form of any animal or human being, and can become invisible at will.[18] The denizens of the spirit world could be peaceable, but also evil and malignant. In the former case it was worth your while to ask for their help and intervention. In the latter case, you needed to do all and everything to protect yourself against them. For that reason, "Soon after a child is born a needle is stuck into its clothing, or an iron charm is fastened on its cap, as it is believed that the jinn will not come near a child which is protected in this way."[19] As a consequence,

> Most Persian villagers, especially in the south, believe in fairies (the *peris*) as
> people who, if properly treated, will help men in this world as much as – if not

---

Through Persia in Disguise (London: Routledge, 1911), p. 232; Anonymous, *Sketches of Persia, from the journals of a traveller in the East* 2 vols. (London, 1828)., vol. 2, p. 77f; and Browne, E.G. *A Year Amongst the Persians* (London: A. & C. Black, 1970), pp. 165, 267; Binning, *A Travel*, vol. 2, pp. 201-02; Klaproth, Julius H. *Travels in the Caucasus and Georgia, performed in the years 1808 and 1808* (London: Henry Colburn, 1814), pp. 290-91 (Caucasus).

[13] Soane, Ely Bannister. *To Mesopotamia and Kurdistan in Disguise* (London: John Murray, 1912 [Amsterdam: Philo Press 1979]), pp. 402-03; Wigram, *The Cradle*, pp. 183-84, 277.

[14] Rice, *Persian Women*, pp. 242-51; see also Wilson, *Persian Life*, p. 145; Donaldson, *The Wild Rue*, p. 168. This was, of course, in line with the Koran (Surah 72 Jinns) that states that some jinns were true believers (also Surah 46: 29-31).

[15] Hale, F. *From Persian Uplands* (New York: E.P.Dutton, n.d.), pp. 140-41.

[16] Hume-Griffith, *Behind the Veil*, p. 166; Rice, *Persian Women*, p. 260.

[17] Adams, *Persia by a Persian*, p. 59.

[18] For information about all aspects of jinns see the article "Djinn," *Encyclopedia of Islam*.

[19] Rice, *Persian Women*, pp. 249-50.

> even more than- God himself; but which, if neglected or treated with a lack of respect, will take their revenge. Many villages have near, or within, their boundaries a sacred tree on which people hang bits or rag and a special copper object, a ghandel, consisting of a sphere with a semi-sphere attached on opposite sides, which is also hung up in the tombs of the Moslem prophets, the Imams. At these sacred trees the fairies meet, and near them the twelve, or perhaps only one or two, Imams have at some time walked. On the whole, the possible positive influence of the fairies for good is immense, fundamental, whilst the Imams, Mahomet and the Koran play the lesser but very useful function of defending man when the fairies are enraged or offended. The tree is often a tamarisk but may be a judas and usually may not be broken without evil results to the breaker.[20]

Villagers in particular clearly believed devoutly in sprites and had a very healthy respect for their powers. "They are real to the village adults and are more important than a mullah's blessing; for the 'little people' have great influence for good and evil. When they have been offended, prayers for protection against their anger are offered to Mohammad, or to his disciples, the Imams, of whom there are nine buried in Iran, and theirs is a saintly intervention."[21] In Gilan, people kept a white rooster for it kept the *peri*s and *div*s away.[22]

There were also many spirits that were malignant. The evil eye (*cheshm-e bad*; *chashm-e shur*, *chashm-e zakhm*, *chashm-e tang*, *nazar*) was the strongest power; it was a malicious, sometimes unconscious, spell that was cast through the eye of a person or animal (*chashm-zadeh*). Sudden disease was often ascribed to the evil eye. Only charms worked against it. "Certain substances are supposed to contain a soul-stuff which will insure protection. Blood is effective; a sheep is often killed so that its blood may be sprinkled on the foundations and doorposts of a new building. Metals such as iron, gold, silver and brass are helpful. For this reason a large pair of scissors or some other steel implement will be placed at the head of the bed during the birth of the child, and will be fastened to its cradle afterwards."[23] Many a woman would "tie a large padlock and two or three keys around her waist, hopeful that the evil influence will be repelled and that she can then become a mother of sons."[24]

---

[20] Merritt-Hawkes, *Persia*, pp. 195 (an example what happened to someone who broke the tree), 203 ("At birth each man has a fairy self, the *homsault*, which must never be harmed, for the evil at once affects its human counterpart."); Millingen, Frederick. *Wild Life Among The Koords* (London: Hurst and Blackett, 1870), pp. 220-22, 232; Sabar, *The Folk Literature*, p. 191 (the story told here is the same as the one related by Merritt-Hawkes, *Persia*, pp. 199-200). Damaging the tree belonging to an imamzadeh also had dire consequences, see Feilberg, *Les Papis*, p. 148; for another example, see Homayun, *Molk-e `Anbir-amiz*, p. 117.

[21] Morton, *A Doctor's Holiday*, p. 57.

[22] Chodzko, "Le Ghilan," p. 293 (A man came crying top Chodzko to help for a *pari* woke him every night and beat his wife mercilessly.); see for other examples, Massé, Henri. *Croyances et Coutumes Persanes* 2 vols. (Paris: Maisonneuve, 1938), vol. 2, pp. 280-86, 351-68. On roosters in Persia in general see Donaldson, *The Wild Rue*, pp. 161-63, 166.

[23] Morton, *A Doctor's Holiday*, p. 209; Rice, *Persian Women*, pp. 243; Sabar, *The Folk Literature*, pp. xvi, 193, 195; Loeb, *Outcaste*, pp. 176, 199, 213-16, 220-21.

[24] Rice, *Persian Women*, pp. 244-45; Morton, *A Doctor's Holiday*, p. 210.

Islamic law sanctioned the belief in the evil eye, because the prophet Mohammad also had believed in the evil eye and the use of charms to avert it. "A woman once asked him: 'O Prophet, the family of Ja'far are affected by the baneful influences of the evil eye; may I use spells for them or not?' His answer was: 'Yes, for if there was anything in the world which would overcome fate, it would be an evil eye.' Another time he said" 'There is nothing wrong in using spells, provided the use of them does not associate anything but God.' The prophet also allowed a spell to be used for the removal of yellowness in the eye, which he said was 'caused by the evil eye.'"[25]

To fight against evil supernatural influences it was necessary to marshal benign powers and elements that could protect against or control evil. Very important in this connection were those animate and inanimate elements that were endowed with extra strong 'life force.'

> Many substances are supposed to contain 'soul-stuff,' which acts as a protection against the evil eye. This soul-stuff is a material conception, and by it is meant something which contains life-power or life-fluid. Blood is an instance; this is sprinkled on the foundations and door-posts of a new house or building, sheep often being killed for the purpose. If a walnut-tree yields a poor crop, you are advised to kill an animal, by cutting its throat, at the base of the tree and then burying it there. Soul-stuff is also found in certain metals, such as iron, gold, silver, brass, lead, also in jade.[26]

The use of 'life force' was not limited to the use of animal blood or metals. There also were persons, who were believed to have this 'life force.' They could use this power to protect people against evil and sickness. Their usual method to do so was by "blowing, spitting and stroking, so as to bring benefit to sick people. The prophet is said to have worked cures by these means."[27]

The third system of medical practice was Prophetic medicine, about which a recent study concluded, "The medical literature attributed to the prophet or to the Imams, was in fact a mixture of old medicine, astrology, aphrodisiac lore, tropical dietics and personal hygiene, embroidered with Galenic concepts and terminology."[28] Prophetic medicine was developed to Islamicize a medical reality that was not. Galenic medicine was pagan in origin, and was mostly practiced by non-Moslems. Folk medicine was pre-Islamic in origin and used many practices that were un-Islamic. It was, of course, impossible to forbid these systems. The medieval Islamic governments had neither the means to do so

---

[25] Rice, *Persian Women*, pp. 244. In general, see the article "'Ayn," *Encyclopedia of Islam*, also Heiler, *Erscheinungsformen*, pp. 180-81 and Donaldson, *The Wild Rue*, pp. 13-23.

[26] Rice, *Persian Women*, pp. 244-45; Churchill, S.T.A. "Sacrifices in Persia," *The Indian Antiquary* 20 (1891), p. 148. On the supernatural power of blood in religious rites see Heiler, *Erscheinungsformen*, p. 190.

[27] Rice, *Persian Women*, pp. 243; Morton, *A Doctor's Holiday*, p. 209. On the apotropaic power of spit and stroking, see Heiler, *Erscheinungsformen*, pp. 190-91, 238-40; see also Donaldson, *The Wild Rue*, pp. 178-80.

[28] Ebrahimnejad, "Religion and Medicine," p. 93.

nor an alternative medical system to offer, and the same held for the olama. The latter therefore decided that if they could not beat the un-Islamic medical practices they could join them. The means to do so was to take control over these foreign bodies, so that they might be brought into the fold of Islam. The best way to do that was to develop a framework that religiously sanctioned such practices and brought them under the all-encompassing notion of their artificial construct called Prophetic medicine. Because the Koran has not much to offer in terms of medical knowledge, apart from having faith in God, recourse was had to the *hadith* literature. The number of medical *hadith*s or traditions was not as numerous as the developers of Prophetic medicine may have liked, while they also were contradictory. The latter was nothing new and experienced olama could live and deal with that, as they had in all other aspects of life. The purpose of the system, after all, was not so much to develop a credible medical system from a scientific point of view, but rather one that offered an Islamic conceptual view of health, well-being and illness. At the same time, it had to incorporate actual medical practices and accommodate their continued existence by providing an Islamic explanation for them. This had both the imprimatur of the prophet and of 'scientific' medicine.[29]

From the above it is clear that, irrespective of which medical system they adhered to, Persians, whether doctor or patient, strongly believed in the supernatural cause, including as manifested by the movement of celestial bodies, of epidemics and other forms of disease. In 1820, people in Shiraz believed that the outbreak of cholera had been caused by the influence of the star Canopus.[30] When in the 1830s, there was a cholera outbreak in Isfahan, the people claimed that this was due to the fact that the governor, Mo'tamed al-Dowleh, had taken away the talisman that protected the town.[31] In 1886, there was a rumor throughout Persia that a white chicken would lay an egg that contained the plague. Within the space of one week all white chickens were killed and all chicklets born from their eggs as well.[32]

The appreciation of what caused disease was also expressed in the terminology used to refer to the various disorders. "An abscess in the leg would be described as 'a devilish wind'; dropsy is considered to be 'wind,' of which at last the sufferer gets so full that he will be wafted up to heaven. The after-effects of small-pox may be spoken of as 'the cold wind of small-pox'; palpitation as 'the flapping of a dove's wings'; a cold as the 'eating of a chill.' Some people think they must have at least one cold a month to relieve the

---

[29] For a detailed analysis see Perho, Irmeli. *The Prophet's Medicine. A Creation of the Muslim Traditionalist Scholars* (Helsinki, Finnish Oriental Society, 1995); see also Bürgel, J.C. "Islamisches Mittelalter," in Heinrich Schipperges, Eduard Seidler und Paul U. Unschuld ed. *Krankheit, Heilkunst, Heilung* (Freiburg-Munich: Karl Alber, 1978), pp. 288-98; Newman, ed. *Islamic medical wisdom: the Tibb al-A'imma*, [compiled by Abd Allah ibn Bistam ibn Sabur and al-Husayn ibn Bistam ibn Sabur] translated by Batool Ispahany (London: Muhammadi Trust, 1991); and Ibn Qayyim al-Jawziyah, Muhammad ibn Abi Bakr, *Natural healing with the medicine of the prophet: from The Book of the provisions of the hereafter by Imam Ibn Qayyim Al-Jawziyya (1292-1350 C.E.)*, translated & emended by Muhammad Al-Akili (Philadelphia, Pa.: Pearl: 1993).
[30] Fraser, *Narrative*, p. 64 ("this star has very extraordinary powers, good and malignant.")
[31] Schindler, A.H. *Eastern Persian Irak* (London: Murray, 1898), p. 125.
[32] Dieulafoye, *La Perse*, p. 106.

brain, otherwise they might go mad."[33] The Bakhtiyaris "attribute all ailments but those of the skin and eyes to 'wind.'"[34]

The use of the term wind (*bad*) in relation to the cause or nature of many a disease is of interest here, because the concept is both found in Islamic-Galenic and folk medicine.[35] The modern Persian term *bad* is derived from the Pahlavi verb *va*, meaning, to blow. *Vata* or *Vayu* (in Latin *ventus*) was the god of the winds in Achaemenid times and sacrifices were made to him. In the later Vedic texts (Upanishads), *Vata*, like *Vayu*, is identified as *prana* (Breath). Originally a supreme deity, *Vayu* acquired two aspects; one that brought good and the other that brought evil winds. These winds were not only atmospheric phenomena, but were also later perceived as being the breath of the soul. It is not clear whether these winds also brought illness as they did during the Islamic period, but it seems likely. The fact that the *Vendidad* associates this demon *Vayu* with the demon of death implies that wind was indeed more than an atmospheric phenomenon.[36] At the same time, Galenic medicine (borrowing from the pneumatic school under the influence of the Stoa) identified wind as one of the major causes of certain diseases. These winds, however, were produced in the body as a result of certain chemical reactions.[37]

All three medical systems recognized, implicitly or explicitly, two classes of remedies (*dava*) against disease. According to the Islamic-Galenic system these were divided into those that preserved (*hefz*) health and those that cured (*raf'*) disease. People were advised to lead a religious blameless and exemplary life and, above all, pray! This was no guarantee, because you could not take the positive impact of divine or supernatural healing for granted. Also, the curative effects were not always visible or even noticeable to the pious Moslem, who therefore still could fall ill. For the curative powers only were effective if the person concerned was aware of them. The Persian physician would nevertheless tell the patient not to despair as yet, because there were still somatic cures.[38] Ebrahimnejad sees a contradiction between the power of prayer (*do'a*) and curative medicine (*raf'*), but it was just another means by which the hidden nature of the cure, that had escaped the patient's perception so far, might be revealed, without him even immediately realizing it. This shows the advantage, if not superiority, of Prophetic medicine over the scientific approach, because in the former everything can be explained, even if you do not get it.

---

[33] Rice, *Persian Women*, p. 127; Donaldson, *The Wild Rue*, pp. 99-100.

[34] Bird, *Journeys*, vol. 2, p. 75; Dehkhuda, *Loghatnameh* (s.v. *bad*); Donaldson, *The Wild Rue*, pp. 99-100.

[35] Polak, *Persien*, vol. 2, p. 232, who adds that in French and German folk medicine the same concept existed (*vents*, *Winden*)

[36] Dehkhuda, *Loghatnameh* (s.v. *bad*); Zaehner, R.C. *The Dawn & Twilight of Zoroastrianism* (London, Weidenfeld and Nicholson, 1961), p. 149; Ibid. *Zurvan, A Zoroastrian Dilemma* (Oxford, OUP, 1955), pp. 82-86; Jayne, Walter Addison. *The Healing Gods of Ancient Civilizations* (New Haven: Yale UP, 1925), pp. 172, 178; Heiler, Friedriech, *Erscheinungsformen und Wesen der Religion* (Stuttgart: Kohlhamer, 1961), p. 50.

[37] See, for example, Gruner, O. Cameron, *A Treatise on the Canon of Medicine of Avicenna* (London: Luzac, 1930), pp. 193-94 (paras. 296-301), 204 (paras 314-17).

[38] Ebrahimnejad, "Religion and Medicine," pp. 95, 105.

In summary, the Islamization of Greek and folk medicine was enabled by Prophetic medicine, which provided the Islamic framework to bring daily practice and reality within the Islamic fold. These three systems co-existed in Qajar Persia, but unlike medieval times there was an almost seamless transition from one to the other. The tension that existed between Galenic medicine and Islam in the Middle Ages was something of the past. Galenic medicine, in fact, had become Islamic medicine and physicians gladly adorned themselves with titles such as Galen of the Age (*Jalenus al-Zaman*) or Hippocrates of the Physicians (*Boqrat al-Hokama*). Taking my cue from Dols, I contend that medicine as practiced in Qajar Persia therefore was a blend of pre-Islamic Persian folk medicine, the Galenic concepts of the humors and temperaments that had entered into popular parlance in urban and rural areas, and the overarching principle of divine or supernatural causation as represented by Prophetic medicine.[39]

An example of the influence of Galenic medicine on folk medicine was the realization that maintaining a proper diet was key to a healthy life. When the American missionary Wilson and his party were picnicking and eating hard-boiled eggs, bread and milk, next to a party of a group of Kurdish women, the women told them that "milk and eggs eaten together would make us ill!"[40]

An example of the influence of folk medicine of Galenic and Prophetic medicine is that it had become not only quite normal, but expected, that the physician trained in Galenic medicine invoked God, the prophet, the Imams and what not, in addition to his efforts to prod the humors, temperaments and qualities. Also, advice based on Galenic principles was now in accordance with the teaching of Islam. Likewise, patients and/or relatives while pursuing a supernatural cause of the disease and course of events of the treatment would also be guided by Galenic concepts as part of the treatment strategy. The type of medical intervention chosen depended on a number of factors such as the seriousness of the illness, the stage of the illness, the status of the patient and his family (wealth and education) as well as their location. In addition, everybody used astrology and other magical lore to influence the correct course of events. In rural areas, in particular for nomads, medical help was less accessible, even if they could pay for it, and thus there was little choice. There does not seem to have been a difference in the type of healing between the adherents of different religions, as had been the case in medieval times. The system of medicine as described above was applied by all religious denominations, and many physicians who catered to the needs of Moslems were non-Moslem (mostly Jews).[41]

---

[39] Dols, Michael W. "Islam and Medicine," *History of Science* 26 (1988), p. 421.

[40] Wilson, *Persian Life*, p. 103. On the importance of the choice of hot and cold food ingredients see Tapper, Richard and Sami Zubaida eds. *Culinary Cultures of the Middle East* (London: I.B. Tauris, 1994); Donaldson, *The Wild Rue*, pp. 190-93, and Shahri, Ja`far. *Tehran-e Qadim* (Tehran: Mo`in, 1371/1992), vol. 5, which volume provides information on, amongst other things, the curative properties of fruits, food plants and potherbs.

[41] Loeb, *Outcaste*, pp. 220-21.

MEDICAL INSTITUTIONAL INFRASTRUCTURE

In most of the rural areas of Qajar Persia, there was no doctor, while in urban areas their number also was limited. Moreover, the majority of the population could not afford the high cost of their of services. Old men and women therefore gave most of the primary health care, the latter in particular to women and children.[1] If this first line of defense was not successful, resource was had to dervishes, other 'holy men,' sayyeds, shrines, and, if the family had some money, a barber or physician. A passing European, or, later in the century in some urban areas, the physicians of the British Legation and the missionary hospitals were often the medical healer of last resort.

In rural areas, "The village barber was their chief consultant, and, even if it was a question of life and death, the treatment he gave them originated from crude and ancient superstition."[2] Barbers were only present in the larger villages, of course. Otherwise and in addition to the barber, there were wandering dervishes, sayyeds and other men, or families who were known to be endowed with healing powers. Faith-cures were not uncommon. There also were itinerant traditional physicians, often Jews, who probably wandered in the rural districts of the town in which they had their home base. Among the Bakhtiyaris, and likely among the other Persian tribes, women healers existed who take care of most of the sick and wounded.[3] If all that failed, there also were the tombs and shrines of dead holy persons as well as the denizens of the nether world that also held out hope for healing. In fact, often the rural people were so desperate that they finally even turned for help to passing Europeans who often did not have the slightest idea about medical science.[4] Fowler, who, in his own words, "scarcely knew a bolus from a plaster," was often called upon for cures and invariably by the fair sex. Because he insisted on seeing the person many women opened by degrees their veil, "and it was amusing to see with what caution I was permitted first to see the mouth, then they eyes, they looking askance at me, laughing at the same time at their shamefacedness."[5]

According to Dr. Häntzsche, referring to the situation around 1860, "there is an extraordinary number of so-called doctors, surgeons, eye doctors, and midwives; on the other hand there are no obstetricians, veterinarians, chemists, pharmacies and hospitals."[6] The British Dr. Clarke and the French Dr. de Fontanelle, referring to the situation in the mid-

---

[1] Shakurzadeh, Ebrahim. `Aqayed va Rosum-e `Ammeh-ye Mardom-e Khorasan (Tehran Bonyad-e Farhang-e Iran, 1346/1967), p. 199; Homayun, *Molk-e `Anbir-amiz*, p. 92.

[2] Forbes-Leith, *Checkmate*, p. 88.

[3] Grant, Asahel. *The Nestorians; or The Lost Tribes* (New York: Harper & Brothers, 1841), p. 97, when among the mountain Nestorians he could not get supplies by offering to pay for them. However, when he offered them medicine and medical services he had no problem getting what supplies he needed. "It was gratifying to find these mountaineers prizing them [his medical services] above their money."

[4] Hasanbeygi, Muhammad Reza. *Tehran-e Qadim* (Tehran: Mansuri, 1377/1998), p. 195.

[5] Fowler, *Three Years*, vol. 1, pp. 57-58.

[6] Häntzsche, J.C. "Specialstatistik von Persien," *Zeitschrift der Gesellschaft für Erdkunde zu Berlin* 1869, p. 442. In Tabriz, in 1869, there were no less than 20 veterinarians (*dam pezeshk*). Javadi, *Tabriz*, p. 227; see also Polak, *Persien*, vol. 2, p. 206 (*beytal*).

1830s, both divided the medical profession in Qajar Persia into three classes: "druggists, barbers, and doctors (hakkim; [sic; *hakim*]) who join a slight knowledge of practical surgery to their other qualifications."[7] This classification is also reflected in a treatise by an anonymous Persian author written in the early 1850s. This author maintained that there were: (i) 'able,' that is high-class physicians usually hired by the nobility; (ii) rank-and-file doctors and/or quacks [who] worked for society at large; and (iii) druggist and grocers who sold simple and compound drugs.[8] Functionally, and expanding on the classification used by Dr. Wills, we may distinguish more categories, to wit:

(i) Spiritual healers
   (a) Dead saints
   (b) Denizens of the spirit world, and
   (c) Magical and prayer doctors

(ii) Islamic-Galenic physicians:
   (a) Internal medicine doctors
   (b) Eye-surgeons, and
   (c) Druggists

(iii) Traditional healers:
   (a) Female healers
   (b) Barbers
   (c) Bonesetters, and
   (d) Surgeons

This classification is less absolute than it seems, because there are no clear-cut divisions between these categories of healers and often they overlapped. Many female healers were both eye doctors and surgeons. The barber usually also was the bonesetter and the surgeon. The Islamic-Galenic doctor also might provide surgical services. However, given the different demands in expertise I have decided to make these distinctions. Moreover, in actual practice this classification proved to be historically correct. I have furthermore added the class of spiritual healers, who are totally ignored by most observers or just classified as quacks (*beytal*).

Ebrahimnejad has argued that it is not possible to make a professional division, because it is a subjective matter, for there was no institutional setting that the historian could rely upon.[9] This may be true for the difference between a professional learned Islamic-Galenic physician and one who was a mountebank. However, Persian patients did distinguish between, for example, a barber (*dallak*), a doctor of internal medicine (*hakim*), an ophthalmologist (*kahhal*), or a druggist (`*attar*), as the terminology also suggests. In fact, Dr.

---

[7] Clarke, "Sketches on the State," p. 708; De Fontanelle, Julia. "Das Apothekerwesen in Persien," *Das Ausland* 1838, p. 119; see also Ts., "Persidskie Doktora,"p. 157 (those who have studied; those who have not but have a good memory; and traditional healers, in particular women using witchcraft).
[8] Ebrahimnejad, "Theory and Practice," p. 171.
[9] Ebrahimnejad, "Theory and Practice," p. 172.

Häntzsche observed that only after many years of residence in Resht and through extraordinary circumstances had he been able to treat surgical cases. "This is due to the fact that Persians still strongly adhere to the old distinction between hekim or tabib, physician, and dscherrah (sic; *jarrah*), surgeon."[10] Polak quotes a witty observation made by a Persian whom he asked to explain to him the difference between a *hakim* and a *jarrah*. His informant told him that, "a *hakim* should know how to read and write, a *jarrah* should not." Polak further reports that when a Persian said about a *hakim* that he was a *jarrah*, then he meant to say that the doctor had no knowledge whatsoever about [internal] medicine.[11] Moreover, it would seem that in popular parlance the *hakim* or doctor was a *tabib-e jasmani* (a doctor of somatic diseases), that is, although he might invoke celestial and divine powers, do incantations and prescribe magical cures, he was not a *tabib-e rowhani*, a doctor of the psyche.[12] The latter as I have discussed above worked as spiritual healers. Therefore, I maintain that this classification of medical healers is not only one that reflects historical reality, but it is also one that is used by the sources, either explicitly or implicitly. In what follows I discuss these various categories of the medical service delivery infrastructure.

---

[10] Häntzsche, "Physikalisch-medicinische Skizze," p. 568; see also Babin, C and Houssay, F. "A Travers La Perse Méridionale," *Le Tour du Monde* 64 (1892), p. 98 (A Persian asked whether Babin and Houssay were doctors [*hakim*] or surgeons [*jarrah*]).
[11] Polak, *Persien*, vol. 2, p. 198.
[12] Tahvildar, *Joghrafiya*, pp. 80-81.

SPIRITUAL HEALERS

The class of spiritual or supernatural healers may be divided into three categories: (i) the dead, (ii) the spirits, and (iii) the living. The dead healers were supposedly holy men or women, including pre-Islamic and Christian ones, whose tombs, relics and its ancillaries allegedly had miraculous curative powers. Sometimes these powers were general in nature, sometimes only for certain kinds of disorders. The spirits were fairies and demons, denizens of the spiritual world that co-existed and interacted with human physical reality, and humans, if they knew what was good for them, had to take their doings and powers into account. The living ones were spiritual healers representing a variety of persons. They included wandering dervishes, certain families, mullahs, wise women, and anybody who was able to pass himself off as being empowered with the breath of soul or *nafas*. Their techniques did not differ much, at least as far as we know.

(i) Dead Saints

The very fact that Persia is plastered with *Imamzadeh*s (male or female descendants of one of the Shi`ite Imams), shrines of local saints (*boq`eh*s, *astaneh*s, *mazar*s), and what not is an indication of a great felt need for divine assistance and intervention. The population, therefore, could address their ills to any of these shrines to find solace if not cures.[1] Being in the presence of such a saint might just result in a cure. There were, of course, differences in the power of the saints, some of whom were even specialized in cures of certain disorders only.

In Persia itself, the major sites of pilgrimage such as that of the shrine of Imam Reza were more powerful than others. Faith-based healing thus played an essential role in the healing process. Stirling recounted the story of an *akhund* or mullah from Mazandaran on pilgrimage in Mashad, who felt ill but did not take the medicine prescribed for him by a physician. "During the night he became worse, but the *Imam* Ruza came to him with a cup and [he] drank the contents, after which he became better and kept awake till the morning. It ought to have been mentioned that he had solicited the good offices of the Imam the day preceding. He asserted that all this was perfectly true, that he was perfectly awake."[2]

---

[1] For an exhaustive inventory of most of these shrines see Mehdi Gharavi, *Aramgah dar Gostareh-ye Farhang-e Irani* (Tehran: Anjoman-e Athar va Mafakher-e Farhangi, 1376/1997), and the cult of saints and pilgrimage see Donaldson, *The Wild Rue*, pp. 55-68. For individual sites see, de Gobineau, *Trois Ans*, vol. 2, p. 101; Watelin, *La Perse*, p. 78 (Ardabil); Feilberg, *Les Papis*, p. 147; Stark, *The Valley*, p. 209 (Sitt Zeinabar); Aubin, Eugène. *La Perse d'aujourd'hui* (Paris: Armand Colin, 1908), p. 55 (Hajji Mir Ya`qub-Khoy), 113 (tomb of Sheykh Safi and Shah Esma`il - Ardabil). For the healing phenomenon of dead saints see Heiler, *Erscheinungsformen*, pp. 428-33, 556-58.

[2] Stirling, *The Journals*, p. 129; Fowler, *Three Years*, vol. 1, p. 61 ("This implicit confidence in the skill of the doctor helps very much to the cure, and is universally entertained in Persia").

It is further interesting to note that a number of particular shrines had a reputation to be able to cure in particular snakebites, and oftentimes also bites by other animals. In fact, it would seem that certain shrines could cure all animal related diseases caused by biting. What is further of interest is that such specialized shrines, with similar curative powers and methods, existed all over the country, in parts that normally did not have much communication with one another (Baluchistan, Azerbaijan, Luristan, Fars). Tate reported that a jackal had mauled a Baluch woman. "The recognized resort in such cases ... is to make up an offering for the shrine of Bibi Dost."[3]

Tate tried to find out why Bibi Dost had such a reputation for curing diseases and wounds. He concluded,

> It was never quite clear why Bibi Dost was supposed to exercise a healing influence on injuries received from rabid animals. The popular idea is that no sooner is a person bitten than he or she is mad-though the disease may not have taken an active form. The visit to the shrine is believed the cure the sufferer-provided of course that it had not been decreed that he is to die in this way. The principal shrine dedicated to Bibi Dost is close to the village of Kasamabad. It is here that the sufferers resort. There are many shrines, offshoots of this, but the efficacy of the cure is most sure at the parent shrine.[4]

At the diagonal other end of the country, in the hills near Tabriz, was a small Imamzadeh, which likewise "was reputed most efficacious in curing persons afflicted with hydrophobia, or bitten by a serpent."[5] In nearby Khoy, Hajji Sayyed Mir Ya`qub had died 40 years ago, Wilson reported in 1896. Allegedly, "by his blessings bandages received power to dispel fever." After his death people therefore built a mosque over his tomb, so as to make sure that such an asset was not lost. As a result, Wilson reported that, "The sick are brought there and laid within its precincts for the operation of the faith-cure."[6]

In yet another part of Qajar Persia, there was "A tomb named the Imam Zadahi Pir Mar, a shrine of great celebrity in Luristan." It was said to have miraculous powers to cure snakebites. "Anybody has been and is close by goes there. His descendants also have inherited these powers. The Lurs believe that the cure is performed merely by the touch of the cold blade of a knife which belonged to the great Pir Mar, and is still preserved in the family; but I saw that the real antidote, which, however, is not a little curious, was

---

[3] Tate, G. P. *The Frontiers of Baluchistain. Travels on the borders of Persia and Afghanistan* (London 1909 [Lahore: East & West Publishing Comp, 1976]), p. 193 (The husband of the woman who had been attacked by a jackal was too poor to make the offering at the shrine. His neighbors raised a subscription and the suffering woman then could be taken to the shrine; also a man bitten by a camel went to Bibi-Dost), Ibid., p. 200.

[4] Tate, *Frontiers*, pp. 200, 204-05 (for a description of the shrine; animal sacrifices; shreds of cloths on sticks and rods).

[5] Browne, *A Year*, p. 62. On the mountain overlooking Tabriz there is a mosque with tombs of two imams. Tablets were disposed there "inscribed with accounts of wonferful cures and other miracles, said to have been performed by the efficacious ashes of the departed Imams." Perkins, J. *A Residence of Eight Years in Persia* (Andover: Allen, Morrill & Wardwell, 1843), p. 211.

[6] Wilson, *Persian Life*, p. 84.

contained in a poultice of leaves and wild herbs kept constantly applied to the wound."[7] In Fars, there is a pre-Islamic tomb with curative powers. It is the well-known tomb of Madar-e Soleyman. "The *ked khoda* of the village wished me particularly to know that the power of her sanctity was a certain cure for the bite of a mad dog."[8]

Generally speaking, whenever a snake or scorpion had bitten somebody, he would be hurried to a holy place renowned for its healing powers. However, these were not everywhere available. Thus, other remedies also had been developed as alternative treatment of bites.[9] In the Bojnord area, old stags were believed to be snake eaters. "They catch the serpents by the tail, dash them about on their antlers till dead, and then swallow them. Hence it comes, he explained, that the exudation from the lachrymal glands is an antidote to snake poison. It is at any rate administered to newly born infants with this object in "a wine-glass full of water.' Another concoction: when the antlers are soft they are boiled down into a jelly and are much appreciated. But these people do not, like the Chinese, use them as a the basis of 'love philters.' For this purpose they use a different part of the stag's anatomy."[10]

Elsewhere, a total different approach was taken. For snake-bite, which was common, the Bakhtiyaris "keep the bitten person moving about and apply the back part of live hens to the wound till the hens cease to be affected, or else the intestines of a goat newly killed."[11] Mme. de Freygang reported that Persians, in general, "Instead of applying oil, the best remedy for the scorpion's venom, they repeat certain prayers, which they consider a sovereign medicine. So persuaded are they of the efficacy of these prayers, that, having gone through them, they will lie down to sleep in the very midst of the reptiles."[12] It is more likely that she referred to certain dervishes, who had trained themselves to be impervious to the poison of certain snakes rather than that this applied to the population at large.

In the tomb of Shehab al-Din at Ahar, Holmes saw a quantity of reeds in an arched widow of the mausoleum.

> We inquired what they were, and were informed, that, if a person suffered from
> pain or disease, he twined a reed with string or rag, prayed over it, and
> consigned it to this holy place, and the people gravely assured us that the malady

---

[7] Rawlinson, Major H. C. "Notes on a March from Zohab ... to Khuzistan," *JGRS* 9 (1839), p. 96; for the same story see Chirikov, E.I. *Putvoj zhurnal russkogo komissara-posrednika po turetsko-persidskomu razgranicheniyu* (St. Petersburg, 1875) translated by Abkar Masihi as *Siyahatnameh-ye Mosiyu Cherikof.* ed. `Ali Asghar `Omran (Tehran: Jibi, 1358/1979), p. 39.

[8] Reitlinger, *A Tower of Skulls*, p. 89. Although it has not been reported that it had curative powers, nevertheless, the tomb of Cyrus was hung with bells and filled with prayer-payers indicating that pilgrims believed it could heal, protect, and bring fortune, see Moore, *From Moscow*, p. 353.

[9] On Persian remedies other than those mentioned in this section see Jozani, *La beauté*, pp. 175-78.

[10] Kennion, *By Mountain Lake*, p. 234.

[11] Bird, *Journeys*, vol. 2, p. 74. Poor Lurs who did not have the means to go to a shrine applied an oak leaf poultice. Stark, *The Valley*, p. 75.

[12] Freygang, *Letters*, pp. 338-339.

> duly passed away. What peculiar efficacy belonged to the reed or the string
> nobody pretended to explain, but every one asserted the fact. This superstition
> resembles the hanging up of rags or offering on the branches of trees near sacred
> spots; a custom common both in Turkey and Persia, and many other countries,
> Ireland and Scotland not excepted.[13]

The dust of the tombs of holy people, or even that of living very revered people, also was believed to have healing powers. `Eyn al-Saltaneh wrote in his Diary, "I left Qom for Tehran. I had malaria (*nowbeh*) and severe shudders (*larz*)." He therefore took female remedies (*dava-ye zananeh*), prayer water (*ab-e do`a*), dust of the fifth Imam ['s tomb], and key-water (*ab-e qofl*; *i.e.*, water that had been poured over the locks of the tomb) and a pill made of the dust of the tomb-railing (*zarih*) of the Ma`sumeh. The cure helped, for later he got somewhat better.[14] The same powers were also described to tombs of famous historic persons such as that of Ebn Sina (Avicenna). In 1866, Lycklama noted that a number of persons, competing with one another, pressed themselves against the tomb to find a cure for their malady.[15] John Malcolm reported some preventive measures taken by nomadic groups. "A few pieces of bread, covered with oil, which were laid upon a rock, as an offering to a saint; and they were told, that they might, by these pieces of bread, compute the exact number of sick in the black tents that were pitched near, as this offering was the usual, and almost the only effort made to obtain their recovery from any disease with which they were attacked." The 'Moslem' saints referred to probably originally were *pari*s or fairies, a subject to which I will turn next.

Similar beliefs also existed among the Jews and Christians in Persia. In Kurdistan, many fruit trees had been planted around Rabbi Samuel, and "whosoever became ill would take a fruit from those trees and say, 'I plead with righteous man who is buried here to cure me,' and his ailment would immediately be healed." If you took the fruit, or pomegranate, without Rabbi Samuel's permission you would become ill with fever.[16] In the Urumiyeh region it was believed that "if you rub dust from a church upon a wart it will disappear."[17]

(ii) <u>Denizens of the Spirit World</u>

The belief that not only God, but also other beings influenced if not controlled your life was in particular strong among the rural population. Many pre-Islamic rituals such as for rainmaking continued to be practiced by the Islamicized population until well into the

---

[13] Holmes, W.R. *Sketches on the Shores of the Caspian, Descriptive and Pictorial*. (London: Richard Bentley, 1845), pp. 18-19; see also E`tesam al-Molk, *Safarnameh*, p. 183 for a description of a non-Moslem (pre-Islamic) idol in the village of Seh-Deh, as if it were an imamzadeh complete with an overseer and women hanging rags and burning candles.

[14] `Eyn al-Saltaneh, *Ruznameh*, vol. 1, p. 312; Feuvrier, J.B.: *Trois ans à la Cour de Perse*. (Paris: F. Juven, 1900), p. 71 (the royal physicians prescribed earth from the tomb of Imam Hoseyn to treat Naser al-Din Shah's diarrhea); Aubin, *La Perse*, p. 313; Polak, *Persien*, vol. 2, p. 236. In general see Donaldson, *The Wild Rue*, pp. 65-67.

[15] Lycklama à Nijeholt, T.M. *Voyage en Russie, au Caucase et en Perse*. 4 vols (Paris-Amsterdam: Arthus Bertrand-C.L. van Langenhuysen, 1873), vol. 3, p. 517.

[16] Sabar, *The Folk Literature*, p. 122.

[17] Knanishu, *About Persia*, p. 187.

twentieth century.[18] Another atmospheric manifestation, thunder and lighting, scared the lights out of Mozaffar al-Din Shah, who strongly believed in jinns and *pari*s. He therefore kept Sayyed Bahrami and his sons at his side. "When the weather changed and became cloudy, or when there was thunder and lighting [this sayyed had to] chant the Greatest Name or other verses, in order to be a shield against nature."[19] The belief that you not only had to protect yourself against any occurrence of contact with the spirit world, but also with the physical manifestation thereof was still strong and acted upon. Edith Benn observed a perfect example of the rural population paying their dues to the representatives of the netherworld and 'buy' their non-interference.

> The subject of charms and amulets reminds me of the seals found by treasure-hunters amidst broken pottery and other indestructible remains of the sites of Persia's ruined cities. Some of these, cut in crystal, agate, chalcedony, and carnelian, are engraved in Kufic characters, others have head of Grecian type cut in intaglio, but the most interesting to me were those representing animals, wild and domestic, which it seems not unlikely were carried by the owners as totems. Some of these display a good deal of 'life.' Relics of animistic beliefs are indeed common among these primitive peoples. At Shusp is a fissured rock which is known as the shrine of Shah-i-Mar, the Shah (or spiritual leader) of snakes. At any time in the heat of the day you could go and see a wicked flat head looking at you from a crack in the rock. The snakes were protected, and, I think, fed by the people of Shusp. Every time we passed through Sushp on our annual migrations to Kain we were delayed by the illness of some member of the family, and my Seistanis believed us to be under the ban of this being. It was then necessary to do *khairat*, which meant the sacrifice of a sheep-and their consumption by the villagers."[20]

These beliefs were not confined to nominally Moslem villagers, but also existed among Jewish and Christian communities in Persia.[21]

People also had recourse to the fairies for cures in case of illness. In a village near Yazd, the village mullah

> Prepared a great fairy feast that the little people might cure his sick daughter. ... These fairy feasts take place in both villages and towns and are of great importance in cases of illness, a coming journey or any major event. The feast, which is completed in three parts, must take place on a Saturday or Tuesday and be presided over by a girl who has not reached the age of puberty, or a woman who has passed the climacteric and who knows the special fairy prayers as well as some of the Moslem prayers.

---

[18] See Floor, *Agriculture in Qajar Iran*, p. 202.
[19] Taj al-Saltaneh. *Crowning Anguish*, p. 235.
[20] Kennion, R.L. *By Mountain Lake and Plain, Sport in Eastern Persia* (Edingburgh-London: Wm. Blackwood & Sons, 1911), p. 40.
[21] Wilson, *Persian Life*, pp. 132-33; Loeb, *Outcaste*, pp. 213-16.

> The mullah had to take a donkey twenty miles to fetch the nearest woman suitably qualified to preside over his feast.[22]

Tying rags to certain sacred trees, a custom that was widespread all over Persia, was another manner in which sufferers could make a demand for a cure or protection from the fairies.[23] A variant of the same method to expiate the spirits and obtain their good will was the amassing of stone cairns as votive monuments, which was also a phenomenon practiced throughout Persia.[24] Women in Kerman made supplications to the Queen of the Fairies to grant them pregnancy.[25]

During his survey of plants and their use in Eastern Persia, Aitchison noted the following superstitions:

> Celtis caucasia [Willd.], Pinus halepensis [Mill.], and Pistacia vera [Linn.] are usually found planted round their holy places or Ziarats, with an occasional Rosa moschata [Rosa brunonii Lindl.] climbing up one of these trees. The stems of the Tamarix, and the Almond, Prunus amygdalus, are valued as hafts to whips, as a protection against snakes; a rod of the almond carried in the hand indicates the priestly office. Peganum harmala [Linn.] and Ferula galbaniflua [Boiss. et Buhse] are supposed to be preventatives of sickness; the former is collected and burnt in heaps to drive away sickness, or hung up in doorways; the latter is hung up in and around dwellings to drive off evil influences, especially during parturition. Amber, and the seeds of Caesalpinia bonducella [Linn.], with pieces of the wood of Celtis, are worn as amulets to keep off evil spirits. The cone of Pinus halepensis is kept by the ladies in their workbags in order to give luck. It is propitious to eat of the fruit of the Date-palm at certain holy feasts.[26]

---

[22] Merritt-Hawkes, *Persia*, p. 197; for a detailed description of the three parts of the feast, and other feasts by the fairies see Ibid., pp. 197-204; Soane, *To Mesopotamia*, pp. 402-03; Donaldson, *The Wild Rue*, pp. 42, 88, 156.

[23] Wigram, *The Cradle*, p. 205 (for not respecting the sanctity of the tree the transgressor and others would pay a price, as an example shows); Ouseley, W. *Travels in various countries of the East: more particularly Persia*, 3 vols. (London, 1819-23), vol. 3, p. 435; O'Donovan, *The Merv Oasis*, vol. 2, p. 25; Watelin, *La Perse*, p. 39; Rivadeneyra, Adolfo. *Viaje al interior de Persia* 3 vols. (Madrid, 1880), vol. 2, p. 212.

[24] Wigram, *The Cradle*, pp. 15, 233; Landor, *Across*, vol. 2, pp. 50, 353; Watelin, *La Perse*, p. 39; Feilberg, *Les Papis*, pp. 19, 131 (photo), 149; Curzon, G.N. *Persia and the Persian Question* 2 vols. (London, 1892 [London: Frank Cass, 1966]). vol. 2, p. 299; Edmonds, C.J. "Luristan: Pish-e Kuh and Bala gariveh," *Geographical Journal* 59 (1922), p. 439; Stark, *The Valley*, pp. 58, 89 (Peri stones); Donaldson, *The Wild Rue*, p. 151; Correspondent, Daily News. "Curious Customs in Kurdistan," *The Indian Antiquary* 10 (October 1881), pp. 288-89.

[25] Sykes, *Through Persia*, p. 96.

[26] Aitchison, J.E.T. "Notes on the products of Western Afghanistan and of North-Eastern Persia," *Transactions of the Botanical Society* (Edinburgh) XVIII (1890), pp. 200-201. See in general Donaldson, *The Wild Rue*, pp. 141-47.

In most cases, soothsayers and other magickers (see next section) were used as intermediary to converse with the denizens of the spirit world. Sykes described the following intervention by a soothsayer. After having uttered cabbalistic phrases he told the family that the patient must have been attacked by jinns, "either from passing along a canal at night without repeating the name of Allah, or else from putting his hand into hot ashes, which disturbs the young Jinns." Although the family knew that the patient had done none of these things they agreed to summon the king of the Jinns. The soothsayer than asked for a basin of water in which all those present were asked to put money in accordance with the love they had for the patient. The soothsayer then uttered the following incantation, accompanied by wild gestures:

> I adjure you, by the name of Allah, those of you who live in buildings, and those who reside in deserts and uninhabited places, that you present yourselves before me to listen to my order and execute it. All of you who are riding horses should appear, accompanied by your kings and princes; and all who are present or who are absent should appear, so that I may see you and speak to you in your own language, and obtain replies from you to the inquiries made from you as regards the treatment of this patient. Help, O Angels Rakyail, Jibrail, Mekiail, Sarfiail, Ainail, Kamsail, in producing these Jinns.

The soothsayer then foamed at the mouth and spoke to Shamburash, the king of the Jinns, who had entered his body. During the discussion with the king the patient was accused of all kinds of offences against the jinns, "such as sitting at night under a green tree without repeating the name of Allah; throwing stones at the heaps of house-sweepings, the usual place of rest at night of Jinns, and their children; throwing a bone, and thereby hurting the Jinns; finishing his meals without leaving anything; or throwing a half-burnt piece of wood without uttering Allah's name." The result of the dialogue was that "a black cock should be sacrificed, and a charm written with its blood and placed underneath the pillow of the patient, who also was ordered to eat its liver raw; but, alas! My dear uncle was dying."[27]

(iii) <u>Magical and Prayer Doctors</u>

In addition to the dead holy men and women as well as the denizens of the spirit world, there also were the living ones, some of who either aspired to become holy or were already on their way towards sanctity. This reputation usually started because some families were believed to possess an infallible remedy for the stings and bites of scorpions and tarantulas, in the shape of certain small stones, which were kept as heirlooms, and handed down from generation to generation as most cherished possessions.[28] This meant that they came close to be promoted to the next level of sanctity, as is clear from Percy Sykes' observation. At Zeinulabad (in Qa'en), "the headman informed me that his ancestors came from Bokhara some six generations ago.

---

[27] Sykes, *The Glory*, pp. 107-08.
[28] Sykes, *Through Persia*, pp. 111-12. On the role of religious leaders in all their manifestations and healing in pre-industrial societies see Heiler, *Erscheinungsformen*, pp. 373-407

On this account they consider themselves saints, able to perform cures, but this did not prevent them from anxiously enquiring whether I had a doctor with me!"[29] The chiefs of a Kurdish tribe, on the border between Persia and Iraq, claimed the power to be able to cure the ague.[30] According to Millingen, "in every tribe, there are a lot of Khodjas and Shekhs [sic] of both sexes, who are considered first-rate mediums, endowed with great spiritual and magnetic powers."[31]

Not only the dust of the tombs of holy people, but also that of living very revered people, was believed to have healing powers. Perkins observed that in Tabriz, "The chief Moollah is so much revered, that the dust where he treads is sometimes collected and administered to the sick as a medicine."[32] Among the Kurdish tribes similar customs existed. The local sheikhs not only managed tribal affairs and dispensed justice, but also medicine and spiritual guidance. Their followers revered these sheikhs, because of their ascetic and spiritual exemplary life. "The devotees eagerly take the water in which their sheik has bathed or washed his clothes, and rub it on their faces, or drink it, for its sanctifying qualities.[33]

One of the reasons that Persians believed in the healing powers of these aspiring saints was that they were allegedly endowed with magical 'life force' (*dom* or *nafas*). Morier, described the importance of a particular kind of charm, one that was reinforced by the 'breath of life' of the person who had made it.

> The Persians have great faith in a charm called the *dum*, or breath, which they say secures them against the bite of snakes and the sting of scorpions; and the courage was remarkable with which those who possessed it encountered those reptiles. We had among our servants one or two who had this charm.... Not long ago at Shiraz lived a man greatly celebrated for his sanctity, who had the reputation to possess the *dum* to such a degree, that he communicated it to *mureeds*, or disciples, who again dispensed it to the multitude. A young Mirza, brother to the then acting Vizier of Shiraz, gave to the Ambassador, as a great present, a knife, which he said had been charmed by this holy man, and if rubbed over the bite of a snake would instantly cure it. One of his disciples was at Shiraz whilst we were there, and he willingly complied with our request, that he would communicate his charm to us. The operation was simple enough. From his pocket he took a piece of sugar, over which he

---

[29] Sykes, Percy M. *Ten Thousand Miles in Persia or Eight Years in Iran* (New York: Charles Scribner's Sons, 1902), p. 396.
[30] Malcolm, *The History*, vol. 2, p. 536.
[31] Millingen, Frederick. *Wild Life Among The Koords* (London: Hurst and Blackett, 1870), p. 232; Hay, W.R. *Two Years in Kurdistan. Experiences of a Political Officer 1918-1920* (London: Sidgwick & Jackson, 1921), p. 38 (The word sheykh in Kurdistan "invariably refers to a man who is holy and venerated either on account of his descent from a sacred origin, or because of a pious life.").
[32] Perkins, *A Residence*, p. 151.
[33] Wilson, *Persian Life*, pp. 103-04 (they also gave written prayers or pills to sick people).

mumbled some words, breathed upon it, and then required that we should eat it, in full belief that neither serpent nor scorpion could ever more harm us.[34]

Another case of the occurrence of *nafas* was in Seistan. Just as there were stones that could prevent diseases there also were those that, if preventive measures clearly had failed, would cure disease. Edith Benn, the wife of British consul in Seistan, related that the headman (*kalantar*) of Iskil (near Nasratabad) had a black healing-stone. When the consul complained about headache, the headman vigorously rubbed Benn's neck, "breathing down his back at the same time, and punctuating his heavy puffs with several Allahul-Allahs and ummed-ba-Khudas (*i.e.* 'In God is our hope')." He told the Benns that he had recently cured his entire family of boils by rubbing them with the stone. When Benn declared that his headache had entirely gone, the headman even more firmly believed in the stone's efficacy.[35] In the same province, Captain Christie, masquerading as a sayyed, had been engaged in "breathing upon necklaces and into children's mouths, that they might derive all the benefit a Syyud could bestow."[36] Among the Kurdish tribes there was great faith in the 'breath of soul' of certain Naqshbandi Sufi sheykhs, who treated those afflicted that came to seek their help by blowing on the patient's shoulder, shoulder blade, or belly. This was referred to as entrusting oneself to the application of *dagh*, which was not a red-hot iron, but it was *qaw* or tinder. The sheikh would blow on it and his 'breath of soul' would penetrate the flesh and blood of the patient and thus heal him.[37] In and around Ardabil there were healers known as *ojaq* or hearth. They treated in particular children's diseases such as diarrhea and vomiting. These healers were mostly old women, in particular from two villages near Ardabil. They would heat an iron in the hearth (*ojaq*) and briefly put the hot iron on the neck of the patient and then rub the warm ashes of the hearth on his forehead. This and other therapies prescribed and applied by folk healers were called *tarkeh-dava* in Ardabil.[38] There were other female healers in the Ardabil region, known as *tikeh-otoran* or 'lump removers.' They would heal people with, for example, intestinal problems by rubbing with their fingers over the sick spot of the patient's body.[39]

The perceived power of a written charm could be significantly enhanced if it became known that another person with the 'breath of soul' also had taken it. When there was a cholera outbreak in Shiraz, Wills visited the house of the high priest (probably the Sheikh al-Eslam) to attend the latter's daughter, who was sick.

---

[34] Morier, *A Second*, p. 101-102. Basir al-Molk, *Ruznameh*, p. 60 (a snake catcher provided him with some pepper and a lump of sugar that he called *dom*. Basir al-Molk ate two grains of pepper and the lump of sugar. The snake catcher told him that since he had eaten the medicine, no snake or similar creature would come closer than 72 paces of anyone who had eaten that *dom* nor would it bite them.)

[35] Benn, *An Overland Trek*, p. 156. On the importance and significance of 'breathing' in general in Persia see Donaldson, *The Wild Rue*, pp. 14, 28, 87, 180-82.

[36] Pottinger, H. *Travels in Baluchistan and Sind* (London, 1816 [Karachi: Indus, 1976]), p. 410.

[37] Soltani, *Joghrafiya*, vol. 1, pp. 537-38.

[38] Safari, *Ardabil*, vol. 3, pp. 495-96.

[39] Safari, *Ardabil*, vol. 3, p. 497.

> He was writing charms against the cholera, I, out of curiosity, asked him for one; it was simply a strip of paper on which was written a mere scribble, which meant nothing at all. I took it and carefully put it away. He told me that when attacked by cholera I had but to swallow it, and it would prove an effectual remedy. ... The next day he called on me and presented me with ... a present. He laughingly told me that my serious reception of his talisman had convinced the many bystanders of its great value, and a charm desired by an unbelieving European doctor must be potent indeed. 'You see, you might have laughed at my beard; you did not. I am grateful. But if I could only say you had eaten my charm, ah – then.'[40]

While traveling through Kurdistan, Fraser observed "a very old woman who happened to pass, and who blew or grunted a prayer over them, and gave them pieces of old rags and coins, which she also blessed, and which were fixed to the caps of the little ones as charms against evil. The Doctor found the Koords, like all mountaineers, very superstitious."[41] Many dervishes traversed the countryside, where they offered their healing services in competition to mullahs, imams, sayyeds and other religious people. These all demanded payment before they would treat patients.[42] Sayyeds claimed special powers, of course, being descendents of the prophet himself, amongst other things through laying their hands upon the sick.[43] In the village of Sayyed Faj al-Din (NW Azerbaijan), most of the population consisted of sayyeds, who claimed, because of their heritage, that their prayers could heal those who had been afflicted by rabies.[44] A new group of faith healers was that of the panegyricists (*rowzeh-khvan*s), which was a growing group in, for example, Isfahan. Under Mohammad Shah their number in Isfahan had been only 10-15 persons, while in 1877 there were more than 100.[45]

The type of treatment described so far was not confined to Moslems only, but was applied too and believed in by all Persians whatever their creed. For example, a Chaldean Christian man with malaria would go to his priest who would pray over him and perform some ceremonies and then tie a string of cotton on his wrist and tell him to come again if he did not get well. The same priest would give a woman with tuberculosis two written "prayers, one to hang around her neck, the other to put in water and rub over and over

---

[40] Wills, *In the land*, pp. 290-91.
[41] Fraser, *Travels*, vol. 1, p. 72; Millingen, *Wild Life*, p. 232.
[42] Olivier *Voyage*, vol. 5, p. 113; Feilberg, *Les Papis*, pp. 151-52 for a description of a faith healing among Lur nomads.
[43] For information about the sayyeds and the various ways in which they made a living see Willem Floor, "The Economic Role of the 'Olama in Qajar Persia," in Linda Walbridge ed. *The Most Learned of the Shi`a* (New York: OUP, 2001), pp. 53-81; Aubin, *La Perse*, p. 313.
[44] De Sercey, Comte. *Une Ambassade Extraordinaire, La Perse en 1839-1840* (Paris: L'Artisan du Livre, 1928), p. 114.
[45] Tahvildar, *Joghrafiya*, pp. 80-81.

until the water is kind of black, then drink it."⁴⁶ It is of interest to note here that sayyeds and other mediums performed the same ceremony for sick Moslems.⁴⁷

More ubiquitous was the numerous "class of Persian physicians, called 'prayer doctors,' which will write prayers or quotations from the Mohammedan sacred books and sell them to the sick."⁴⁸ This class writers of prayers (*do`a-nevis*) consisted of dervishes, sayyeds, mullahs, and wise women. De Windt reported that, if purging and bleeding failed, "a dervish is called in, and writes out charms, or forms of prayer, on bits of paper, which are rolled up and swallowed like pills."⁴⁹ These prayer texts were thus prepared before the illness had even struck and were therefore carried by persons who bought them for the eventuality that they might feel indisposed. Korf, for example, related that Qa'emmaqam, Mohammad Shah's grand vizier, did not feel well and put such a prayer text in water, which, with the torn up text, he drunk in his presence.⁵⁰

In addition to wandering dervishes, sayyeds and mullahs, there also were professional prayer-writers who had a shop in the bazaar. Their number was limited. In 1925, there were 20 shops with 18 master prayer-writers (*do`a-nevis*) in Tehran, a city with more than 220,000 inhabitants at that time. These prayer-writers were unequally distributed over the city. There were three shops in the Bazaar quarter, eight in `Owdlajan, one in Sharq, two in Mohammadiyeh, six in Sangalaj quarter.⁵¹ In 1869, in Tabriz there were 50 prayer-writers.⁵²

As to the prayer charms, either "the writing washed off into water and swallowed, or the whole taken as a pill, or some form of prayer or incantation, are common; also propitiatory sacrifices, and, in case of the rich, money given to the poor, or to holy men."⁵³ Charms that were used to prevent disease also could be used as a medicine. Prayer, reciting verses from the Koran, and casting lead into a basin of water all were cures to extirpate fever in which people strongly believed.⁵⁴ Although a missionary with strong religious beliefs, Perkins did not have faith in the offer made by a sayyed to write a cure

---

⁴⁶ Sargis, "Persia and Her Doctors," p. 585.
⁴⁷ Massé, *Croyances*, vol. 2, p. 336; Millingen, *Wild Life*, p. 232. According to the *Borhan-e Qate`*, the string was known as *reshteh-ye tebb*. To be effective it had to have been strung by a maiden.
⁴⁸ Cochran, "Treatment," p. 106; Anonymous, "Ärtze und Arzneiwissenschaft," p. 97.
⁴⁹ De Windt, Harry. *A Ride to India across Persia and Baluchistan* (London: Chapman & Hall, 1891), p. 178; Polak, *Persien*, vol. 2, pp. 213-14 (*beytar*); Sykes, *Through Persia*, p. 46; Aubin, *La Perse*, p. 313. In Ardabil, there was a group of old women who were known as *chopchi* and *boghaz* who were engaged in prescribing these 'paper' medicines. Safari, *Ardabil*, vol. 3, p. 497.
⁵⁰ Korf, *Safarnameh*, p. 113.
⁵¹ Baladiyeh, *Dovvomin Salnameh*, pp. 82-83. On *do`a-nevisi*, augury, omen-taking and other supernatural practices, see Ahmad Kasravi, *Pendarha* (Atehran: Gutenberg, 1337/1958).
⁵² Javadi, *Tabriz*, p. 227. For facsimiles of various *do`as* for different disorders and explanation, see Homayuni, Sadeq. *Molk-e `Abir-amiz. Farhang va Mardom-e Fars, "Sarvestan"* (Shiraz: Beh Nashr, 1377/1998), pp. 347-62.
⁵³ Wills, *Persia*, pp. 86-87; Collins, *In the Kingdom*, p. 108; Nweeya, *Persia*, p. 87 ("prayer-water," obtained by soaking a prayer in water till the native ink is dissolved; if the patient will swallow the pulpy paper as well as drink the water, the remedy is quicker.")
⁵⁴ Millingen, *Wild Life*, p. 232.

for his ill son that would heal him, after having eaten the written text. Nevertheless, it was a useful and enlightening experience to him. "This incident explains a circumstance, that was a ludicrous enigma to us, when we first opened our medical dispensary at Oroomiyah. The sick, when receiving their doses, often inquired whether they should swallow the *paper* enclosing the medicine, as well as the medicine itself, -and some actually swallowed the prescription. And strange to tell, it does actually effect cures."[55] Because of the strong belief in faith healing, dervishes and sayyeds were much sought after. In urban areas, they usually did not make house calls, for patients came to them. Sometimes a strange utterance was enough to have the desired effect.[56] This was also brought home to European physicians, such as Hume-Griffith who noted the effective cures that placebos brought about.[57] Dr. Lichtwardt commented: "Let us not scorn this ancient system of psychotherapy, based upon a rational faith in an omnipotent God and necessitated by an isolation from scientific medical assistance. There are many less scientific and less effective systems even in countries which consider themselves enlightened."[58]

Although there were cheaters, such as Wolff's servant Hoseyn, who "pretended to cure diseases by saying Duas (charms),"[59] most of the providers of the faith-healing remedies were firm believers in their efficacy as well the seriousness of their task. In 1927, Norden saw in the square of Kazerun a man [a dervish] squatted on the ground, who wrote something on a strip of paper. He did not reply to Norden's question what he was doing. When he had finished his task, he told Norden's servant: " 'Your master should not have spoken. He almost broke the spell. I was writing for the girl who stands beside you. She wishes to become a mother.' He now handed the paper to the girl. She gazed reverentially at that panacea for her trouble, the cure for her barrenness; then she folded it and tucked it somewhere inside her dress. Another suppliant came. He wished to be healed on an infirmity. ... The faith of these simple folk was of a piece with that of the rest of the world, and who shall estimate what healing may be wrought because of faith?"[60] So strong was the belief in the Word of God that when treatment did not help a reader, sometimes a man, sometimes a woman, was sent for to read the Koran over their sick relatives in the hope to cure them.[61]

---

[55] Perkins, *A Residence*, p. 380.
[56] Serena, *Hommes*, p. 136.
[57] Hume-Griffith, *Behind the Veil*, p. 152.
[58] Lichtwardt, "Ancient Medicine," p. 81.
[59] Wolff, *Researches*, p. 280.
[60] Norden, Hermann. *Under Persian Skies* (Philadelphia: McCrea Smith, n.d.), pp. 134-35.
[61] Malcolm, *Children*, pp. 58 (with picture), 86.

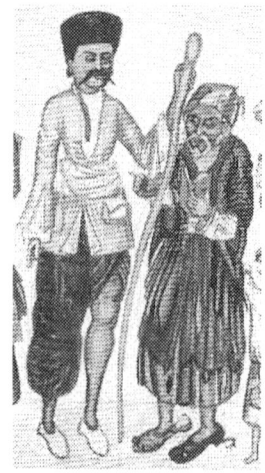

Figure 2: A Jew divining from his book for a muleteer.

There were also other professionals who provided cures, protection, and above all hope to the desperate and credulous population.[62] In 1869, in Tabriz, there were no less than 50 magicians and soothsayers (*jadugar va falbin*) and 20 geomancers (*rammal*), as well as 150 dervishes, who all catered to a needy clientele.[63] In Isfahan, there were physicians' families who of old were engaged in astrology, magic, and charms.[64] Among the Jews and Christians, similar customs existed and some rabbis made a living from writing amulets just as their Moslem counterparts.[65]

Because the human world is co-habited by demons and fairies, who could cast the evil eye, cause illness and other misfortunes, Persians had great belief in protective amulets (*telesm; ta`vidh*) and consequently they were bedecked with them as if they were highly decorated soldiers in the war against disease and misfortune. "There is scarcely, perhaps, an individual in the country, who does not carry one; some indeed are covered with them, and they positively attach these things to the necks of brute animals. These charms are scraps of paper or parchment with inscriptions, or stones carefully enclosed in little bags."[66]

---

[62] Donaldson, *The Wild Rue*, pp. 194-202.

[63] Javadi, *Tabriz*, pp. 227-28; Sheykh-Reza'i and Azari, *Gozareshha-ye Nazmiyeh*, pp. 88, 134, 236 (*tale`bin; do`akhvani*), 283 (*falbaz*). In the rural areas of Khorasan it were in particular gypsy women (*qereshmaliha*) who offered their services to see into the future and the past. Shakurzadeh, *`Aqayed va Rosum*, pp. 249-57. As to the belief in witchcraft see also Knanishu, J. *About Persia and its People* (Rock Island, Ill. 1899), pp. 81-83. Jews also were engaged in this occupation, see Loeb, *Outcaste*, pp. 215-16; Malcolm, *Five Years*, frontispiece; `Eyn al-Saltaneh, *Ruznameh*, vol. 2, p. 1387.

[64] Tahvildar, *Joghrafiya*, pp. 80-81.

[65] Sabar, *The Folk Literature*, p. xxxvii.

[66] De Freygang, Madame. *Letters from the Caucasus and Georgia* (London: John Murray, 1823), p. 345; Brugsch, *Im Lande*, pp. 207-08; Polak, *Persien*, vol. 1, p. 346; Ts., "Persidskie Doktora," p. 169.

The art of making charms and amulets was known as *jafr*, although the term normally referred to arithmomancy or divination by means of numbers.[67] Both animals and people were given amulets. There were amulets against all maladies, but there were also those that would bring about good things. Merchants hung them on their shops to attract buyers.[68] Charms were made of a variety of materials. The most powerful ones were made of metal or jade, inscribed with magical incantations, which were supposed to provide extra protection. The incantations could be the inscription of Koranic verses, mystical astrological signs, or of constellations that supposedly were possessed of magical power.[69] No Persian man left his house without a piece of cold iron in his pocket, "and a magnet is considered specially powerful in this way. A more common form of iron to carry is an iron chain, which is useful for driving mules and donkeys and beating off savage dogs."[70] Persians in particular believed that a diamond worn at the neck provided strength and annulled fear, while it was also an antidote against epilepsy.[71] Charms written on precious stones were not only powerful because of their innate properties, but also because the inscribed text did not easily fade.[72] Persian women believed that various colored stones (in particular, turquoise and blue ones) possessed healing properties, and they wore them round their neck against sickness.[73] Not only blue beads, but also tiny shells were effective against the evil eye. Women often tied one or more to their long plaits. A tattoo also attracted the evil eye and having one might just save you from harm.[74] A tiny bag with the scented earth of Karbala also served as a charm, while "if

---

[67] Schlimmer, *Terminologie*, p. 36, who also reported that the *Makhzan al-Adviyeh* recommends putting red coral (*marjan*) on a small child's stomach to take away all fear. Ibid., p. 157, and that onyx or *hajr-e babaghouri* was imported from Soleymaniyeh to be used as amulet. Ibid., p. 20. For some of the desired ingredients of an amulet see Vambéry, Arminius. *Voyages d'un Faux Derviche dans l'Asie Centrale* (Paris: Hachette, 1865), p. 37; Khan, Mesrop Nevton. "Talismanic Superstitions of Persia," *Gunter's Magazine* VI/2 (September ,1907), pp. 179-93. On Islamic amulets in general see Schienerl, Peter W. *Dämonenfurcht und böser Blick. Studien zum Amulettwesen* (Aachen: Alano, 1992), on the situation in Persia see Donaldson, *The Wild Rue*, pp. 203-08, 113-19, and on magical formulas and amulets in general see Heiler, *Erscheinungsformen*, pp. 340-43.

[68] Eichwald, *Reise*, vol. 1, pp. 446-47; Polak, *Persien*, vol. 2, pp. 213-14. The Bakhtiyaris had great faith in amulets and charms, and in chewing verses of the Koran in case of illness, according to Bird, *Journeys*, vol. 2, pp. 74-75.

[69] Morton, *A Doctor's Holiday*, p. 212; Rice, *Persian Women*, pp. 245; Eichwald, *Reise*, vol. 1, pp. 446; Lichtwardt, "Ancient Medicine," p. 83. In the case of Jews or Christians the text was, of course, of biblical origin. Sabar, *The Folk Literature*, p. 190; Loeb, *Outcaste*, pp. 213-15; Wigram, *The Cradle*, p. 329.

[70] Malcolm, Mrs. Napier. *Children of Persia* (Edinburgh: Oliphant, Anderson & Ferrier, 1911), p. 60; Malcolm, *Five Years*, p. 122. Klaproth, *Travels*, p. 43 reported that a mollah in Daghestan did not want to sell an old copper coin at any price, because he wore it as an amulet.

[71] Serena, *Hommes*, p. 135; see also Sykes, *Through Persia*, p. 112.

[72] Eichwald, Eduard. *Reise auf dem Caspischen Meere und in den Caucasus Unternommen in den Jahren 1825 1826*. 2 vols. (Stuttgart und Tübingen: J.G. Cotta, 1834), vol. 1, pp. 446-47. The text often was: There is no God but God, [and Mohammad is his prophet], or the names of Hasan and Hoseyn. Knanishu, *About Persia*, p. 83. In general see Donaldson, *The Wild Rue*, pp. 148-54.

[73] Sykes, Ella. *Persia and its People* (London: MacMillan, 1910), p. 336.

[74] Rice, *Persian Women*, pp. 245; see also the articles "Kardakkan" and "Tamima," *Encyclopedia of Islam*.

rubbed on the eyelids it is said to cause the eyes to shine brightly."[75] The right eye of a sheep that had been offered in sacrifice at Mecca also offered powerful protection.[76]

However, "The most common charm consists in a verse of the Koran enclosed in a tiny silver or tin box, worn at the throat."[77] Indeed, many if not most people had a part or the entire Koran with them. This was facilitated by the fact that the Koran could be had in a tiny and very popular two-inch hexagonal edition, written in a minute script known as *ghobar*, which could easily be, and in fact was, made into a charm. They were "sewn up in two little round or hexagonal cases, each containing half," worn on the arms. The small cases were made of plain leather or cloth, often green, because green was the sacred color, or they were "more elaborate and ornamental, or silver cases may be used with texts from the Qoran engraved upon them."[78] The use of silver metal added to the power of the amulet.

Morton rightly observed in this connection that, "This indicates, of course, that to some the Koran itself is a fetish. A miniature copy is placed on the head of a new-born infant. The 94th and 105th chapters, if read at morning prayer, will keep away toothache. The 13th verse of the 22nd chapter is a cure for headache. Its recitation on occasions of birth, death, or marriage is a cardinal necessity."[79] However, Islam had this veneration of the Holy Book in common with all other religions. Given the fact that most people (95%) were illiterate, the act of writing itself was magical and the Holy Book, having been written, or being written in the case of an amulet, was in and by itself supernatural. As such, the Koran had a powerful influence not only on the spirit, but also the body of the believer, if he really believed, of course.[80]

If you fell ill despite the fact that you carried the Koran or leaves from it with you could be very handy indeed. Merritt-Hawkes observed in the household she was visiting two children. "The younger boy was wearing on his arm a beautifully-engraved small square

---

[75] Malcolm, *Children*, p. 60.
[76] Nweeya, Samuel K. *Persia and the Moslems* (St. Louis, 1924), p. 86; Rice, *Persian Women*, p. 246; Lichtwardt, "Ancient Medicine," p. 84.
[77] Benn, *An Overland Trek*, p. 157.
[78] Malcolm, *Five Years*, p. 122; Stileman, Rev. Charles Harvey. *The Subjects of the Shah* (London: CMS, 1902), p. 49; Malcolm, *Children*, pp. 58-59 (a charm in the form of a little cloth camel, Abraham's camel, sewn on the cap). Tears shed during Moharram were collected as "charms to ward off sickness and evil influences." Perkins, *A Residence*, pp. 209-10; Donaldson, *The Wild Rue*, p. 178 ("Formerly there were to be seen numerous tear-bottles with long crooked necks and an opening of an eye bath, which were used to catch the tears which were shed for the martyred Husain."). Rice, *Persian Women*, p. 69 also mentioned, the wearing of the tiny Koran charm "in a small filigree gold or silver box, sometimes set with precous stones, or ornamented with the husband's photograph." For more details on charms see Ibid., p. 126.
[79] Morton, *A Doctor's Holiday*, p. 211; Rice, *Persian Women*, p. 246. In general see Donaldson, *The Wild Rue*, pp. 130-40.
[80] On the holy character of the Holy Book in various religions see Heiler, *Erscheinungsformen*, pp. 340-43.

box used to hold a piece of the Koran; but it was empty, as he had had a stomach ache two days ago and the Koran had been swallowed to ease the pain."[81]

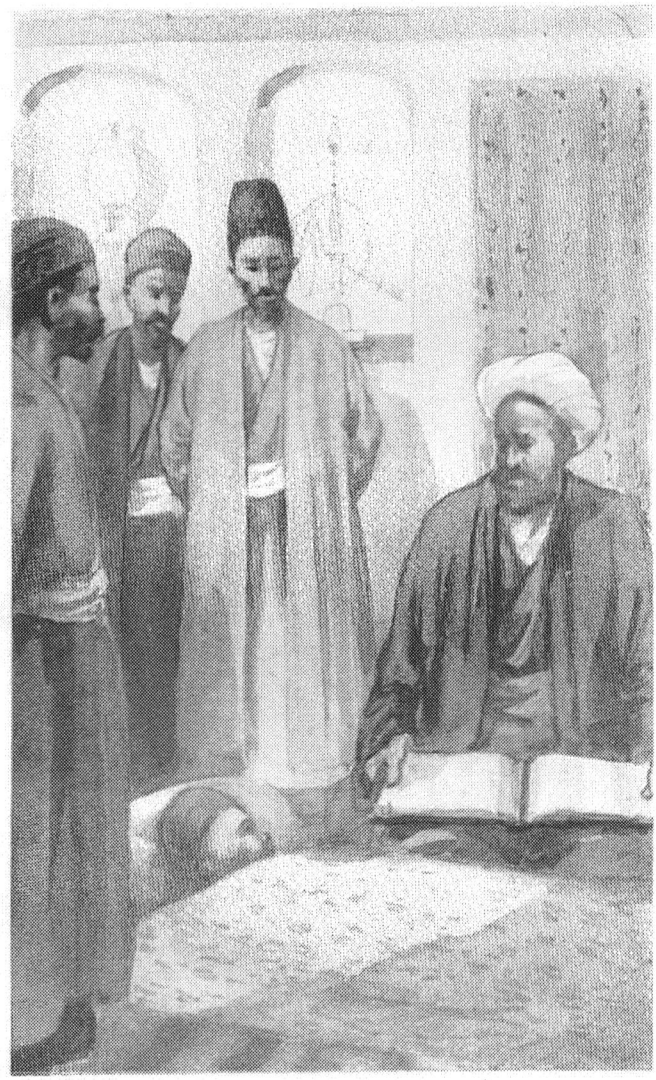

Figure 3: Reading the Koran to heal a sick child.

Most often, charms would be written on a small piece of paper, sewed on a child's hat or at the back of its coat. However, it also happened that relatives or well-meaning friends made an incision in a person's arm and inserted a blue bead or a paper prayer and then bound up the arm. Often infection was the result.[82] People, when they were ill, put these

---

[81] Merritt-Hawkes, *Persia*, p. 16.
[82] Morton, *A Doctor's Holiday*, pp. 212-13; Linton, *Persian Sketches*, p. 78; Lichtwardt, "Ancient

amulets on the front of their head, or close to the heart, and then would heal their malady, they hoped. Many people carried as many as six to eight amulets sewed to a ribbon as a bracelet, or carried it in a small box or case with them. They never put them off, and even kept them on their body while taking a bath.[83] Talismans were not only worn, but it seems they were even more powerful if they were put into the fire. They were also put into sweets (tea or sherbet) and buried with hidden treasure, for protection.[84] If an amulet inadvertently cracked, its wearer would be convinced that this was because somebody had cast the evil eye on him, but that fortunately the charm had counteracted and consequently had cracked. Otherwise worse would have happened to him.[85]

Pregnant women and babies were in particular the target of demons and the evil eye, and hence a strict system of do's and don'ts was adhered to during the last few months of pregnancy and the first 40 days after birth. The use of amulets formed an essential part of these procedures. Charms against the demon *Al*, who attacked women in childbirth, were in particular important. This demon already existed in Babylonian times (then known as *Lamashtum*) and remained part of the Persian cultural heritage. Amulets dating from that period are still extant. Given the fact that childbirth was and is dangerous the threat of the demon *Al* received special attention. The danger of *Al* and what to do about it was even described in popular Persian literature, for example, in the well-known *Kolthum-nameh*. There were even lithographed charms against the *Al* as well as invocations against it in the published texts concerned.[86] However, as important, if not more so, than written invocations against the *Al*, was the use of metal implements that contained the necessary powerful 'life force' to provide protection. "On this account a large pair of scissors, or some other steel or iron implement, is put at the head of the bed during the birth of a child, and kept there, or fastened to its hammock cradle afterwards."[87]

Once a child had been born, one of the women assisting at childbirth threw a bunch of iron keys into the basin in which the baby had been washed, then muttered a religious invocation and blew three times into the water, as a protection against the evil eye.[88] The preparatory arrangements having been completed,

---

Medicine," p. 83; Knanishu, *About Persia*, p. 83 (These "prescriptions are bound in a triangular form."). For pictures of children with their amulets and clothes with amulets see Feilberg, C.G. *Les Papis* (Copenhagen: Nordisk, 1952), pp. 117, 124, 126.

[83] Eichwald, *Reise*, vol. 1, pp. 446-47.

[84] Rice, *Persian Women*, p. 245 (charms were also fastened to valuable jewelry); Knanishu, *About Persia*, p. 186.

[85] Stileman, *The Subjects*, p. 49.

[86] Eilers, Wilhelm. *Die Al, ein persisch Kindbettgespenst* (Munich, Bayerische Akademie der Wissenschaften, 1979) (with pictures of the amulets); Merritt-Hawkes, *Persia*, p. 203; Donaldson, *The Wild Rue*, pp. 28-31.

[87] Rice, *Persian Women*, pp. 244-45; Churchill, "Sacrifices in Persia," p. 148. On practices at childbirth in general see Donaldson, *The Wild Rue*, pp. 24-34; see also Omidsalar, Mahmoud. "Childbirth in modern Persian folklore." *Encyclopaedia Iranica* V, pp. 404-407.

[88] Shabaz, *In the Land*, pp. 78-79; Khanishu, *About Persia*, pp. 82-83 ("When a child is born to a bride they stick needles in her clothes and let them remain there for forty days so that no demons may approach or touch her.").

they hang about the child's neck, or sew to its cap, a bangle, the colour of a turquoise, which they look upon as the most fortunate, and serves to annul the glance of an evil eye. They also insert paragraphs of the Koran into little bags, which they sew on the child's cap, or on its sleeve, esteeming them as great preservatives against sickness. If a visitor should praise the looks of a child, and if afterwards the child should fall sick, the visitor immediately gets the reputation of having an evil eye; and the remedy is, to take part of his clothes, which, with the seed of Ispedan*, they burn in a chafing-dish, and walk around and around the child. Him who has the reputation of having the evil eye, they keep at a distance.[89]

Persian women feared the evil eye more than anything and covered up their young babies out of fear that a stranger might admire them and have the evil eye.[90] "They bind the eyes of a child very tightly with a kerchief for the first ten to fifteen days. This they suppose, protects them from nervousness caused by seeing the light for the first time" Baby girls were not taken outside for 40 days and baby sons not for about 90 days, "because they believe illness will be caused by the expression of surprise from people that see them for the first time. Again their eyes must be always filled with khol, a black powder, which they think keeps them from becoming sore and makes them pretty when they are grown."[91] If, however, a child were stricken by the evil eye the mother would go to a holy man, a mollah or seyed, to have him remove the spell. "This holy man, whose breath, sanctified by the constant repetition of the name of the deity, has acquired a supernatural healing power, proceeds to make a series of mysterious breathings on the face of the child, accompanied by the imposition of his hands." He further prescribed drinking water mixed with some holy words written by him, or to tie the text to the child's arm, and to put another text under the child's pillow during the night, and he would be free from the evil eye.[92]

But not only were prayers or invocations written on paper to effect cures. Mme Serena reported that boiled eggs on whose shell an invocation to God had been written, and which was held for 24 hours under one's armpit, should prevent all internal pain.[93] Eggs with invocation written on them were also used to heal animals. In the Hazar Chal valley, the mollah of the village of Dizan had written Koran verses on two eggs which were to be broken over a sick mule's head.[94] In case a child had convulsions, its relatives would get a piece of silk or calico the length of the child, then would ask a mullah "to write a prayer

---

[89] Morier, *A Second*, p. 108 (note * is the seed of cresses). Blue colored-turquoise was indeed an effective antidote against the evil eye, but so were European shirt-buttons. Stileman, *The Subjects*, p. 49. For a similar rite practiced by Jews see Loeb, *Outcaste*, p. 220.
[90] Malcolm, *Children*, p. 60; Yonan, *Persian Women*, p. 25; Ts., "Persidskie Doktora," p. 170.
[91] Yonan, *Persian Women*, p. 25.
[92] Shabaz, Absalom D. *Land of the Lion and the Sun* (Madison, Wis., 1901), pp. 79-80, 137 (for other methods to achieve the same), Knanishu, *About Persia*, p. 83 ("Formerly when a child was born they would not carry with a coin or piece of gold because that would make the child become sallow.").
[93] Serena, *Hommes*, p. 135; Knanishu, *About Persia*, p. 81 (an egg "contains vital energy. This spell lasts for forty days but after that it must be renewed again.").
[94] Stark, *The Valley*, p. 285.

on it exactly the right length, and strap it down the child's back."[95] According to Ella Sykes, "the chief stock-in-trade of a Persian doctor is a brass bowl the outside of which is elaborately incised with the signs of the Zodiac and texts from the Koran. The inner surface is engraved with short prayers to suit all diseases, and the doctor has merely to make a feint of unlocking with a key the prayer that alludes to his patient's complaint, and when the sick man has drunk the water with which the basin is filled he will speedily recover."[96]

Apart from clear somatic medical problems, witchcraft was also a phenomenon that required the assistance of one or more curative health practitioners. According to Ella Sykes, "If witchcraft is suspected, one method is to bake eggs on the hearthstone of the patient's room, calling each by the name of some possible enemy. The egg that cracks first reveals the name of the wizard, and in order to free the sick man from his power the egg must be thrown into running water. Another plan is for the wife of the patient to beg bits of bread from the whole circle of acquaintance, as [sic; and] if he can eat the food of the man who has bewitched him he will be cured."[97] A variant of this method was known as *Aligi Salmakh*, a treatment applied by certain old women in the Ardabil region. The term refers to a shaved tall, thin, and conical spindle-like piece of wood. On top, where the end was in the middle of the balance, they fastened a thread, which was used for spinning or twisting wool and cotton threads. This instrument was used in the case of those patients, who according to these old women, was possessed by a dead person who had made him sick. This was manifested by fever and trembling followed by weakness of the entire body. The old woman would take the *aligi* in her hand and kept it still and quiet as a plumb line. Then one of the patient's relatives would name the names of deceased relatives one by one. If he mentioned the person who had taken hold of the patient the *aligi* would move. The same person then would name the foods that they ate and once again if the food was mentioned that the dead man liked the *aligi* would move. In this manner the name of the dead person and the food item that he liked had become known, both necessary elements to make the dead person depart from the patient's body.[98]

In addition to defensive apotropaic rites and symbols such as discussed above there also were eliminatory rites that aimed to achieve the same objective. It was achieved by transferring the illness to another being or to transform the nature of the illness to one less serious. Ussher observed a case of disease transfer in 1864 in Isfahan. The Imam Jom'eh had been suffering for a long time of an unknown ailment. During Ussher's visit a man came with a black sheep, "which was dragged forward by the horns, and with many pious ejaculations, led twice round the religious dignitary, after which it was taken away and given to some wretched and poverty-stricken people in the court below, who were eagerly waiting for the prize. The object of this strange ceremony was, that a disease

---

[95] Nweeya, *Persia*, p. 87.
[96] Sykes, *Persia and its People*, p. 339 (also for example, when given a safety pin by a European lady; it worked like a charm!); Sykes, *Through Persia*, p. 46.
[97] Sykes, *Persia and its People*, pp. 337-38; Brugsch, *Im Lande*, p. 207. On the use of various forms of magic by Kurdistani Jews see Sabar, *The Folk Literature*, pp. 85 (necromancy), 95-98, 172, 178, 194; Loeb, *Outcaste*, p. 216.
[98] Safari, *Ardabil*, vol. 3, p. 498.

under which the holy man had for some time laboured, should pass from his body into that of the sheep, which had been presented by one of his most faithful followers, with the design of thus relieving his spiritual director from his ailments."[99] Churchill confirmed this custom. He reported that when a member of the family was sick it was customary to kill a sheep to propitiate fate and avert danger from the sick person. "Should a goat or any animal die during the illness of any member of the household, it is held as a sure sign of the recovery of the patient, as it is thought that Fate has been satisfied by the substitution of the goat or other animal in the place of the patient."[100] The French traveler De Hell reported a case of disease transformation, which, he maintained, was an often-used 'cure.'

> Another presumption, which has its really comical side, that reigns generally in Persia, is to believe that each person, stricken by a chronic disease, is as if cured from that disease when any other disease manifests itself. Thus the shah, who suffers severely from the gout since a number of years, one day believed that he had a cold in the head, at a time that M. Labat was still his physician, it was a serious event, which was a source of satisfaction among the court and the people. Everybody congratulated the king with his cold in the head, as if something very felicitous had happened to him, and M. Labat received magnificent presents to have brought about such a remarkable change in the condition of his august patient.[101]

---

[99] Ussher, *A Journey*, pp. 591-92.
[100] Churchill, S.J.A. "Sacrifices in Persia," *The Indian Antiquary* XX (April 1891), p. 148; see also Bricteux, A. *Au pays du lion et du soleil (1903-1904)* (Brussels, 1908), p. 207.
[101] De Hell, X. Hommaire *Voyage en Turquie et en Perse*. 2 vols. (Paris: P. Bertrand, 1856), vol. 2, p. 62.

ISLAMIC-GALENIC PHYSICIANS

How to Become a Doctor

In principle, anyone could become a doctor (*hakim, tabib, pezeshk*). There was no school that provided formal training, nor was there an agency that certified the ability of a physician or licensed him to practice. A physician's education consisted of what he had learned from commentaries on the ancient, classical medical textbooks of Galen, Hippocrates, Razi, Avicenna, and the like. This meant that all diseases were classed as hot or cold, moist or dry.[1] According to the French traveler Olivier, who was in Persia during 1796-97, each physician had a number of apprentices who learned the art on the job. The master gave them some general instruction on the human body, the range of diseases that afflicted man, as well as their symptoms and causes, based on Galen and Avicenna. Most attention was paid how to distinguish between the various drugs, to know their properties, how to make opiates, electuaries, and syrups, in short, what remedies to prescribe. However, there was no interest to examine the biological properties of plants or the physical one of minerals.[2] Most physicians learned the medical practice as an apprentice to a physician, in particular, the son learning the art from his physician-father, according to Wills, writing some 80 years later.[3] Gilmour, writing in 1924, confirms the existence of this doctor-apprentice system, although he mentioned that it existed in the past. The apprentices had to learn Arabic, because most medical treatises were in Arabic. Once they had mastered that and had been in the doctor's service for some time they would be allowed to assist during examinations and the treatment of

---

[1] Mostowfi, *Sharh*, vol. 1, p. 527; Ts., "Persidskie Doktora," p. 158; Sykes, *Through Persia*, pp. 111-112; Serena, *Hommes*, p. 135; Bélanger, *Voyage*, vol. 2, pp. 218-19 ("They were the disciples of Galen, Avicenna, and supersition, and therefore were in need of development."); Morier, *A Second*, p. 191; Hasanbeygi, *Tehran-e Qadim*, pp. 197-98.

[2] Olivier, *Voyage*, vol. 5, pp. 109-110; see also Good, "The Transformation," p. 67; Polak, *Persien*, vol. 2, p. 193.

[3] Wills, *Persia*, p. 90; see also Haqiqat, `Abdol-Rafi`. *Tarikh-e Semnan* (Tehran: Farmandari-ye Koll-e Semnan, 1352/1973), pp. 536-37, 546-47, 550-52; Zarrabi, `Abdol-Rahim. *Tarikh-e Kashan*. ed. Iraj Afshar (Tehran: Ebn Sina, 1342/1963), pp. 400-03 (all the sons and grandsons of the doctors mentioned were also doctors); Moshtaq Kazemi, *Ruzgar*, p. 12 (doctor Mo'addeb al-Dowleh Nafisi was the son of doctor Nazem al-`Olama); Sepehr, *Mer'at al-Vaqaye`*, p. 217; Aubin, *La Perse*, p. 313; Nafisi, Sa`id. "Doktor `Ali Akbar Nafisi Nazem al-Atebba," *Yadgar* 3/4 (1325/1946), pp. 52-55; Qasemi, *Danesh*, p. 22; Dieulefoy, *La Perse*, p. 436; Good, Byron J. "The Transformation of Health Care in Modern Iranian History," in Michael E. Bonine and Nikki Keddie eds. *Modern Iran. The Dialectics of Continuity and Change* (Albany: State University of New York Press, 1981), pp. 62, 67; Ghani, *Yaddashtha*, vol. 1, pp. 188-89; Pirzadeh, *Safarnameh*, vol. 1, pp. 39, 48; Anonymous, "Ärtze und Arzneiwissenschaft in Persien," *Mitteilungen der K.K. Geographischen Gesellschaft* XLVIII (Vienna, 1905), p. 97; Lichtwardt, "Western Medicine," p. 237. Sometimes the sons did not follow in their physician-father's footsteps, see Afzal al-Molk Kermani, Gholam Hoseyn. *Tarikh va Joghrafiya-ye Qom*. ed. Hoseyn Modarresi Tabataba'i (Qom, 1396Q/1976), p. 145; Nezam al-Saltaneh Mafi, *Khaterat va Asnad*, vol. 1, p. 265; Safari, *Ardabil*, vol. 3, p. 475; and sometimes a doctor's father was not a physician but, for example, a confectioner (*qannad*), see Asaf al-Dowleh, *Asnad*, vol. 2, p. 237.

the sick. It was the task of the apprentices to copy the doctor's prescriptions for the different diseases, of which they learned to recognize the various signs and symptoms. They also weighed and mixed the herbs when preparing medicines. After having worked for two or three years in that manner the doctor would give his apprentice a certificate stating that he had the necessary competence to practice this art.[4] The students of medicine did not read the classics of Islamic-Galenic medicine, such as the *Qanun* of Ibn al-Sina, but mainly read commentaries on commentaries on commentaries of the classics. These included texts such as the *Nazir-e Qanun va Shafa'*, *Tohfeh-ye Hakim-e Mo'men*, *Barabar al-Sa`ah*, *Tebb al-Sadeq*, *Makhzan al-Adviyeh*, *Tebb al-Reza*, and possibly the handwritten notes of their teacher detailing his own experience with diagnostic and therapeutic results.[5]

However, the new doctor's knowledge still was quite limited. "Anatomy is quite unknown, and no such thing as necropsy is ever permitted."[6] An anonymous mid-nineteenth century Persian author stressed that, "very few [Persian] doctors existed who were able to distinguish between diseases with similar symptoms or to cure dangerous maladies."[7] Another Persian author, Mohammad Shafi` Qazvini, wrote about 1880, that

> "[Persian doctors] should be qualified, have experience and should have taken the government's tests. If they are qualified, they should treat people according to the instructions, which prevail in European countries. It happens that a lot of them kill people. Uneducated doctors and druggists (`attar) who have no religious beliefs have killed a lot of people over the years." They were unlike doctor Qazvini, Mirza Abu Torab, who was well-known and qualified, having all the required characteristics. He had cured many people and always maintained, "that people because of their poverty go to these inexperienced doctors and the patient comes close to death and then they come to me and I enter to see the patients with the Angel of Death together, but fortunately I prevail and the patient gets well, with the help of God."[8]

---

[4] Gilmour, *Rapport*, p. 33; Good, "The Transformation," pp. 66-67.

[5] Hasanbeygi, *Tehran-e Qadim*, p. 198; Ts., "Persidskie Doktora," p. 162. The *Tohfeh-ye Hakim-e Mo'men* was published in 1851 and was much used by doctors, as is clear from Schlimmer's many references to this book. At the time of its publication it cost 15,000 dinars, see Government of Iran, *Vaqaye`-ye Ettefaqiyeh*, vol. 1, pp. 188, 216; `Oqeyli Khorasani, *Makhzan al-Adviyeh* (Calcutta, 1844 [Tehran, 1355/1976]). According to Lichtwardt, "Western Medicine," p. 237 they had a "few textbooks (some written in beautiful quatrains!)." Lichtwardt referred to texts written by, for example, Yusef b. Mohammad, *Tebb-e Yusef*, written in Herat in 1511, "his still-popular book of therapy." Lichtwardt, H.A. "Ancient Therapy in Persia and England," *Annals of Medical History* 6 (1934), pp. 280-84 in which he presents some of Yusef's quatrains in versified English.

[6] Wills, *Persia*, p. 90; Clarke, "Sketches, p. 708 ("A man to be seen dissecting would be taken for a ghoal, and he would be shunned as a degraded being."); Drouville, Gaspard. *Voyage en Perse pendant les années 1812 et 1813*. 2 vols. (Paris, 1819 [reprint Tehran: Imp. Org. f. Social Services, 1976), vol. 2, p. 164; Ts. "Persidskie Doktora," p. 162. For the preceding era see Savage-Smith, E. "Attitude towards Dissection in Medieval Islam," *Journal of the History of Medicine and Allied Sciences* 50/1 (1994), pp. 67-110.

[7] Ebrahimnejad, "Theory and Practice," p. 171.

[8] Qazvini, *Qanun-e Qazvini*, pp. 124-25.

This is not surprising given the nature of medical knowledge available to Persian doctors as well as the way in which many acquired it. According to Dr. Carr, a Church Missionary Society (CMS) physician, "if a man wishes to become a doctor he buys a book in the bazaar, reads it for a few weeks, learns what diseases are said to be hot and which are cold, and the same with regard to food and medicine, and then he is ready for practice. He knows nothing of the circulation of the blood."[9] According to Hume-Griffith, "with this knowledge, plus a few Persian medical books and an appropriate turban, the native quack sets up as a doctor."[10] Adams was even more negative and wrote that, "Native doctors require no other diploma to enter the profession of medicine than a supply of infinite assurance."[11] This approach excluded knowledge of manual procedures such as bleeding, which were learnt through apprenticeship, and generally were not done by doctors, but by barbers and surgeons.[12]

The critics who maintained that anybody could get a smattering of medical knowledge by simply buying and reading a medical text were right. Professional doctors as well as amateurs copied existing older texts and turned them into short practical compendia for use by laymen (`avam). As Ebrahimnejad has rightly pointed out this delivery system ensured the adoption of Galenic concepts into social life.[13] For example, Freya Stark related that she discussed the cuckoo bird with a man in the Alamut region. The man disagreed with her that it was a useless bird, arguing: "If your eye is diseased, and you smear ointment made from the cuckoo's eyes upon it, it will heal. Allah makes all things useful. This is written in a book called *The Peculiarities of Beasts*. It is true. You can buy it in the bazaar."[14] Nezam al-Saltaneh Mafi consulted both Persian and European medical texts when several physicians had been unable to cure him of his problem of blood loss (*nazf al-dam*). He was in particular familiar with the Persian pharmacopoeia *Makhzan al-Adviyeh*.[15] In fact, according to Polak, every family (he undoubtedly meant those that were well-to-do) had a medical text among its store of books. Whether man or woman, those familiar with the medical text, felt obliged to be the medical counsel for the family and beyond.[16]

---

[9] Stileman, *The Subjects*, p. 47; Sargis, "Persia and Her Doctors," p. 586 ("as a rule the profession of a man has descended to him from his ancestors for many hundred years"); Qarib, `Abdol-Karim. *Gorgan* (Tehran, 1363/1984), p. 48 (Mirza Mostafa Khan Mostowfi, when he retired as an accountant in Astarabad, provided free-of-charge medical advice that he obtained from books such as *Tebb-e Yusefi* and *Majmu`eh al-Kobra*.); Polak, *Persien*, vol. 2, p. 193.

[10] Hume-Griffith, *Behind the Veil*, p. 160; Rice, *Persian Women*, p. 253; Good, "The Transformation, " p. 66; Ts., "Persidskie Doktora,"p. 169.

[11] Adams, *Persia*, p 59. This opinion was shared by Linton, *Persian Sketches*, p. 78, who wrote that because his father and grandfather had been a *hakim*, no qualification was necessary, for this was conferred on him by heredity. "He may not be able to to read or write, but he is hakim by birth, and so he can practise."

[12] Drouville, *Voyage*, vol. 2, p. 165.

[13] Ebrahimnejad, "Theory and Practice," p. 173.

[14] Stark, *The Valley*, p. 181. The text referred to probably was *Khavass al-Hayavan* by Mohammad Taqi Tabrizi, a dictionary of the medical properties of animals, based on Damiri's *Hayat al-Hayavan*.

[15] Nezam al-Saltaneh Mafi, *Khaterat va Asnad*, vol. 1, pp. 69, 141.

[16] Polak, *Persien*, vol. 2, p. 195.

PERSIAN DOCTORS ENJOYED HIGH STATUS

Although Europeans considered most Persian doctors superstitious medicine men rather than physicians, these doctors nevertheless occupied a high status in Persian society.[17] This was bound up with the fact that medicine was a science that was imbued with a supernatural dimension, and like the primitive medicine man, gave the doctor a 'magical' aura.[18] However, this respect was not sufficient to protect the doctor if the patient died, because the doctor was blamed. For if he had not interfered the patient would not have died, or so was the belief. Doctors therefore withdrew from the case when they realized that the patient's end was near. If he was unlucky to be present at the death he ran the risk to be being beat up by the womenfolk and the rabble. To avoid such an event doctors (including Polak) had informants to apprise them about the patient's condition.[19]

Some physicians even reached high social and political status. Mirza Nazar `Ali Hakim-Bashi-ye Qazvini, married Mohammad Shah's half-sister and in vain tried to become grand vizier.[20] In 1824-25, Fath `Ali Shah's physician (*tabib-e khasseh*), Hajji Mirza Ebrahim-e Shirazi, who was known for his stylistic skills, was appointed royal chancellor (*monshi al-mamalek*) with the honorific Mo`tamed al-Dowleh.[21] There were also minor Qajar princes who had become physicians.[22] Other doctors held in addition to their practice as physician also government posts. One, Mirza Abu'l-Qasem Tabib, had to estimate conversion prices (*tas`ir*) for government grain and Mirza Kazem Hakim-Bashi had been hired by Asaf al-Dowleh, governor of Gilan, to construct a road between Enzeli and Pir-e Bazar.[23] Leading Persian doctors often had many interests other than medicine.[24] Indeed, Mirza Salman Tabrizi, who was a well-known philosopher, also was a well-respected doctor.[25]

Apart from the fact that a Persian doctor was a learned person, and was the harbinger of help and hope, if not cure, the fact also, as Perkins put, that "this profession is usually

---

[17] Wills, *Persia*, p. 90; Hume-Griffith, *Behind the Veil*, p. 160; Olivier, *Voyage*, vol. 5, p. 109; Drouville, *Voyage*, vol. 2, p. 164; Jaubert, *Voyage*, p. 249; Bird, *Journeys*, vol. 1, p. 325; Hasanbeygi, *Tehran-e Qadim*, p. 198.

[18] Adler, *Jews in Many Lands*, pp. 189-90; Ebrahimnejad, "Religion and Medicine," p. 91 (he also stresses the religion-medicine relationship). That attitude is still the same irrespective of the location of any given society on this planet.

[19] Polak, *Persien*, vol. 2, p. 216.

[20] Varjavand, Parviz. *Simay-e Tarikh va Farhang-e Qazvin* 3 vols. (Tehran" Ney, 1377/1998), vol. 2, pp. 1244-47. Physicians also belonged to the local elite of Semnan and Kermanshah. Haqiqat, `Abdol-Rafi`. *Tarikh-e Semnan* (Tehran: Farmandari-ye Koll-e Semnan, 1352/1973), pp. 526-27, 544-45, 550-52; Soltani, Mohammad `Ali. *Joghrafiya-ye Tarikhi va Tarikh-e Mofassal-e Kermanshahan*. 3 vols. (Tehran, 1370/1991), vol. 1, pp. 532-33.

[21] Fasa`i, *Farsnameh*, vol. 1, p. 727, 739.

[22] Nezam al-Saltaneh Mafi, *Khaterat va Asnad*, vol. 1, pp. 179, 255, 275.

[23] Asaf al-Dowleh, *Asnad*, vol. 1, pp. 82, 137; vol. 2, pp. 86, 93. These extra-professional activities could be a very enriching experience, according to Polak, *Persien*, vol. 2, p. 195.

[24] See, for example, Taqi, Mir. *Pezeshkan-e nami-ye Fars* (Tehran, 1361/1982); Safari, *Ardabil*, vol. 3, p. 475.

[25] De Gobineau, *Les Réligions*, vol. 1, p. 112.

united with the clerical, in some of the inferior Moollahs," may further explain this high social status.[26] This was not only because doctors dressed and comported themselves like mullahs (including the use of a walking stick), but also the result of the fact that medicine was part of the curriculum of religious students (*talebeh*) in addition to religion, grammar, mathematics, philosophy, etc. Some of the popular compendia, such as the *Qavanin-e `Alaj* (Compendium of the rules of treatment) explicitly catered to religious students.[27] In Maragheh, in 1921, of the 11 herbal doctors three had been trained as mullahs.[28] In this connection the 'biography' of Mo`ezz al-Din Mahdavi's father is of interest. Mahdavi Sr. had studied both exegesis (*feqh*) and first principles (*osul*), but was not interested in spending his life as a religious professional and turned down the offer of the prestigious function of *pishnamaz* of the Royal Mosque in Isfahan. Because he also had studied medicine and mathematics he had practiced as a doctor when he was young. After having practiced for some time, he abandoned this line of work, because ethically he was not convinced that he was a good physician and he therefore became a teacher of mathematics. Nevertheless, Mahdavi Sr. strongly believed that he was at the same level of medical knowledge as his fellow student Hajji Mirza Mohammad Baqer Hakim-Bashi, a famous physician and trainer of a new generation of medical doctors.[29]

As in other major towns, in Kerman doctors also belonged to the elite. Until about the mid-nineteenth century there were only doctors of the Hakimiyan and Nafisi family, thereafter a few others also started to practice in that town. Apart from medicine, all of these doctors also had studied other subjects and some even were known to excel in poetry, for example.[30] Likewise, in Qom, physicians belonged to the town's elite and the same held for rural districts such as Arasbaran (Azerbaijan).[31] In the first half of the nineteenth century some of the doctors in Kermanshah were so renowned that people from other parts of Persia sought their treatment and healing.[32] In Ardabil, in addition to

---

[26] Perkins, *A Residence*, p. 390. Rasooli, Jay M. and Allen, Cady H. *The Life Story of Dr. Sa`eed of Iran* (Grand Rapids: Grand Rapids International Publications, 1958), pp. 19-20; Zarrabi, *Tarikh*, pp. 400-03; Balaghi, Sayyed `Abdollah. *Ketab-e Ansab-e Khandanha-ye Mardom-e Na'in* (Tehran, 1369Q/1949-50), pp. 24-25 (Sadat-e Hakimi family who were both physicians and *ahl-e menbar*); Ghani, *Yaddashtha*, vol. 1, pp. 188-89. A Russian doctor stated that in Persia doctors were either barbers or clergymen, see Anonymous, "Ärtze und Arzneiwissenschaft," p. 97.
[27] Ebrahimnejad, "Religion and Medicine," p. 99; Nezam al-Saltaneh Mafi, *Khaterat va Asnad*, vol. 1, p. 276; Ts., "Persidskie Doktora," p. 158.
[28] Good, "The Transformation," p. 68.
[29] Mahdavi, Mo`ezz al-Din. *Dastaha'i az panjah sal owza`-ye ejtema`i-ye nim-qarn-e akhir* (Tehran, 1348/1969), p. 6.
[30] Vaziri, Ahmad `Ali Khan, *Joghrafiya-ye Kerman* (Tehran, 1346/1967), pp. 51-52; Nafisi, "Doktor `Ali Akbar Khan," pp. 56-58. As in other towns, the leading physician of each city quarter had the title of *hakim-bashi*, while the doctor taking care of the work of the Sanitary Council was known as *hafez al-sehhah*. Mirza Bozorg, who had studied medicine in Paris, was engaged in spiritual medicine (*yadubeyza*) and manual medicine (`amal-e yadi)
[31] Afzal al-Molk Kermani, *Tarikh*, pp. 145-46 (one was even a brother of the town's governor); Beyburdi, Sarhang. *Tarikh-e Arasbaran* (Tehran: Ebn Sina, 1341/1962), p. 225.
[32] Soltani, *Joghrafiya*, vol. 1, pp. 531-33; Fasa'i, Hajj Mirza Hasan Hoseini. *Farsnameh-ye Naseri*. 2 vols. ed. Mansur Rastgar Fasa'i (Tehran: Amir Kabir, 1378/1999), vol. 2, p. 995.

Moslem doctors, there also were a few Armenian ones, one Christian Assyrian, and one Jewish doctor, who was much respected in particular.[33]

In Zarrabi's *History of Kashan* the doctors are classed in one chapter together with the old elite families of olama and government officials. The doctors were not only famous for their knowledge of natural science (*hekmat-e tabi`i*), medicine (*tebb*) and their experience (*tajrebeh*), but also for other sciences. This held, in particular for the Jewish doctors, the most famous of which was a very learned religious scholar, a superior stylist, who had an outstanding hand of writing, and excelled at orthography (*emla'*), eloquence (*fasahat*), rhetoric (*balaghat*), and Arabic. He also was well versed in the Jewish and Islamic religions. Moreover, the Jewish doctors of Kashan, unlike their Moslem colleagues in the same town, were renowned for their knowledge of natural science (*hekmat-e tabi`i*), knowledge (*`elm*), and manual practice (*`amal-e yadi*) such as surgery (*jarrahi*), ophthalmology (*kahhali*) and chemistry (*dava-sazi*), in which subjects they were without peers.[34] Brugsch also noticed that both Moslem and Jewish doctors practiced medicine in Hamadan province. He opined that they had a kind of veterinarian approach to medicine, which unavoidably resulted in many mishaps.[35] Lycklama noticed that in the large village of Kengavar there were 15 Jewish families, who were all druggists and doctors. In the next village, Sa`adatabad, there was only one Armenian and 12 Jews, all of whom were also druggists and doctors.[36] In 1907, Aubin noted a Jew who had come to the village of Vertcheh to practice medicine, whom he considered to be representative of the Jewish physicians who dominated the supply of medical service the rural areas of `Iraq-e `Ajam.[37] There also were quite a few Jewish doctors practicing in Tehran, two of whom treated Mohammad Shah for some time and later also Naser al-Din's crown prince.[38]

Not every Persian was happy with the dominant role of Jewish healers in certain towns, however. Mohammad Shafi` Qazvini, for example, opposed the dominance of these Jewish doctors, because they came too much into contact with Moslem women and, to make his point 'convincing,' for he had no other 'evidence,' he did not eschew a bit of stereotype anti-Semitism.

---

[33] Safari, *Ardabil*, vol. 3, pp. 477-79; vol. 2, p. 80.
[34] Zarrabi, *Tarikh*, pp. 402-03; see also Fasa'i, *Farsnameh-ye Naseri*, vol. 1, pp. 393, 460, 496, 553, 555, 996; vol. 2, 1005, 1007, 1012, 1020-21, 1053, 1135, 1159, 1165, 1167. As to Nur Mahmud Hakim as he was know to Moslems, but Rabbi Nahurai to his co-religionists, "his European colleagues of the most advanced type respect as infirntely superior to the ordinary native Hakim. In fact they regard him as a mine of empirical knowledge. He possesses a fine little library of Persia, Arabic, and Hebrew manuscripts, mostly medical." Adler, *Jews in Many Lands*, p. 188.
[35] Brugsch, *Reise*, vol. 2, p. 17.
[36] Lycklama, *Voyage*, vol. 3, pp. 493, 498.
[37] Aubin, *La Perse*, p. 312. Polak, *Persien*, vol. 2, p. 194 stated that Jewish doctors had a quasi-monopoly of medical assistance in Kurdistan and Turkistan.
[38] Elgood, *Medical History*, p. 494; Polak, *Persien*, vol. 1, p. 194 (Hak Nazar); see also Nezam al-Saltaneh Mafi, *Khaterat va Asnad*, vol. 1, pp. 149, 167; Adler, Elkan Nathan. *Jews in Many Lands* (Philadelphia: Jewish Publication Society of America, 1905), p. 188 (Nur Mahmud Hakm or Rabbi Nahurai also treated Mozaffar al-Din Shah).

Presently the custom in Persia is that Moslem women do not stay away from Jewish men and every day they go back and forth to fifty Jewish houses for different transactions, especially with three groups of these people:

First the Jewish priests (molla) who deceive the women; Tehrani women all have problems, either their husband has another wife (*huv*) or their husband has relations with another man or a prostitute, which has made the wives unhappy (*siyah-bakht*), and those devils tell a lot of lies to Moslem women. They waste the money (*mal*) of Moslems and also they risk their chastity. God and his prophet have ordered that Moslem women should stay away from Jewish women. It is for this reason that, in their home at night, Jewish women will tell their husband the qualities of Moslem women and change his thinking to bad thoughts. God was not satisfied with this behavior and ordered his Angel Gabriel to announce that Moslem women should stay away from the Jews. I seek refuge with God from the obliteration of Islam, because all distinguished women of Tehran are in the office of a Jewish doctor every morning, and these pure women have to be treated by Jewish doctors.

Besides these cases, those Jews, who go around the city peddling and do business with Moslem women have insisted on [using] invocations … such as 'by the split [head] of Morteza `Ali,' (*beh farq-e shekafteh*), on Fatemah's hair (*beh gisu-ye Fatemeh*), or say 'by the blood of the martyr of martyrs.' They have agreed amongst themselves to use these three invocations because of their animosity towards Moslems. In our religion, the taking of these important names by a Moslem in the presence of a Jew is very disrespectful, and they should not take the names of these pure ones."[39]

NOT EVERY DOCTOR WAS A PHYSICIAN

The opaque situation of a Persian doctor's training and credentials made it impossible for Persian patients, or even the professionals themselves, to distinguish between a real physician and a quack, if there was such a distinction. However, apart from word-of-mouth information about the expertise of a doctor, there also was an effort by doctors themselves to set themselves apart from those whom they considered to be quacks or at

---

[39] Qazvini, *Qanun-e Qazvini*, pp. 123-24. Agha Najafi, the leading religious leader of Isfahan between 1880-1910 actually enforced a ban on access by Jews to the *enderun*s in 1907 for a while, until the government intervened. Aubin, *La Perse*, p. 296. It is unlikely that Jewish doctors actually had access to the harems. See, however, Hardy, Arthur Sherburne. *Things Remembered* (Boston: Houghton Mifflin, 1923), p. 94 (he was American Minister in Persia 1898-1900) who reported that "I saw an Armenian merchant from the bazaar, laden with silks and velvets, coming out of the door [of the harem] I was not privileged to pass. "So mere man," I said to His Excellency [Moshir al-Dowleh], "sometimes crosses this threshold." "Bah!" was his half-laughing, half-scornful reply, "an Armenian is not a man." Most of the doctors' patients were indeed women, according to Polak, *Persien*, vol. 2, p. 195.

least undesirable competitors. In the rank-conscious Persian society, physicians therefore also followed the general trend by trying to obtain high-sounding honorifics and titles to distinguish themselves from their less fortunate, but not necessarily less qualified, colleagues. As in other sectors of Qajar society, for a person to obtain a leading post and title with commensurate high income was more due to whom you knew than what you knew. Irrespective of whether a doctor had been able to obtain an official court title, after 1854 they all wanted to have the title 'doctor' in front of their name, a title bestowed on those who graduated from the medical course of the *Dar al-Fonun*. Those that had obtained the title of doctor, rightly or wrongly, tried to deny others who had not been so lucky the use of the same to mark themselves off against these automatically lower-classed physicians.[40] Also, doctors dressed up and behaved as if they were well-off so as to project an image of success, which enhanced their reputation.[41]

It did not convince Perkins, who was aware of the good standing doctors enjoyed, but he also pointed out the down side of this situation. "The medical profession, in Persia, is a most flagrant system of quackery. Naturally superstitious and supremely devoted to the body, the people have great reverence for physicians; and much as they suffer from empiricism, they are never tired of seeking relief from imposters."[42] John Malcolm put quackery in perspective when he wrote "in this country, as in all others, there are many quacks in medicine, who obtain money or respect by pretending to cure all complaints."[43] Because Persian physicians were not accessible or not able to provide effective treatment, the desperate Persian sick turned to anything or anybody that held out hope for relief, if not cure. European charlatans in Persia also took advantage of them, because the people had no notion of medical science at all. Korf, a member of the Russian Mission in Tabriz related, that when he was in Tabriz there was a German who made beer. It was a bad batch and nobody wanted it. Because he had to make money to live, the German brewer set himself up as a doctor. He had a box with instruments and another with bottles filled with remedies. He hung them on his belt and off he went in search of patients.[44]

LOCATION OF A DOCTOR'S PRACTICE
As in any profession you had physicians who just started their calling, others who had already established their reputation and then those who were in between those who had experience, but did not yet have the reputation they aspired to. Most physicians were urban based, although a few would also travel to small towns and large villages in the district of the district's chief town in which they lived. Mostowfi, for example, related

---

[40] Ebrahimnejad, "Theory and Practice," p. 172; Sepehr, *Mer'at al-Vaqaye`*, p. 217 (in this case the son obtained his father's title); Linton, *Persian Sketches*, p. 81. According to Afzal al-Molk, *Afzal al-Tavarikh*, p. 198 the sons of many of the leading Islamic-Galenic doctors acquired western training and in addition to their traditional title also added the title of 'doctor' to their name.
[41] Ts., "Persidskie Doktora," pp. 158-59.
[42] Perkins, *A Residence*, p. 390.
[43] Malcolm, *The History*, vol. 2, p. 534. This situation has not changed either as indicated by the growth (or rather the revival) of so-called alternative medicine, in all its manifestations.
[44] Korf, *Safarnameh*, pp. 230-31; Perkins, *A Residence*, p. 390 (Europeans also offer their services as quacks).

that his sister had been treated for a heart problem a few times in Nayeh, his family's village. The first time, an itinerant Jewish doctor treated her, and the second time another Jewish doctor did.[45] These itinerant doctors demanded payment up front. What they lacked in medical knowledge they made up for in self-assurance. They had a small sack with a limited number of medicines and some instruments. They prescribed electuaries, concoctions, and they did cautery, bleeding, cupping, without having the least idea why they did so, according to Olivier.[46] Adams also reported that Persian doctors "are generally itinerants who go from village to village and announce their profession on arriving. Extraordinary remedies are given. Having prescribed, the physician decamps before the results become perceptible, aware that a common sequence is death. Fortunately, for the practitioners, this result is generally quietly accepted as the fiat of Kismet or Destiny."[47]

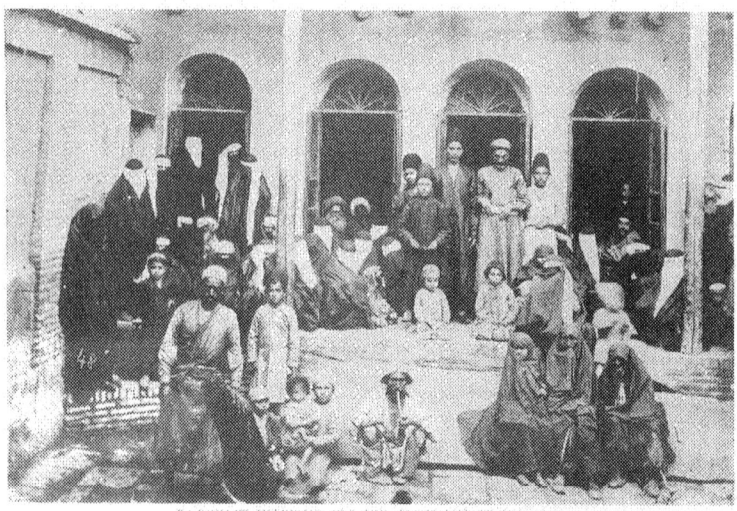

Figure 4: Patients waiting at the doctor's office.

Other physicians had their office, which was referred to as *mahkameh*, in the bazaar or at home. Dr. Bélanger, for example, mentioned many of such cases in the bazaar of Tabriz, some of whom had their lodgings and an apothecary in a caravanserai.[48] This may have occasioned the remark made by Waring that "medicine is a trade with them."[49] The floor of the doctor's office was covered with a felt, while some shelves against the wall were filled with jars and bottles bearing labels with Latin script that contained syrups, elixirs

---

[45] Mostowfi, *Sharh*, vol. 1, p. 527 (both times with a medicine that they had ready-made in their pouch); Aubin, *La Perse*, pp. 312-13.
[46] Olivier, *Voyage*, vol. 5, pp. 112-13.
[47] Adams, *Persia*, pp. 59-60.
[48] Bélanger, *Voyage*, vol. 2, pp. 195, 336; Polak, *Persien*, vol. 2, p. 195; Wishard, *Twenty Years*, p. 198 picture of the physician's shop in the bazaar. E'tesam al-Molk, *Safarnameh*, p. 115-17 ("In the sanctuary of Imam Reza I went to the doctor's office [*hojreh*]."); Hasanbeygi, *Tehran-e Qadim*, p. 197.
[49] Waring, *A Tour*, pp. 48-49

and pills.⁵⁰ These were not beginning physicians, but experienced men with some reputation. The latter was the most important qualification for a physician, as is clear from the case of illness that fatally struck `Eyn al-Saltaneh's servant. The servant, Mohammad Taqi, died after four days of diarrhea (*eshal*) and general weakness in Shemiran.

> I told him, 'let's return to the city, for there are good doctors there.' 'No,' he said, 'here they are better.' He thus put himself in the hands of bad doctors. For example, `Abdollah Khani, the Armenian, does not know anything about medicine. He gave him this unlucky fellow one garlic per day with some *krt* (?); how can you treat typhoid fever (*hesbeh*) that way? I wrote for good doctors to come, they could not heal him either. Now he took garlic and died.⁵¹

There were also less successful or beginning doctors who sat in mosques waiting for patients. They were considered second-rate doctors, for having no office, sitting in mosques and having no good clothes did not inspire much confidence among the potential patients. Even if, objectively speaking he were a good doctor, few people would believe that given the image that he projected.⁵²

During the 1835-45 period or thereabouts, there were more than 150 physicians, both well-known and less well-known, in Isfahan. By 1877, that number had decreased, both important and less important ones, to 25 or 26, not more.⁵³ According to Höltzer, in 1890, or thereabouts, there were 65 traditional physicians (*hakim*) in Isfahan and 34 surgeons (*jarrah*). The best new physicians, at least according to Höltzer, were those that had received practical training from European physicians (mostly in France) or had been trained in Tehran. The rest still very much adhered to the traditional methods, because the majority of the population and in particular the mollahs did not want it any other way. Höltzer wrote, "They do not desire any progress, although they have accepted some European medicines such as quinine and opium. The situation of the surgeons is still rather lacking in change. They form a substantial number, but few of them have any good education or reliability. In fact, there are quite a large number of cases that have been badly handled, although the climate is very propitious as far the healing of wounds and fractures is concerned."⁵⁴ Prior to the Russian conquest of Eastern Armenia (Erevan Khanate) in 1828, there were only four physicians/surgeons in the town of Erevan (one Moslem, three Armenians) and three in the *mahall*s (two Moslems, one Armenian).⁵⁵ A Russian sources states that no country has so many doctors as Persia, in particular in the province of Mazandaran. Most doctors in Tehran came from the town of Tonakebun in that province.⁵⁶ In Tehran, 18 physicians were

---

⁵⁰ Polak, *Persien*, vol. 2, p. 195.
⁵¹ `Eyn al-Saltaneh, *Ruznameh*, vol. 1, p. 144.
⁵² Ts., "Persidskie Doktora," pp. 158-59.
⁵³ Tahvildar, *Joghrafiya*, p. 80.
⁵⁴ Höltzer, *Persien*, p. 21. In the Meydan-e Gosfand quarter in Qazvin there were three doctors (*tabib*) in one of its seven neighborhoods. Sadvandian, "The Inhabitants of Meydan-Gusfand," p. 53.
⁵⁵ Bournoutian, George A. *Eastern Armenia in the Last Decades of Persian Rule 1807-1828* (Malibu: Undena, 1982), p. 203.
⁵⁶ Ts., "Persidskie Doktora," p. 157.

mentioned by name around 1880, but there were, of course, many more.[57] In Tabriz, in 1869, there were 50 doctors (*pezeshk*).[58] There were two physicians in Zenjan in 1901, but none in 1828 in Kazerun.[59] In 1919, there were three doctors in Sabzavar.[60] In 1921, there were 13 medical practitioners in Maragheh, two were *hakim*s, and 11 were herbal doctors.[61] In 1900, or thereabouts, there were only 20 Western educated Persian physicians in 12 of Persia's major towns, according to Dr. Sargis.[62]

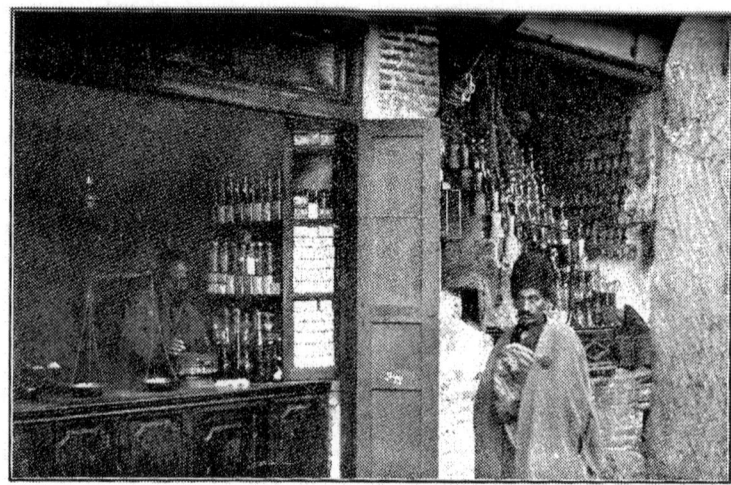

A PERSIAN HAKIM'S (DOCTOR'S) ESTABLISHMENT.

Figure 5: A doctor's office in the bazaar.

As in other parts of the world, the physician either received his patients in his office or he made house calls (*ejadat*). The choice depended on the relationship with, or the social and financial standing of, the patient. Some had a waiting room; others just received all patients in the same. Of course, men and women would sit or stand apart, and the women would be behind a screen.[63] Physicians, of course, did not serve the poor. However, those who could pay were welcome, and they were even willing to make house calls. Most distinguished families had a family doctor who took care of all their illnesses, whether master or servant. In fact, Aubin called the doctors in the homes of the rich and mighty "trustworthy employees." But even those would consult more than one physician, if the case required, and the family physician was not able to cure the patient. Also, during the

---

[57] Sheykh-Reza'i and Azari, *Gozareshha-ye Nazmiyeh*, Index q.v. *Hakim* and *Tabib*. I was too lazy to tally all the *tabib*s mentioned in the three published census documents of Tehran, which would have yielded a more correct and higher figure as a glance at the documents already suggests. Sa`dvandiyan, Sirus and Ettehadiyeh (Nezam-Mafi), Mansureh. *Amar-e Dar al-Khelafeh* (Tehran: Nashr-e Tarikh, 1368/1989).

[58] Javadi, *Tabriz*, p. 227.

[59] `Eyn al-Saltaneh, *Ruznameh*, vol. 2, p. 1509; Stirling, *The Journals*, p. 43.

[60] Ghani, *Yaddashtha*, vol. 1, pp. 188-89.

[61] Good, "The Transformation," p. 68.

[62] Sargis, "Persia and Her Doctors," p. 588.

[63] Ghani, *Yaddashtha*, vol. 1, p. 43; Polak, *Persien*, vol. 1, p. 195.

night one did not dare to disturb the important physicians. In that case, a junior doctor would be summoned. He would prescribe something that the elders of the family would throw away in the morning. They would then send for a well-known physician. But the junior physicians remained on call in the hope to make a name for themselves.[64] It is clear from this that the patients also expected that a well-known doctor with a reputation knew better than a young one, even if it were not true. In case of illness of an important patient everybody who had a political interest to know what was going on sent his own doctor to assist the afflicted person. As a result there would be a group of physicians who had to recommend the best treatment. This was not always possible, for despite reference being made to one medical text or the other there might be dissent, in which case the patient took an omen (about which later) to determine which counsel to follow.[65] Large wealthy establishments such as that of `Abdol-Hoseyn Mirza Farmanfarma, which housed 215 people and where an additional 486 external staff and dependents worked, had a live-in physician.[66]

DOCTOR'S ACCESSIBILITY

Most Persians only consulted a physician, if they could afford one, and if there was one within easy access, when their disorder had reached severe degree. But before doing so, they first started doctoring themselves, giving the patient all kinds of concoctions, "except in smallpox, when they say it is dangerous to give any medicine."[67] Money was an obstacle to consult a physician. This became quite clear to Frey Stark, when she fell ill herself in the Alamut valley in 1932. The nearest doctor or chemist was three stages by mule. When finally a doctor was found at a five hours' ride distance. He refused to come for a ten hours' ride for less than five tomans, which was very expensive for villagers.[68] In fact, a Russian observer stated that the first-class doctors only tended to the needs of the rich.[69]

It was not only the fee, but also the cost of entertaining the doctor. Persians, being a very hospitable people, felt obliged to offer the visiting physician(s) something nice. "The physician is honored with an hour's social chat before the ailments of the caller-in are

---

[64] Mostowfi, *Sharh*, vol. 1, p. 528; Ehtesham al-Dowleh, *Khaterat*, p. 11 ("Feylosuf al-Dowleh Malek al-Atebba Reshti, who was our family doctor"); Amanollah Khan Ardalan's family physician was Entezam al-Saltaneh. `Eyn al-Saltaneh, *Ruznameh*, vol. 2, p. 1058; Fakhr al-Atebba was `Aziz al-Soltan's doctor from his infancy. `Eyn al-Saltaneh, *Ruznameh*, vol. 1, p. 796; Moshtaq Kazemi, *Ruzgar*, p. 12; Hasanbeygi, *Tehran-e Qadim*, p. 199; Aubin, *La Perse*, p. 312; Nezam al-Saltaneh Mafi, Hoseyn Qoli Khan, *Khaterat va Asnad*. 2 vols. eds. Ma`sumeh Nezam-mafi, Mansureh Ettehadiyeh (Nezam-Mafi), Sirus Sa`vandiyan, and Hamid Ram Pisheh (Tehran: Tarikh-e Iran, 1361/1982), vol. 1, pp. 62, 64-65 (consulted two physicians), 149 (family doctor of Amin al-Soltan).
[65] Nezam al-Saltaneh Mafi, *Khaterat va Asnad*, vol. 1, p. 69; Polak, *Persien*, vol. 2, pp. 196-98; Ts., "Persidskie Doktora," p. 160.
[66] Farmanfarma, `Abdol-Hoseyn Mirza. *Siyaq-e Ma`ishat dar `Ahd-e Qajar*. 2 vols. eds. Mansureh Ettehadiyeh and Sirus Sa`dvandiyan (Tehran: Tarikh-e Iran, 1362/1983), vol. 1, p. 156.
[67] Brugsch, *Reise*, vol. 2, p. 17; Malcolm, *Children*, p. 85; Morton, *A Doctor's Holiday*, p. 224; Hasanbeygi, *Tehran-e Qadim*, pp. 195-97.
[68] Stark, *The Valley*, pp. 122, 183, 208, 213, 218 ("the village people usually brought their cases in the last and hopeless stages. And his rates were not exorbitant, even for these poor folk").
[69] Ts., "Persidskie Doktora," p. 157.

mentioned. He is expected in return to make himself comfortable in the parlor for a prolonged tea-drinking before being inducted into the sick-room."[70] Foreign doctors were also a bit taken aback by the custom, because rather than attending to the sick person they first had to relax for half an hour with the patient's friends and relatives, before anybody thought it necessary to recall the reason for the doctor's visit.[71] This social custom was an obstacle for the poor to seek help from a doctor, because they could not receive him properly. "Sometimes this deters the very poor from calling even the mission doctor, who, they know, would treat them free. It was a great relief to more than one poor person, when it was discovered that the mission ladies were fond of boiled turnips, for a plate of turnips was within the reach of the poorest, costing only about a halfpenny. The news spread, and several sick people were able at once to have a doctor."[72] But even when money was not a major obstacle, Persians "will consult the beads as to whether to send for the doctor, and again, after he has come, to see whether they should buy the medicine he prescribes, they consult them once more before deciding whether the patient shall take the dose."[73] Consequently, the *hakim* was not the patient's family first choice for medical assistance. In fact, several European observers mentioned that Islamic-Galenic doctors had to face stiff competition from the traditional faith healers and folk medicine men.[74]

A VISIT TO THE DOCTOR

Bedside manners were, of course, vital for any doctor's appreciation. It did not matter whether the physician was in his office in the bazaar or at the patient's home. With some exaggeration, Bélanger described how the Persian physician in Tabriz, received his patients in his shop with gravity. "Without changing from his seat he examined the urine that they have brought, examines their tongue, their pulse, and asks them some questions, writes a recipe and gives it to a young boy or apprentice in charge of the sale of drugs. These are always available, as is the formula: you owe that much!"[75] Hume-Griffith described, or rather caricaturized, the house call by a Persian physician. "His impudence and native wit are inexhaustible; he will cheer his patients with extracts from Hafiz and Ferdosi, talk learnedly of vapours, and have a specific for every mortal ailment. The quack physician is amusing, and probably confines himself to fairly harmless compounds."[76] Arnold, a traveler who had made use of the services of a Persian physician, opined that, "The ideas of a Persian doctor are few. He relies most conspicuously upon the aid of Allah, whom he invokes every minute, and at every step in his proceedings."[77] Drouville reported that Persian physicians uttered mysterious words, irrespective of the condition of the patient, which they then asked the patient to repeat as much as they were able to.

---

[70] Wilson, *Persian Life*, p. 243; see also Malcolm, *Children*, pp. 87-88 ("I asked for the sick child, and was told I should see her after tea").

[71] Malcolm, *Children*, p. 88; Rice, *Persian Women*, p. 263.

[72] Malcolm, *Children*, p. 88.

[73] Malcom, Napier. *Five Years in a Persian Town* (London: John Murray, 1905), pp. 119-120; Ts., "Persidskie Doktora," p. 160.

[74] Aubin, Eugène. *La Perse d'aujourd'hui* (Paris: Armand Colin, 1908), p. 312; Lichtwardt, "Western Medicine," p. 237.

[75] Bélanger, *Voyage*, vol. 2, p. 195; see also Dieulefoy, *La Perse*, p. 436.

[76] Hume-Griffith, *Behind the Veil*, p. 160; Polak, *Persien*, vol. 1, p. 194.

[77] Arnold, A. *Through Persia by Caravan* (New York: Harper & Brothers, 1877), p. 261; Drouville, *Voyage*, vol. 2, p. 164.

Then they would apply skinned dogs or cats to certain parts of the patient's body, or snakes, toads or similar animals with a view to destroy the disease's 'spell.'[78] In short, a doctor never said that the illness was not serious, that it would be over soon, but if it was he made much 'ado about nothing,' because patients liked to feel that their case was important.[79]

Urban women in elite families had less access to medical help, because of their cloistered life in the harem. If a doctor was allowed to visit a sick woman in a harem his mode of operation was limited and strictly prescribed. "Accompanied by the chief eunuch, with numerous attendants guarding the way, the doctor stalks cautiously in, and nothing meets the eye but a series of hands, poked out from under a screen, and covered each with a gauze glove. [...], many of the ladies feigning illness just to have a sight of the doctor, equally amused with himself at the passing scene." However, if the doctor insisted to see the patient given her condition this was denied, "he would send her to 'Jehannum' first." In this particular case the woman died.[80] This kind of attitude still existed in the 1930s. Freya Stark reported that a friend of hers, an enlightened man, "refused the chance of saving his dying daughter when the doctor came, because she could on no account be seen by so improper a creature as a man; all that he had been allowed to do was to send her a dose of Epsom salts."[81]

With the advent of more European doctors and better acquaintance of European medicine, some of the harems or *enderun*s in particular the royal one, became more accessible to the physician.[82] The visits were not only to diagnose indispositions and illnesses, but also to provide variety to the monotony of the cloistered life of the harem women. "Husbands and brothers in the company of their wives and sisters used to sit with the hakim sahib in the anderun gossiping."[83] His visit to the harem, often served only to divert the women with a new face.[84] However, this was an exception and physicians in general could not treat women. They were not even allowed to feel their pulse.[85] Later in the century, women of the elite came to see European doctors incognito, because they did not want it be known that they visited a foreign doctor.[86] In life-threatening cases some women were operated upon, but it was rare. Polak mentioned that he operated on nine women in the 1850s who had stones.[87] The arrival of female physicians and nurses as of around 1890 made therefore a big difference. Moslem husbands usually did not oppose

---

[78] Drouville, *Voyage*, vol. 2, pp. 164-65.
[79] Ts., "Persidskie Doktora," p. 169.
[80] Fowler, *Three Years*, vol. 1, pp. 61-62.
[81] Stark, *The Valley*, pp. 217-18.
[82] Polak, *Persien*, vol. 2, pp. 208-09.
[83] Sheil, Lady. *Glimpses of Life and Manners in Persia* (London, 1856 [New York: Arno, 1973]), p. 213 (see also engraving opposite to this page showing "women seated on a carpet gossiping outside the Doctor's door.").
[84] Wills, *Persia*, pp. 80-86; Ibid., *The land*, pp. 38-42.
[85] Yonan, *Persian Women*, pp. 120-21.
[86] Collins, *In the Kingdom*, pp. 162-63.
[87] Polak, *Persien*, vol. 2, pp. 319-20. He did not state whether these were Moslem or non-Moslem women, but he implies that they were women of high-ranking Moslem families, see Ibid, vol. 2, p. 202.

that their womenfolk consulted a lady doctor or nurse. The fact that these female medical providers could physically examine their patients often made a major difference in the life of many a woman.[88]

What also struck some Europeans was the openness with which rural Persians discussed the most intimate details of their disease in public without any shame or inhibition. Binning related his interesting experience in Daleki, where people came to see him for treatment. "Three women honoured me with a visit, soliciting advice. They all complained of not being blessed with any family, for certain very satisfactory reasons, which they unfolded at length, in the plainest and broadest terms. Nor were they deterred from speaking thus freely, by the presence of several of the male sex, who crowded into my cell, bound on similar errands, to obtain relief from real or imaginary complaints. One young man, in his turn, quite unabashed by the presence of the females, communicated a detail of weakness, which he laboured under, and which in more civilized societies, a man would be studious to keep concealed."[89] They were disappointed that he could not heal them on the spot. On the other hand, Shahri creates the impression that urban people, in his case Tehranis, were less prepared to share their ills with the world, because many of them would whisper their complaint in the ear of the roadside healer, for example.[90]

START OF TREATMENT

The standard reaction of a Persian doctor to the occurrence of illness was to purge the patient. Purging (*tanqiyeh kardan*), principally by means of calomel (mercurous chloride used as a purgative or *moshel*), was "the almost universal commencement of treatment; for the Persian, like the sailor, thinks little of medicine unless it be heroic. This is followed by bleeding to at least twelve or eighteen ounces; this latter is generally repeated several times. The hakim now leaves his patient very much to nature, prescribing merely placebos, such as syrup of violets, or sugar-candy and water; and, as the Persian has a strong constitution, he often survives, the credit of the physician being in direct proportion to the violence and the novelty of the remedies he has employed."[91] Another, more often used, purgative was castor oil, which, just like in Europe, was in widespread use for a range of disorders. When E`temad al-Saltaneh, for example, had been afflicted by a bleeding (*khuni*), his doctor, Soltan al-Hokama, gave him a purging of cassia (*folus*) and castor oil. It helped and stopped the complication (*pich*) and the blood.[92] It was in particular much used in the rural areas and Wilson noted that it was "administered by the

---

[88] For an example see Rice, *Mary Bird*, p. 119.

[89] Binning, *A Journal*, vol. 1, pp. 164-65. Good, "The Transformation," p. 66 states that in Maragheh, male "patients would gather and sit in a circle before him [and discuss their problems with him]. Women at times would not enter, but would present their complaints and receive their medicines through a small window in the wall behind the hakim."

[90] Shahri, *Tarikh*, vol. 4, p. 330.

[91] Wills, *Persia*, pp. 87; Polak, *Persien*, vol. 2, p. 221; Schlimmer, *Terminology*, p. 477 (q.v. purger).; Safari, *Ardabil*, vol. 3, p. 484. Calomel with antimony was also given in case of fever by Stirling, *The Journals*, p. 190. Calomel was also known as mercurous chloride. It was also used in bleaching and freckle creams. The FDA banned it in 1973, because it slowly decays into a metallic mercury product.

[92] E`temad al-Saltaneh, *Ruznameh*, pp. 893, 907 (his mother took castor-oil), 381 (Amin-e Aqdas drank castor-oil).

glassful to village infants."[93] Castor oil, which was a warm drug, was therefore used in case of disorders of a cold type, and it was "followed by boiling water containing sugar."[94]

The diagnosis was usually arrived at without examination. At best, and then only later in the nineteenth century, the doctor would feel the pulse, visually inspect a swelling, or palpate the abdomen for tumors. Examination and treatment took place in public.[95] This is also clear from a description of a doctor's visit by Adler. He was allowed to sit by the side of one of Nur Mahmud Hakim's sons (the father was a highly respected Jewish doctor in Tehran) when he saw his patients.

> He sat on the floor by the window in European garb, but with the high black Persian conical cap on his head. In front of him was a short of chessboard with ointments and little phials. His doorkeeper brought the patients up to the window, and then ensued a whispered conversation which generally ended in the patients' receiving a minute dose. To my uncultured eye it seemed that all the doses came from the same miraculous cruse, though evidently some were intended for internal application and others for external. Most of the clientèle were women, Shiite women, not Jewesses. They rarely unveiled, but it was funny to sea a lean arm or a tiny tongue projecting from the Yashmak, and blindly seeking inspection![96]

A Russian observer questioned whether the feeling of the pulse and the looking at the tongue had any medical merit. Most doctors did not even know what information the pulse could provide, they did not count time, and they looked sometimes very long at tongues, creating the impression that it was posture rather than a means to arrive at a diagnosis.[97]

Once a Persian physician had diagnosed the nature of the disease he would write a prescription (*noskheh*), which usually could contain three types of information, according to Safari. The doctor would prescribe one or more medicines, a diet, and/or behavioral guidelines. The prescription of a strict diet varied with the nature of the illness.[98] The doctor handed the prescription to the patient's relatives to produce the necessary ingredients, if he had prescribed drugs, after he had explained the mode of preparation and dosage. The relatives would take the prescription to the druggist (there were no apothecaries in the European sense of the term in Persia) who would prepare the required ingredients. He then would give both the ingredients and the prescription to the client, whose family would prepare the medicine. It also happened that the doctor had his own drug store, in which case his apprentice would weigh and mix the prescribed drugs.

---

[93] Wilson, *Persian Life*, pp. 107 (he also "found the remedy worse than the disease it is designed to cure," after he had tried a dose once).
[94] Sykes, P.M. and Khan Bahadur Ahmad Din Khan. *The Glory of the Shia World. The Tale of a Pilgrimage* (London: MacMillan and Co., 1910), p. 103.
[95] Good, "The Transformation," p. 66; Ts., "Persidskie Doktora," p. 163; Ghani, *Yaddashtha*, vol. 1, p. 43. About feeling the pulse (*nabz didan*) see Polak, *Persien*, vol. 2, p. 236-37.
[96] Adler, *Jews in Many Lands*, pp. 189-90.
[97] Ts., "Persidskie Doktora," pp. 163-64.
[98] Safari, *Ardabil*, vol. 3, p. 484.

Schlimmer considered this a rather useful practice. He had assisted many times at the consultations of Persian doctors and knew that the patient (or their relatives) would tell the physician what remedies they had experienced already, sometimes since their infancy. The physician would be able to study all these prescriptions and thus form an opinion about the medical history of the patient. Schlimmer raised the question whether it would not be a good idea to do the same thing in Europe.[99]

The physician would tell the patient's family that the disease was treatable, but he would tell the patient's friends that this case was one of the most difficult in his practice, and that it was untreatable and that the patient would possibly die. If the patient died the doctor excused himself *vis à vis* the family for having kept silent about the severity of the illness, out of respect for them. However, he had told their friends the true state of affairs. If the patient recuperated, he would tell the family, 'I told you so!' while to their friends he would be the hero, because he had saved his patient in an impossible situation. Meanwhile, the patient had to suffer a horse physic.[100] Dr. Wishard related another strategy. He treated a patient, who had come to him after the Persian doctor "had refused to attend the case longer, as he feared he would be blamed if the patient died. In their distress, they had consulted the astrologer, who, after making the *istakharreh*, advised them to try, as a last resort, one of the foreign doctors."[101]

If the patient was rich, he would be reminded of his sins by the illness, and he or his relatives would invite the poor, who were fed and feted and received alms. These would send prayers to heaven that he might heal quickly and remain one of mankind's benefactors.[102] For example, Na`eb al-Saltaneh, governor of Tehran and one of Naser al-Din Shah's sons, had fallen from his coach and had lost conscience. He then ordered to give 4,000 tomans in alms to the poor.[103] When Naser al-Din Shah, despite his treatment with leaches, still had vertigo, the major princes [his sons] gave money to be distributed among the poor.[104] If the patient would get better he would continue living as before without further caring about the poor, of course. Nevertheless, thanks had to be given and gratitude might take various forms. A popular form was to organize a *rowzehkhvan* (panegyric), or even a *ta`ziyeh* or a passion play. In 1833, Mirza Abu'l-Hasan Khan, the Minister of

---

[99] Schlimmer, *Terminologie*, p. 482 (q.v. recette); Government of Iran, *Vaqaye`-ye Ettefaqiyeh*, vol. 1, p. 237 (nr. 45, 17 Safar 1268/12 December, 1851); Good, "The Transformation," p. 68; Safari, *Ardabil*, vol. 3, pp. 488-91(with examples of the text of the various original prescriptions). It is some interest here to note that the word *noskheh* also could refer to a talisman, see Vambéry, Arminius. *Voyages d' un Faux Derviche* (Paris: L. Hachette et Cie, 1865), p. 37. Sometimes the physician would prescribe drugs for a long period in case the patient was traveling, in which case the medicine was prepared at the halting place, see Nezam al-Saltaneh Mafi, *Khaterat va Asnad*, vol. 1, p. 63.

[100] Brugsch, *Reise*, vol. 2, p. 17; Ts., "Persidskie Doktora," p. 169.

[101] Wishard, *Twenty Years*, p. 198; see also Dieulefoy, *La Perse*, p. 436. According to Linton, *Persian Sketches*, p. 77 the Persian doctor (*hakim*) was a man out to make money first and "that medical practice was merely a means to that end."

[102] Brugsch, *Reise*, vol. 2, p. 17.

[103] E`temad al-Saltaneh, *Ruznameh*, p. 144.

[104] E`temad al-Saltaneh, *Ruznameh*, p. 313. For a similar case of the heir-apparent's sick son see Ghaffari, *Khaterat va Asnad*, p. 329.

Foreign Affairs, financed a *ta'ziyeh* presentation that lasted 14 days to give vent to his happiness about his son's cure of an illness. During the presentations no less than 48 very expensive *Reza'i* shawls were used and many jewels with a value of half a million tomans, some borrowed from the royal harem, were displayed.[105]

Missionary doctors were much surprised by patients' requests to give the second medicine first. "It appears that the people think, with how much truth I cannot say, that their doctors give first a medicine to make the patient worse and then one to make him better. [...] It must surely have been in the minds of the friends of one patient who came to the missionary, and said their friend was worse every time she took her medicine, and they wanted some more, it was doing her so much good"[106] Persian who frequented Mission dispensaries or hospitals often attended a Bible reading session, "partly out of politeness and partly because there is a belief among the Persians that those who profess an interest in Christian doctrines get superior medicines to those who do not."[107]

In addition to this, there was much prescribing of traditional medicines.[108]

> The system of medicine in vogue in Persia is a pure empiricism. Diseases and remedies are divided into two classes, *hot* and *cold*; a hot disorder being treated by the administration of cold remedies, and *vice versa*. Diagnosis is not attempted; and if the ailment does not give way under the one class of drugs, the native practitioner simply tries the other. When the patient has obtained the prescription, he, after repeating a prayer, opens his Koran haphazard; and looking at the first passage to his right, or at some other part of the page that is previously decided on, he determines whether he shall act on it or not. Should the omen prove favourable, he swallows the dose, however large (a quart is a common quantity) or nauseous, in perfect faith, having previously fixed on a fortunate hour. This important point is settled by the astrologer, who is much consulted in this country, no important affair being undertaken without his advice, or commenced save at the particular moment that he may choose as fortunate. Prior to calling in the medical attendant, a list of the principal practitioners is gone through, and each one is tried with an omen as described, from the Koran, till he whose name coincides with some especially lucky verse is selected.[109]

Thus, the patient before taking the medicine first would check the omens (*estekhareh*). The patient would look into the air, say a short prayer (often the *Fatihah*, the opening chapter of

---

[105] Chodzko, Alexandre, *Théatre Persan. Choix de Téaziés* (Paris: Leroux, 1878 [Tehran, 1976]), pp. xxi-xxii.
[106] Malcolm, *Children*, p. 87; Morton, *A Doctor's Holiday*, p. 212 and Rice, *Persian Women*, p. 260, reported the same belief.
[107] Ross, Elizabeth N. MacBean. *A Lady Doctor in Bakhtiyari Land* (London: Parsons, 1921), p. 79.
[108] Cochran, "Treatment," pp.105-06; Saad, *Sechzehn Jahre*, p. 184.
[109] Wills, *Persia*, p. 86; Olivier, *Voyage*, vol. 5, p. 110; Brugsch, *Im Lande*, p. 204; Binning, *A Journal*, vol. 1, pp. 220-22. In 1869, there were seven astrologers (*monajjem*). Javadi, *Tabriz*, pp. 227-28. On astrologers see also Höltzer, *Persien*, p. 21; De Lorey, *Queer Things*, p.321-25; and Browne, *A Year*, pp. 158f.

the Koran), breathe the spirit of the prayer on the rosary and then take hold of any bead. The rosary has 99 beads, each representing one of the names of God. It is further divided into three sections of 33, separated by a bead of a different kind, size or color, which may be called pointers. From there he would count the beads, *i.e.*, in groups of three, till the end of the rosary. If one bead remained then it would be a good sign, and the taking of the medicine promised to yield a good result. If two beads remained, however, then the result would average. Not good, but not bad either. If three beads remained, then the patients would not take the medicine under any circumstance. If the omen were positive, even then the Persian might not be satisfied, and would wish to have of 'second opinion' to know whether it would be bad if he would not take the medicine. If the answer were, 'No', then he would not take the medicine, despite the earlier positive omen.[110] The patient still had another alternative. For if the omen was not to the patient's liking, "the beads may be taken again in the mosque, and the answer in the mosque takes precedence of that in the house. If, however, the answer is still the same, there is a third method. For a small fee a mulla will do the same sort of thing with the Qoran, and the text selected overrules the two previous answers."[111] The patient could, of course, decide not to take the advice of his doctor for whatever reason. An *akhund* from Mazandaran, who clearly disagreed with his doctor's diagnosis, decided not to do so, "considering that his illness arose from a warm habit, and not a cold disposition of the body."[112] The taking of omens, when a physician had prescribed a medicine, might also take other forms. The Koran was "opened anywhere, then seven pages are counted backwards, and guidance is taken from the seventh line."[113]

If the taste of the medicine were not to the liking of the patient he would not take it and the doctor to keep his patient happy, had to prescribe something that was more to the taste of the patient. Another obstacle might be if the cure had to start on an unlucky day, in which case the patient would refuse to take his medicine. If everything were propitious the patient would finally start the treatment, but if he sneezed once before doing so then nothing would move him to take his medicine. If he would sneeze a second time he would be more than willing to take his medicine, for that was a good sign. The treatment could still be problematic, if the patient listened to the advice of family and friends, who would suggest other medicines. Thus it might happen that the doctor had prescribed a laxative or a calming drug, while the patient also would take a non-laxative or an excitant at the urgings of friends.[114]

---

[110] Brugsch, *Reise*, vol. 2, p. 18; Rice, *Persian Women*, p. 248 ("Next one bead is grasped and the user counts towards the pointer, repeating the expressions, God, Muhammad and Abu Jahal, or Adam, Eve and the serpent. If the count terminates with the first, the decision is good; if with the last, it is bad; and if with the middle one, it is uncertain and is generally taken again"); Aubin, *La Perse*, p. 313; de Hell, *Voyage*, vol. 2, pp. 60-61; Saad, *Sechzehn Jahre*, p. 185; Ts., "Persidskie Doktora," p. 160. When the sick vizier of Shiraz wanted to smoke the water pipe his chief physician first took an omen, which fortunately for the vizier was favorable, and only then his doctor handed him the pipe. Money, Journal, p. 76.
[111] Malcolm, *Children*, p. 61.
[112] Stirling, *The Journals*, p. 129.
[113] Rice, *Persian Women*, p. 247; Morton, *A Doctor's Holiday*, p. 212.
[114] Ts., "Persidskie Doktora," pp. 160-62.

Persian Medical Remedies

According to most European observers, Persian doctors had no idea of disease, and thus were unable to prescribe proper and effective remedies. Rubies and pearls in particular had a place in Persian pharmacology. They were considered to be good remedies against an upset or weak stomach. "They often prescribe real pearls, which they take aside to pound, put in their own pocket and replace them with pounded mother-of-pearl."[115] Persians mixed these with jelly (*ma'jun*) and enjoyed the medicine without any apparent problem. Many times, middlemen (*dallal*s) in Isfahan and Tehran offered Brugsch small bags with similar "Cleopatra-tidbits" for his upset stomach with the assurance that it would totally cure his problem.[116] Ella Sykes also reported that Persian physicians often administered "the powder of rubies or emeralds as a tonic, and a ground-up pearl is occasionally resorted to when the patient is believed to be at the point of death."[117]

According to Eichwald, Persians often gave much opium to treat diseases, as a kind of *passe-partout*.[118] Another kind of universal cure, according to Waring, was China root (*Radix chinae*) or sarsaparilla. "I have known them to give it for violent colds, and for diseases which result from too free an intercourse among the sexes."[119] Dr. Clarke confirmed Waring's report some 30 years later, writing that China root was used for about every disorder, "inflammatory, asthenic, or chronic." It was strongly believed that nothing could withstand its healing power. However, the patient when taking this drug had to stay in a room, "with the door and windows closed and all external air excluded. He was then given a strong decoction' clothes are heaped upon him till he has the burthen of a camel, or till a profuse diaphoresis is produced, when he is allowed to eat."[120]

Korf, a member of the Russian mission in the 1830s, who mentioned the cold-hot system guiding Islamic medicine, did not reject it out of hand. However, he questioned its scientific basis when its practitioners could not make clear why the cock was hot, but the hen cold, which he considered to be ridiculous. However, Persian patients disagreed. In the English missionary hospital in Jolfa (Isfahan), patients who thought that they were suffering from a hot disease, refused to take chicken broth that the hospital served them, "until they were satisfied that it was made from a cock and not a hen."[121] It was the trial-and-error approach of Islamic medicine that put off Europeans, who insisted on the

---

[115] Eichwald, *Reise*, vol. 1, p. 372.

[116] Brugsch, *Reise*, vol. 2, p. 79.

[117] Sykes, *Persia and its People*, p. 337; Ibid., *Through Persia*, pp. 111-12.

[118] Eichwald, *Reise*, vol. 1, p. 373.

[119] Waring, Edward Scott. *A Tour to Sheeraz*. (London, 1807 [New York: Arno, 1973]), p. 48 (the rootstock of various kinds of the Smilax genus). There also were books on China root such as *Kefayeh-ye Mansuri va Resaleh-ye Chub-e Chini* (Lucknow, 1306/1888) and *Resaleh-ye Chub-e Chini* (Lucknow, 1306/1888).

[120] Clarke, H.T. "Sketches on the State of Medical Knowledge in Persia," *London Medical and Surgical Journal* 2 (1837), p. 709; Waring, *A Tour*, pp. 48-49 ("When they administer it, the patient is confined to a room, where the smallest breath of air is to be carefully shut up, and the poor man not only suffers from his complaint, but also from the intense heat").

[121] Korf, *Safarnameh*, pp. 230-31; Stileman, *The Subjects*, p. 47; Rice, *Persian Women*, p. 259 ("Lump sugar is cold and moist sugar is hot. Persians appreciate foreign doctors, who appear to recognize their prejudices in such matters"); Ts., "Persidskie Doktora," p. 164.

reiterative and verifiable process of modern science. Many of the therapies prescribed by Persian doctors were indeed just ridiculous, of course. What to think of treatments "such as the placing of a live pigeon or disemboweled fowl or lamb to the feet of a dying patient, or such a plan as burying the patient in a hotbed of fermenting manure [that] are in high repute."[122] According to the American physician, Cochran, "For croup, a child's forehead is scarified, and, if possible, a turtle is held in front of the patient's mouth and tormented till it sticks its head out and hisses or breathes into the child's throat. For certain forms of swellings a frog is cut in two and bandaged over the part. For jaundice, a few ounces of a child's urine are administered, in addition to dieting and remedies to produce biliary discharges from the bowels."[123] Wolf dung mixed with white wine allegedly healed colics; however, when mixed with honey it allegedly healed angina.[124] No wonder that Rice concluded that the combination of ignorance about basic hygiene, "and the foolish treatment of illness or accidents causes an immense amount of needless suffering."[125]

In addition to the rather odd therapeutic treatments proposed by Persian healers, there were among their bags of tricks treatments that were indifferent or even helpful. For example, on Qeshm Island "The leaves of a tree called Murt are powdered and applied to the skin for prickly heat."[126] Browne, himself a trained physician, noted the following herbs with therapeutic characteristics. "Kasni, was 'cool' and good for the liver; from it is prepared a spirit called araq-e kasni; razdaneh or fennel said to be an analgesic; shah-tareh, accounted 'hot and moist'; a decoction of it, taken in the morning on an empty stomach, is said to be good for indigestion and disorders of the stomach; shavij, a 'hot' umbelliferous plan; gashnij a 'cold' umbelliferous plant."[127] The knowledge about the medicinal characteristics of the various plants and herbs were transmitted from mother to daughter, and from father to son.[128] Antidotes or *taryaqat*, in particular fresh human feces

---

[122] Wills, *Persia*, pp. 90; Saad, *Sechzehn Jahre*, p. 186.

[123] Cochran, James P. "Treatment of the Sick and Insane in Persia," The American Journal of Insanity 56 (1899), pp.105-06. According to Sargis, "Persia and Her Doctors," pp. 585-86, in case of "pnemonia, they use cupping on the neck and head, bleeding first days and often branding. In jaundice, frightening, making the patient go around the fireplace seven times a day, and bleeding."

[124] Serena, *Hommes*, p. 136 (see here also for other remedies and treatments); Adams, *Persia*, p. 59 (for other fantastic remedies); Morton, *A Doctor's Holiday*, p. 213 (for some amazing treatments); Schlimmer, *Terminologie*, p. 103 (q.v. canis lupus). Fowler, *Three Years*, vol. 1, p. 564, reported a patient eating pills, or rather chicken dung. "Album nigrum or mouse dung (*fazleh-ye mush*) is used to irritate the uretrum, introducing it into that canal in case of dysury to provoke the flow of urine. It is a useless exercise, though damaging, which I have never seen to be successful." Schlimmer, *Terminologie*, p. 24; Ts., "Persidskie Doktora," p. 167. Mirza Abu'l-Hasan Khan told Sir Gore Ouseley that, "most Iranian doctors prescribe assess' milk for complaints of the chest." Mirza Abu'l-Hasan Khan. "A Persian," p. 94.

[125] Rice, *Persian Women*, p. 127.

[126] Floyer, *Unexplored*, pp. 134-35.

[127] Browne, *A Year*, p. 424. See also Stirling, *The Journals*, p. 178 who mentions oxymel (*taranjabin*) and kaksheer (probably *shirkhesht* or *gapshir*), two species of manna and rhubarb (*revand*), which were used mainly to treat fevers. On the various kinds of manna see Floor, *Traditional Crafts*, pp. 370-75.

[128] Zargari, 'Ali. *Giyahan-e Daru'i* 3 vols. (Tehran: Daneshgah, 1361-62/1992-93); Jazayeri,

(*stercus humnane recens*) in high dosage and in liquid form was used, *e.g.*, in case of people who had taken an over dosage of opium to suicide. The theory was that the remedy was so awful that the patient would vomit all that he had swallowed.[129] In case of deafness they would pour two drops of toad's blood or three drops of onion juice into the patient's ear with a large syringe. If that did not cure the patient he was told that there was nothing to be done for him.[130]

Also less controversial was the wide use of mercury; probably the most used medicine in Persia according to Polak. It was used for any and all diseases: skin diseases, eye diseases, syphilis, gonorrhea, cancer, etc. In Tehran, the expression *hobb khordam* (I ate pills) only meant mercury pills. Despite the dangerous nature of mercury, of which Polak was aware, he only saw positive results and he became a frequent prescriber of the ingredient.[131]

According to Polak, if a Persian felt unwell he would diet, take a digestive (*monzej*), followed by a purgative (*karkon, moshel*) as well as one or more enemas (*emaleh*).[132] This is borne out by the description of a typical case of treatment of a case of fever. The patient ate some oxymel (*teranjebin*). Then he applied an enema (*emaleh*) from rocket seeds (*khakeshi*) and salt, after which he ate a simple soup (*ash*). The next day Basir al-Molk took a digestive (*monzej*), ate a simple soup and had a visit from his physician. Basir al-Molk also reported the treatment of another case, not his own, of fever. A physician came; he wrote a prescription (*noskheh*) and gave a digestive and an enema of rhubarb (*revand*). Basir al-Molk gave his son Mansur three pills of quinine (*ganeh ganeh*) when he ran a fever and had him rubbed with bitter almond oil. In the afternoon, the fever had broken.[133] The enema instrument was a high funnel with a rounded off circumjacent end. Polak considered this instrument simple, easy to clean and to use, in short, much better than the instrument that was used in Europe. Each house had such a funnel, which was usually made of glass, but of silver in the homes of the well-to-do. The enema usually consisted of: reed sugar from Mazandaran (*shekar*), crystal salt (*namak-e Torki*), ricinus oil (*rowghan-e karchak*), manna (*shirkhesht*), rhubarb (*revand*), senneh leaves (*sehheh-ye Makki*), and to

---

Ghiyath. *Darman-e Giyahi* (Tehran: Hamgam, n.d.); Amir Hoseyni, Karim Nikzad. *Shenakht-e Sarzamin-e Char Mahall* (Isfahan, 1357/1979), pp. 38-44.

[129] Schlimmer, *Terminologie*, pp. 44, 297 (q.v. gardeniae), 555 (q.v. vomitifs). For cases of suicide by opium, see Hume-Griffith, *Behind the Veil*, p. 158, Ghani, *Yaddashtha*, vol. 1, p. 49, and Häntzsche, "Physikalisch-medicinische Skizze," p. 566. For statistics on suicides in Tehran in 1922-23, see Gilmour, *Rapport*, p. 65. For a case of poisoning and the use of an emetic, see Wills, C.J. *Behind an Eastern Veil* (London: William Blackwood & Sons, 1894), pp. 333-38.

[130] Anonymous, "Ärtze und Arzneiwissenschaft," p. 97. Hadadian, Azar. "History of deaf education in Iran." in: R. Fischer & T. Vollhaber, with H. Zienert eds. *Collage: works on international deaf history* (Hamburg: Signum, 1996), pp. 117-23. (Mainly an account of the work of the kindergarten teacher Jabar Baghcheban (1885-1966), who began Iran's first formal educational work for deaf children in 1924 at Tabriz and who later founded a school at Tehran, and contributed original methods and approaches to teaching deaf children).

[131] Polak, "Ueber den Gebrauch," p. 564. Other doctors reported cases of mercury poisoning, however (see infra).

[132] Polak, *Persien*, vol. 2, p. 218.

[133] Basir al-Molk, *Ruznameh*, pp. 170-71, 195.

make it more powerful, but also more dangerous, cassia fistulosa (*folus*) would be added. A variety of ingredients was used as digestive and as purgative.[134]

In case of an infectious disease, the family was quite fatalistic about the possible course of events. "If a child it to have it, he will have it; it is *kismat*, and nothing that you can do will make any difference. If the child is to live it will get better; if it is to die, what is the use of doing anything to try to prevent it? What difference will it make?"[135]

Apart from drugs, a strict diet was usually prescribed. Sykes reported that the physician after having made "the most minute inquiries, ordered that all pickles and all white foods, such as milk, cheese, or curds, should be given up; and he prescribed a broth of meat, vegetables, and rice all boiled together. He added that it was most important that the meat should be cut from the neck of the sheep."[136] The prescribed diet would be carefully respected, and particular things would be forbidden, not so much for any harm they might do, but according to Brugsch, to give the physician a scapegoat should his treatment fail.[137] A very common custom, among those who were rich, was that the patient was rubbed during the night by a number of attendants so that he might sleep.[138] It was also done, because the fever was strong and the patient was perspiring, in which case "the legs of the patient were fumigated and mustard was rubbed in."[139]

CONVALESCING?
During the course of the illness, chances of recovery were "diminished by friends who smoke, drink tea, talk, never leaving him, day or night, until he is dead or convalescent. They consult with the patient, whether he is in state fit to do so or not, on the expediency of following his physician's treatment, and nothing is administered without the approval of the majority of the bystanders. As the disorder increases in intensity, so do the friends, neighbours, and passers-by increase in number, till, at the decease of the patient, it is no uncommon thing to find eighty people in the room, and two to three hundred in the house."[140] Visitors would tell the patient that he looked good; that he was not really sick, and that the problem would be over quickly. They also would suggest different medicines

---

[134] Polak, *Persien*, vol. 2, p. 218-20 (for details on these ingredients). For some of these ingredients also see Floor, *Agriculture*.
[135] Rice, *Persian Women*, pp. 259-60.
[136] Sykes, *The Glory*, p. 103.
[137] Wills, *Persia*, p. 87. The Persian calendar or almanac (*taqvim*), which was offered for sale in a new version every year by the bookseller just prior to *Nowruz* contained, amongst other things, an indication of which days were lucky and unlucky, when you should take a bath, when to do circumcision, etc. Brugsch, *Im Lande*, pp. 205-06.
[138] Speer, *Hakim Sahib*, p. 272. Massaging was also done for 'medical' reasons. For example, `Eyn al-Saltaneh's daughter had pain in the neck and middle and suffered from cholic (*qowlanj*). She was therefore rubbed with oil. `Eyn al-Saltaneh, *Ruznameh*, vol. 1, p. 545. There were specialized persons, both men and women, who applied massage of the joints, and were known in Azerbaijan as *badchi*.
[139] Sykes, *The Glory*, p. 103.
[140] Wills, *Persia*, p. 89; Malcolm, *Children*, p. 87; Morton, *A Doctor's Holiday*, p. 221; Rice, *Persian Women*, p. 263 ("but if people did not come and show their interest in this way it would be considered unkind"); Wishard, *Twenty Years*, p. 199; de Hell, *Voyage*, vol. 2, pp. 61-62.

or medical treatment than the one suggested by his doctor.[141] "When people are very ill their friends give them food and medicine (if a *Hakim* be attainable), till, in their judgment, the case is hopeless."[142]

Another danger was the giving of medicines in bulk, for the patients might swallow them in one go. Because they believed that it would cure more quickly than three times a day for a number of days.[143] If the disorder proved to be obstinate, "the bystanders each prescribe a remedy more or less ludicrous; and, save in the case of the very rich, or until the patient is *in extremis*, the European practitioner is seldom called in."[144] It also happened that another doctor was called in, for a second opinion, which usually gave rise to altercation between the physickers as to the diagnosis and the treatment to be followed.[145]

A complication that was usually overlooked in case of villagers was that they sometimes had to walk for miles to get treatment every day, which did not help the healing process.[146] Also, as Forbes-Leith found out too late, when having prescribed a liquid diet as a result of which the patient was getting better, that relatives would interfere with the treatment. In this case the patient's mother said "how can a man live on that and killed a lamb and gave him a meaty dish and the patient relapsed." Despite this mishap the patient recuperated, but then he got a case of endocorditis. Forbes-Leith then found that his family had made him walk on his weak legs every day as a result of which he died.[147]

When the patient was dying, or they despaired of recovery, the patient's relatives would give him poison or opium, the last soup or sherbet as it was called, and kill two chickens that were "applied warm to the patient's feet, as a restorative."[148] The family also would turn the dying person's bed into the direction of the *qebleh*.[149] When the patient had died finally, his friends would tell the family that indeed he must have been very ill.[150] If you were informed about somebody's death, or you expressed your sympathies (*sar-e salamat*) then you should not forget, out of respect, to express a wish for the well and hail of the person addressed. The higher ranking the person the more emphasis had to be put on this wish.[151]

---

[141] Brugsch, *Reise*, vol. 2, p. 18; Ts., "Persidskie Doktora," p. 160.

[142] Bird, *Journeys*, vol. 1, p. 324.

[143] Forbes-Leith, *Checkmate*, pp. 94-95; Heinrich, *Auf Panthersuche*, p. 40.

[144] Wills, *Persia*, p. 87.

[145] Sykes, *The Glory*, pp. 104-05.

[146] Forbes-Leith, *Checkmate*, pp. 95-96 for examples.

[147] Forbes-Leith, *Checkmate*, pp. 97-98.

[148] Serena, *Hommes*, p. 138; Malcolm, *Children*, p. 86; Wishard, *Twenty Years*, p. 199.

[149] Ehtesham al-Dowleh, *Khaterat*, p. 11; Höltzer, *Persien*, p. 37; for details on the funeral customs and ceremony see Sykes, *The Glory*, pp. 109-18.

[150] Brugsch, *Reise*, vol. 2, p. 18. For a description what happened after a patient died see Rice, *Persian Women*, pp. 263-66.

[151] Brugsch, *Reise*, vol. 2, p. 18.

THE DOCTOR'S FEE

According to Mostowfi, doctors did not have a special rate for their treatment. Patients of modest means put five or ten *shahi*s wrapped in the previous day's prescription and offered it to the doctor. He also maintained that, as a rule, doctors did not expect payment from people who could not afford it. The doctors did not keep their offices open necessarily to receive patients and collect fees. Keeping the practice open was a way to pay dues for their other income. It was a good practical training, while it also allowed them to earn spiritual points (*thavab*s) by providing free medical care to the poor, occasionally.[152] However, according to Eichwald, if you did not belong to the well-to-do class the physicians would ask much money for their visits, and agree on the sum to be paid beforehand. The patient's relatives would have to pay already part of that sum during the first two or three visits. "Tout comme chez nous," Eichwald wistfully commented.[153] Dr. Häntzsche confirmed Eichwald's experience. In fact, he stated that, "there is not a fixed doctor's fee, and the physician either insists on payment beforehand, or is indemnified through the sale of his own medicine."[154] The fact also that so few people had access to physicians was not only due to their limited number, but also, above all, because people could not afford the cost of medicines and treatment.[155] Even if the doctor did not charge a fee for his advice he did charge for the drugs that he prescribed, and it was in this way that he was recompensed for his trouble.[156] When doctors made house calls, in case of patients who could not be moved, the cost of transportation by droshke, for example, was paid by the patient's family. In Ardabil, a fee, known as *haqq al-qadam*, was paid, and it could be twice the cost of the transportation cost.[157] If desperate the poor sold all their possession and put themselves in debt, in particular if it was to save the breadwinner.[158] Rural doctors asked 3 to 4 *qran*s per consultation, while those in towns accepted what was given them, often in kind, and made their money on the sale of drugs.[159] Dr. Emmeline Stuart had a rather low opinion of her Persian colleagues. She wrote, "No Persian doctors took to the profession from philanthropic motives, or were actuated by a desire to lessen the sufferings of their fellow creatures. They were, as a

---

[152] Mostowfi, *Sharh*, vol. 1, p. 528; Hasanbeygi, *Tehran-e Qadim*, p. 199; Ebrahimnejad, "Theory and Practice," p. 174.

[153] Eichwald, *Reise*, vol. 1, p. 373; Fowler, *Three Years*, vol. 1, p. 57 (the physician hinted to my attendant what would be agreeable him in the way of 'peishcush.'). Babin and Houssay, "A Travers," p. 98 stated that Persian doctors were expensive.

[154] Häntzsche, "Specialstatistik," p. 442; Ibid., "Physikalisch-medicinische Skizze," p. 561 ("Very numerous are also the so-called Persian doctors who are motivated by greed for money"); see also Mirza Fathollah Akhundzadeh, *The Vazir of Lankuran. A Persian Play*. Transl. by W.H.D. Haggard and G. le Strange (London: Trübner & Co, 1882), pp. 69-70, who wrote: "My brother was sick: they said, 'This is a doctor:' I gave him three tomans." This shows that it was indeed quite common to pay the doctor's fee upfront. For a similar case see Wills, C.J. *Behind An Eastern Veil* (London: William Blackwood & Sons, 1894), pp. 333-36.

[155] Forbes-Leith, *Checkmate*, p. 99; Ts., "Persidskie Doktora," p. 158 (the doctor tries to get as much money as he can).

[156] Good, "The Transformation," p. 66.

[157] Safari, *Ardabil*, vol. 3, p. 483.

[158] Wishard, *Twenty Years*, p. 200; Polak, *Persien*, vol. 1, p. 195 (the patient paid cash when he received the prescription).

[159] Aubin, *La Perse*, p. 313.

class, filled with the greed of gain, and their chief idea was to enrich themselves at the expense of credulous patients."[160]

According to Mostowfi, who belonged to an important and rich bureaucratic family, it was not customary to pay a doctor for a house call. If the patient died, the physician would be too embarrassed to even ask for money. If the patient was treated and cured, depending on the number of calls and the gravity of the case, a fee would be sent to him. The financial means of the patient was of great importance, of course.[161] However, as is clear from Basir al-Molk's experience, for example, physicians did not hesitate to ask for their money. It may have been that Basir al-Molk did not employ a family physician, of course.[162] Physicians also often received homespun fabrics, a shawl, and money, especially if the family was rich or the doctor's service important. A regular fee, often a quantity of wheat, would be sent for the services of the family physician without any previous agreement. Both sides were considerate and generous, without any problems between them. If the master happened to neglect the physicians, a simple reminder to one of the members of the family would settle the matter.[163]

Vambéry en route from Zenjan to Tehran was overtaken by a physician returning from visits to his patients in the neighborhood. He had a servant with him with a mule "so heavily laden that it well-nigh sank beneath the weight of its load. The poor beast was carrying the fees collected in kind by the physician, such as dried fruit, corn and so forth. This loquacious disciple of Aesculap dwelt, during the whole time, upon the miraculous cures he had accomplished, and gave vent to his unbounded astonishment at the impudence of the Frengis (Europeans) who dared to appear as physicians in the home of *Ali Ben Sina* (Avicenna). He unceasingly dilated upon the efficacy of his amulets and talismans, and how he had driven devils out of his patients, made the dumb speak, the blind see and the deaf hear."[164]

EUROPEAN APPRECIATION OF PERSIAN DOCTORS
Europeans in general, and European physicians in particular, did not write in glowing terms about the traditional Persian physician. They considered them quacks, who, at best, were pure empiricists (*i.e.*, acted by trial-and-error) and at worst snake doctors. After some 30 years having lived in Persia and Basrah at the end of the eighteenth and the beginning of the nineteenth century, the British ambassador Brydges-Jones gave as his opinion, "as to her [Persia] medicine and surgery, God help the patient!"[165] As to the

---

[160] Stuart, Emmeline M. *Doctors in Persia* (London, CMS, n.d.), p. 7.
[161] Mostowfi, *Sharh*, vol. 1, p. 528; Hasanbeygi, *Tehran-e Qadim*, p. 199; Farmanfarma, *Siyaq-e Ma'ishat*, vol. 1, pp. 67 (payment of a modern doctor based on an invoice), 74 (payment of traditional doctor in a discrete manner); see also Dieulefoy, *La Perse*, pp. 436-37; Polak, *Persien*, vol. 2, pp. 215-16.
[162] Basir al-Molk, *Ruznameh*, p. 275; Ghani, *Yaddashtha*, vol. 1, pp. 194-95.
[163] Mostowfi, *Sharh*, vol. 1, p. 528; Aubin, *La Perse*, p. 313.
[164] Vambéry, Arminius. *His Life and Adventures* (London: Fisher Unwin, 1884), p. 67. According to Hasanbeygi, *Tehran-e Qadim*, p. 199 and Saad, *Sechzehn Jahre*, p. 183, patients usually paid in kind rather in cash.
[165] Brydges-Jones, *An Account*, p. 436.

theoretical foundation of Persian medicine he was even more dismissive. "'Necessity is the mother of invention,' and, perhaps, when our incestors [sic; ancestors] knew little more on this subject, than that if a pitcher was dipped into a well, it would fill itself, the Persians were acquainted with many of the most powerful properties of this blessed and most extraordinary fluid."[166] There were some exceptions to this rule, but these were far and between. Likewise, Persians in general were not initially impressed with European physicians either.

These opinions were not necessarily based on fact, and more often than not based on some prejudice, religious or otherwise in nature. Both attitudes are understandable. Europeans had abandoned the Galenic medical system for a more scientific approach and were reminded by what they saw in Persia of their own not so distant past.[167] Wills, a British physician in the service of the Anglo-Indian Telegraph Department, expressed this sentiment when he wrote, "Some of the remedies of the native physicians recall the strange old medieval and classical plans."[168] You did not want to be reminded of your own similar recent past, because it would diminish your position, and more importantly, your perception of superiority. Rather than trying to understand the other it was easier to stereotype them. Despite this feeling of intellectual and scientific superiority it did not mean that Western medicine had all the answers, or that Western doctors were better healers and knew what they were doing.

Persians were not better, of course. Many of them believed that Christian doctors would kill them, or that it would impair their piety and purity, because Christians were impure.[169] Eichwald related the experience with his Moslem secretary, who fell ill. He refused to consult a Russian doctor, or to try Eichwald's medicines. As a *hajji* he rather would die than to take medicines from Christians. Eichwald commented, "Only those poor Persians who have not been to Mecca do so. The secretary called for a Persian doctor, a Shi'a who only prescribed pulverized sandalwood, which his stomach could not stand. In addition he received opium." As a consequence, Eichwald's secretary died.[170] Kotzebue, a member of the 1817 Russian mission to Persia, related a case that concerned the treatment of a Cossack, who was a Moslem, and spurned the Russian embassy doctor's treatment. He insisted on the help of a Persian doctor, who "appeared, looked grave, and prescribed for the patient, who was labouring under inflammatory fever, a large quantity of ice, which the poor wretch swallowed with extacy-he died on the third day."[171] Morier, the secretary of the 1809 Ouseley embassy, related a similar story. "Our

---

[166] Brydges-Jones, Sir Harford. *An Account of the Transaction of His Majesty's Mission to the Court of Persia in the Years 1807-11* (London, 1834 [Tehran: Imp. Org. f. Social Services, 1976]), p. 436; Ts., "Persidskie Doktora," p. 162.

[167] Collins, *In the Kingdom*, p. 168 ("Medicine in Persia is much in the condition in which it was in England previous to Sydenham's time.")

[168] Wills, *Persia*, pp. 90-91.

[169] Saad, *Sechzehn Jahre*, pp. 182-83, 187; Dieulefoy, *La Perse*, p. 436. There is no Islamic interdiction to use the services of a non-Moslem doctor and, as will be clear in what follows, Persian Moslems were patients of Persian Jewish and Christian doctors, it may be that the resistance had to do with a particular fundamentalist point of view.

[170] Eichwald, *Reise*, vol. 1, pp. 371-72.

[171] Kotzebue, *Narrative*, p. 148.

head Persian writer was long laid up with a fever, which brought him to the point of death. He was bled copiously six times in six days. These people put no faith in our medicines, and therefore he would not allow the physician of the mission to visit him. At length, however, he was persuaded by a '*fall*' which he took in Hafiz, and which pointed out, that he should 'trust in a stranger.'" He did not take the advice anyway; the royal physician prescribed watermelon, and he recovered.[172] Even when towards the end of the nineteenth century visits by Persian Moslems to Western missionary dispensaries and hospitals as well as house calls made by missionary medical staff had become normal "extensive ablutions would be gone through by the patients and their friends to cleanse them from the defiling touch of infidel hands."[173]

Contrariwise, Europeans had less of a problem in seeking the advice of Persian physicians during the first part of the nineteenth century, and, occasionally thereafter, to try out Persian traditional medicine. Jaubert, a member of the French diplomatic mission (1807-09), when he was ill, sought the skills of Persian physicians. They felt his pulse, but did not talk to him.

> The one said to the other: 'I know what it is. The fever is continuous; the skin is dry and the pulse high and frequent. The indication of the remedy is easy; he needs to take cold and acid seeds, to have the patient observe a strict diet, and above all to ban the use of bread. For each liquid he uses he needs to use oxymel [sekanjebin], granate and lemon juice, and for all food, pilau, bitter herbs, raw cucumbers and green fruits. He also needs to strictly avoid sleeping before his meals; soon, God willing, and with the refreshing regime, he will recover. If the paroxysms continue we will prescribe bleeding.' When I asked some question the physician was very surprised by my doubts re his knowledge and looking at me with a indignant air he said: do you know that you talk to one, who is considered generally as the Hippocrate of Iran, who looks after the Shah's health. I know your illness perfectly well.... The physician of the harem was less pompous and very old. He knew blood circulation, use of quinine and emetic, and inoculation, but he considered them dangerous innovations. He strongly believed in amulets, talismans and prayers.[174]

Similarly, the British missionary Wolff, en route to Bokhara to try and obtain the freedom of the imprisoned Stoddard, twice fell ill and each time had himself bled by a Persian practitioner. At Deh Molla, "I felt very unwell, I got a barber to bleed me." He nevertheless, had no high opinion of Persian medicine. The manner in which they had treated Mohammad Shah, who had the gout, did not impress him at all. The shah's "quack physician" had prescribed brandy for the shah's condition. As result, so opined Wolff, the shah "was victimized, not by hydropathy, but brandypathy."[175] When Wolff on his return from Bokhara once again and fortuitously was indisposed at Deh Mollah, he "was bled

---

[172] Morier, *A Journey*, p. 230 ("If the patient is supposed to suffer from much heat they bleed him beyond measure; if from cold, they give him cathartics in the same proportion.")

[173] Stuart, *Doctors in Persia*, p. 11.

[174] Jaubert, *Voyage*, pp. 337-38. Jaubert added that the doctors always made us camp on hills, and where possible in orchards with running pure water. Ibid., p. 341.

[175] Wolff, Joseph. *Researches and Missionary Labours* (London: James Nisbet & Co., 1835), p. 120.

almost every day, and took a medicine which they have in Khorassaun called Sheer-khishk, a kind of powerful manna."[176] Fowler had himself treated when struck with ache and diarrhea, and although the Persian doctor did not want to touch him, because he was a Christian, he prescribed a strict diet for him that worked.[177] Burgess who had lived in Persia for 20 years and had used British physicians in case he needed medical advice, nevertheless also used Persian remedies, at times. May be this was the influence of his Persian Christian wife, for he wrote that "after trying almost all the European medicines such as rhubarb magnesia soda etc without much success I found much benefit from the Persian treatment viz astringent acids particularly pomme-granites and I now continue taking this delicious fruit occasionally although I have little occasion for it medicinally."[178]

The British Colonel Baker, on a tour in Khorasan in the 1870s, fell ill; he was feverish and exhausted, with his tongue blistered and cleaving to his mouth. Ya`qub Khan, at five miles from Mashad, advised him

> to use a Persian medicine common in the bazaar, which he presented to be the most efficacious in dysenteric affections. As I had consumed all my own medicines without producing any effect, I agreed to try his remedy; which consisted of a small seed, somewhat resembling linseed and called in Persia *barhang*, made into a tea like linseed tea, with the additional tea-spoonful of oil of sweet almonds. My diet was restricted to rice and a mash made of almonds and sugar, not unpalatable. The effect was marvelous. In two days I improved immensely; and, though I had recurrences of the disease, by immediately flying to *barhang* I managed to continue my journey.[179]

Brugsch, the cultural counselor of the Prussian embassy in 1860-61, had no high opinion of the Persian medical profession. However, when he felt indisposed and feverish and a Persian doctor in Qazi'un (near Pasargardae) offered his service, he accepted his advice. The 'physician' was a rural quack, and dressed as a nomad. He was honest enough to tell Brugsch that he did not know much about medicine. He looked at Brugsch's tongue and felt his pulse. He told Brugsch, "the disorder was serious and many people had died of it, but there also had been people who had gotten better, he consoled Brugsch." He prescribed watermelon water of which Brugsch had to drink as much as he could. "Normally, I would have rejected this as dangerous, but in the desperate situation I was in I started to drink the liquid."[180]

Later in the century, with the progress of medical science in Europe and the larger presence of a number of European physicians in Persia, Europeans were less interested to seek the services of Persian physicians. As Mary Sheil put it, "The dreadful practice of the Persian doctors is quite enough to drive the fair dames of Tehran to an English

---

[176] Wolff, *Researches*, pp. 143, 308.
[177] Fowler, *Three Years*, vol. 1, pp. 55-57.
[178] Schwartz, *Letters*, p. 114 (in 1852).
[179] Baker, Valentine. *Clouds in the East* (London: Chatto & Windus, 1876), pp. 190-91. Baker referred to the *barang*, the seed of a *Plantago*, see Aitchison, "Notes," p. 22.
[180] Brugsch, *Reise*, vol. 2, pp. 131-32.

physician. I am told they give the most nauseating draughts, in immense quantities, to their patients-two or three quarts at a time."[181] She exaggerated here somewhat, and the novelty of the European physician had as much to do with the fair ladies' interest in European medical practitioners as the possible need for medical assistance. Also, these ladies were members of the privileged rich aristocratic families; the same choice was not open to other women. As far as the large size of the draughts were concerned that was as much the doctor's fault as the demand by the patients. At Sarbizan (Kerman) Percy Sykes's party was accosted by nomad women who wanted medicine, "but our tabloids were not at all favourably received, the idea that anything so small could be potent being rejected with scorn. In fact, so much was this the case that our visitors were not mollified until a bottle of some concoction, mainly water, was mixed for their edification. The whole business reminded me of a Cape doctor, who said that if you gave a Boer less than a quart of medicine, he would decline to pay the fee."[182]

What did not help either was the jealousy and competition that was created by having representatives of two different kinds of medical traditions vie for the same market. This market initially was very limited, viz., the shah and/or one of the prince-governors. This jealousy was even felt towards European physicians who passed through and thus posed no threat whatsoever to the position of the Persian court physician. Dr. Bélanger recorded his meeting with the personal physician of the governor of Erevan in 1825. The Persian physician was jealous, and asked Bélanger what he had prescribed for the governor. He did not even wait for the reply, and commented, "Undoubtedly mercury (*jiveh*) like the British doctors." The Persian doctor told Bélanger that he had prescribed a cold treatment, because the governor had a hot illness.[183] Bélanger then asked the Persian doctor to show what drugs he had. He saw amongst other things quinine, whose use was rather unknown in Persia at that time. The Persian physician told Bélanger that the ignorant Christian who had given it him had told him to give it in powdered form at the interval of the start of intermittent fever. The Persian physician then shared his appreciation of this advice with Bélanger. "This ass, I will use it at the very beginning. But it is no good, the temperature rises, and some even die."[184] Bélanger reported this

---

[181] Sheil, *Glimpses*, p. 213. According to Malcolm, *Children*, p. 86, medicine was given "not in little teaspoonfuls, but in nice big bowlfuls, and the nastier it is the more good they think it will do."

[182] Sykes, *Ten Thousand Miles*, pp. 210-11; Binning, *A Journal*, vol. 1, p. 165 ("The Persians are surprised at our small doses of medicine; for their own physicians administer their drugs in large bowlsfull."); Wigram, *The Cradle*, pp. 173-74.

[183] Bélanger, *Voyage*, vol. 2, p. 216; Morier, *A Second*, p. 192 (cases of Persian doctor's interferece). Dieulefoy, *La Perse*, p. 436 reported that Persian doctors would not allow their patients to see European doctors, and only then when they were on death's doorstep, implying that they wanted to shift the blame onto the latter. The vizier of Shiraz was ill. "His ignorant physicians give him no medicine; and they beg him not to call in our Doctor, praise each other before his face as so many Iphlatoons, Iphlatoon [i.e., Plato] being celebrated as a great medical man." Money, Journal, p. 77.

[184] Bélanger, *Voyage*, vol. 2, p. 217. Quinine, a toxic plant alkaloid made from the bark of the Cinchona tree in South America was used to treat malaria more than 370 years ago. Jesuit missionaries in South America learned of the anti-malarial properties of the bark of the Cinchona tree and introduced it into Europe by the 1630s and into India by 1657. The Dutch established Cinchona plantations in Java (Indonesia) in the mid-1800s and soon had a virtual monopoly on

entire story as an example how backward Persian physicians were. Dr. Wills summed up his appreciation of Persian medicine that there was not much to be learnt from Persian medicine, "save the great attention to dietetic rules which is invariably practiced."[185] Dr. Malcolm, who in general also had a negative opinion of Persian physicians and medicine, nevertheless concluded her remarks with the statement: "There are exceptions, and I have met Persian doctors, who not only had real knowledge of medical treatment, but had some of the true doctor's spirit of pity and self-sacrifice. Especially I would mention the brave Persian doctor who stayed at his post in Shiraz in the cholera epidemic of 1904, and fought that terrible disease instead of yielding to the panic that had seized his fellow countrymen."[186]

However, in general, Europeans agreed with Dr. Collins who couched his appreciation of Persian medicine in the famous words of the seventeenth century Dr. Lettsom, who summed up his own manner of medical practice as follows:[187]

> When the patients come to I
> I physics, bleeds, and sweats 'em;
> Then if they choose to die,
> What's that to I? I lets 'em

Dr Lichtwardt who wrote an article comparing the *Tebb-e Yusefi* by Yusef b. Mohammad a text written in 1511 with that a John Wesley's *Primitive Physick* published in London in 1772 concluded his article with a wise word to those who may have felt (or still feel) the need to crow about Persian doctors' ignorance. "Thus, we note that the Persian therapy of the sixteenth century was not much different from the European therapy of the eighteenth; whilst we, gloating in our modern knowledge, skill, and ability, will in a few generations probably be rated as ignorant and backward and ridiculous, in the light of discoveries which will be made in the next century."[188]

Druggists

I have mentioned the role of the druggist (`attar*) to provide the ingredients for the physician's prescriptions. The druggist in Persia was the closest thing to the institution of a pharmacy, which did not exist in Qajar Persia. The only ones of that kind were those managed by European physicians and were private in nature. The exception was the pharmacy established by Mirza Sadeq in the late 1830s, who had learnt the profession through collaboration with the British physician Dr. Charles Bell (physician of the British Mission during 1835-45). However, he left Tehran in 1845 to study medicine in Great Britain, having abandoned a lucrative chemist's practice. Although he had been promised the function of the shah's personal physician after his return to Persia, nothing is known of

---

quinine.
[185] Wills, *Persia*, p. 91.
[186] Malcolm, *Children*, pp. 89-90. Usually, like other peole who could afford it, would flee. Ghani, *Yaddashtha*, vol. 1, p. 188.
[187] Collins, *In the Kingdom*, p. 168.
[188] Lichtwardt, "Ancient Therapy," pp. 280-84.

his life after he had left Great Britain.[189] Persian doctors prescribed the drugs that they believed were required, the druggist supplied them as is, and the patient's relatives made themselves the necessary infusions, decoctions, pills, pastilles, electuaries, etc. The druggist also sold distilled water.[190] Druggists wrapped their products in reject pages of printed books, including of Korans supplied by print shops. In 1851, the government banned this practice in Tehran, as being un-Islamic, and forbade printers (*basmehchiyan*) to print Korans.[191] The druggists also offered their service as healers to those who could not afford a doctor.[192]

The druggists (`*attar*) only existed in towns and had small shops spread out over the main bazaar and the small bazaars in the city quarters. They retailed their wares to all and sundry.

> The greater part of their stock consists of dried herbs and plants, for making decoctions, fomentations, and infusions; the three most lucrative branches of their business: though of late years they have introduced from Georgia small quantities of European chemicals, principally from the Moscow fabriques; such as sulphate of iron and copper, sulphate of quinine, Peruvian bark, alum, borax, bitarbrate of potass, carbonates of soda and potash, and tartatic acid. Calomel occasionally, which they call 'white powder;' and occasionally, though more rarely, antimonial preparations, though these are not be found at every druggist's. They have also euphorbium (Persian variety highly poisonous) elaterium, the ricinus, senna, rheum, tartaricum, gums, and other aromatic herbs which grow wild on the mountains. The dispensatory in common use, which is, like all other works, in manuscript, is that by Nour'odin Mahomet Abdalla hakkim Ain el Melek Shiragi, in which will be found a list of useless and innocuous substances, which have evidently been compiled from the work of the Greek, Latin, and Arab authors. Of the former they have translated Hippocrates, Kitab I Pocral if Mehatm; Galin, Paracelsus, and Pliny, of the Arabs, Rhazes, Abo Senna, Ibu Senna; the canon of Abo Senna Abinsoar, &c. and others of inferior note.[193]

---

[189] Wright, *The Persians amongst the English*, pp. 76, 141-42. Adamiyat, *Amir Kabir*, p. 327 mentioned that he had been appointed as chief surgeon of the army in Azerbaijan. According to Polak, *Persien*, vol. 2, pp. 215 several attempts to open European-type chemist shops had failed due to lack of confidence and the innovation of selling drugs cheaper than customers were accustomed to.

[190] Schlimmer, *Terminologie*, p. 216 (q.v. droguiste); Wills, *In the Land*, p. 182 (his dispensary); Serena, *Hommes*, p. 138; Eichwald, *Reise*, vol. 1, p. 373; Grothe, Hugo. *Wanderungen in Persien* (Berlin, Alg. Verein f. Deutsche Literatur, 1910), p. 207 (primitive apothecaries in the bazaar of Hamadan); Neligan, "Public Health," part III, p. 742; Safari, *Ardabil*, vol. 3, p. 487.

[191] Government of Iran, *Vaqaye`-ye Ettefaqiyeh*, vol. 1, p. 68 (nr. 14, 7 Rajab 1267/8 May, 1851). Paper was scarce in Persia, and old and discarded paper was therefore used to wrap various retail products, see Floor, *Traditional Crafts*, p. 276.

[192] Hasanbeygi, *Tehran-e Qadim*, p. 203; Saad, *Sechzehn Jahre*, p. 182.

[193] Clarke, "Sketches," p. 708 ("to be seen engaged in chemical experiments would argue a correspondance with the Devil, and he would be magnified into a magician; so that their own prejudices prevent them from making any advancement'). De Fontanelle, "Das Apothekerwesen," p. 119 is in agreement with this; see also Polak, *Persien*, vol. 2, p. 215.

According to Clarke, the druggists were also accomplished poisoners who served as passive agents of their princes. He provided a description of the making of one poison, although the secret of the making of the others was tightly kept. Other drugs kept and promoted by the druggists were China root (*chub-e chini*), coffee, and tea.[194] Häntzsche was astonished by the fact that mercury was for sale without any restrictions while Persian surgeons also much used it (in particular in cases of syphilis) leading to many cases of poisoning. Polak had a less negative opinion about the use of mercury, and even saw many advantages.[195]

The druggists also had various prophylactics such as bezoar stones, holy stones from Mecca, and *padzahr*, which all were alleged to be effective against poisonous bites. These were very expensive up to 20 to 30 tomans (£10 to 15). They also had curative medicines. "The vesical calculi are frequently made use of, but are considered an imposition by the druggists, the true tusoan of the Persians following an intestinal concretion, or else a deposition of calcareous matter at the inner canthus of the eye of the stay. The latter is considered most valuable from its rarity, though the former fetches also a considerable sum, even if it be a triple phosphate, where it is likely to be taken for vesical calculi, which cut little, and are considered spurious."[196] A druggist who had tusoan applied it to a patient bitten by a scorpion. He took "it from his breast, and with heated breath applied it, dripping in new milk, to the puncture. The solemnity of the action was further hightened, and the value of the article enhanced, by the pompous manner in which he repeated his supplicatory prayer."[197]

Sometimes the druggists had sarsaparilla, which they called sarsa or cascarilla. They also received occasionally from Tiflis small quantities of lunar caustic, or hell's stone (*hajr al-jehenna*), because of the pain it produces during its application. They also received from English and other travelers small quantities of pulvis, ipecacuanha, and antimony tartarizat or tartrate, which they sold to their neighbors at an enormous profit.[198] The druggists also sold a variety of preparations to women as abortives. Clarke examined one such product, which he found to be "a weak solution of bichloride of mercury, in rose-water, coloured with the juice of red poppy, papaver rhoeas." According to the druggists it was a great beautifier of the skin. Clarke noticed that it had a strong needling effect on the skin, and "the vessels of the cutis become extremely vascular. And 24 hours after the application of this solution the old epidermis falls off, leaving a fine delicate deposition of new epidermis beneath." Clarke also noticed the application of henna to the skin and eyelids. "It is of so irritating nature, that after the age of 25 or 30, you rarely see a Persian women who is not affected with lippitudo." But women want to be attractive and thus nothing will change their mind, Clarke opined.[199]

---

[194] Clarke, "Sketches," p. 709; also De Fontanelle, "Das Apothekerwesen," p. 119; Häntzsche, "Physikalisch-medicinische Skizze," p. 561.
[195] Häntzsche, "Physikalisch-medicinische Skizze," pp. 565-67; Polak, "Ueber den Gebrauch," pp. 564-68.
[196] Clarke, "Sketches," p. 709; also De Fontanelle, "Das Apothekerwesen," p. 120.
[197] Clarke, "Sketches," p. 709.
[198] Clarke, "Sketches," p. 709 (two grams of tartar emetic cost 2*s*. 6*d*.); De Fontanelle, "Das Apothekerwesen," pp. 119-20.
[199] Clarke, "Sketches," pp. 709-10.

The quality of the products sold by druggists was not guaranteed. According to Dr. Häntzsche, the druggists "sold medicines that are unreliable, because they are usually impure and neglected, and often deliberately adulterated."[200] In fact, one Persian author accused them of "selling rotten and corrupt medications."[201] This was, for example, the case in Bandar `Abbas where in 1910, the British medical quarantine officer had to get supplies from the British consulate, because the stocks of the druggists in the bazaar were rotten or too old to be used.[202] It also happened that they gave the patient the wrong product instead of that which the doctor had prescribed.[203]

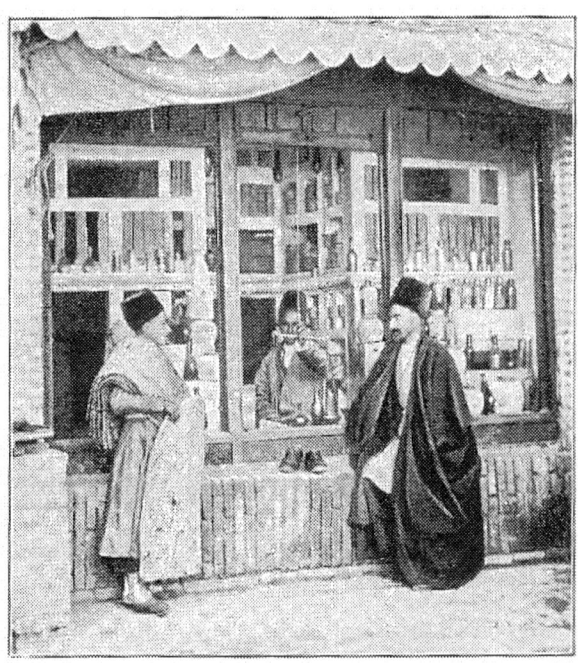

Figure 6: Traditional drugstore.

According to Höltzer, there were only 17 drugstores (`attari`) in 1890 in Isfahan.[204] However, some 15 years earlier, Tahvildar, a fellow Isfahan townsman, stated that, "their shops are spread out of the province and are numerous."[205] Höltzer may only have referred to those in the central bazaar, for in 1920 there were about 120 drugstores in Isfahan.[206] In Tabriz, in 1869, there were

---

[200] Häntzsche, "Physikalisch-medicinische Skizze," p. 561; Polak, *Persien*, vol. 2, p. 215.
[201] Ebrahimnejad, "Theory and Practice," p. 171.
[202] Sadid al-Saltaneh, Mohammad `Ali. *Bandar `Abbas va Khalij-e Fars*. Ahmad Eqtedari ed. (Tehran: Amir Kabir, 1342/1963), p. 169.
[203] Government of Iran, *Vaqaye'-ye Ettefaqiyeh*, vol. 1, p. 237 (nr. 45, 17 Safar 1268/12 December, 1851)
[204] Höltzer, *Persien*, p. 20 (they paid 700 tomans in guild taxes per year. Ibid., p. 40). Allegedly there was only one herbalist in the entire khanate of Erevan, which does not seem right. Bournoutian, *Eastern Armenia*, p. 203.
[205] Tahvildar, *Joghrafiya*, p. 94.
[206] Janab, *Ketab*, p. 79.

120 drugstores and confectioners (`attari va qannadi`).²⁰⁷ The number of drugstores, indeed, was large as table 3 demonstrates. However, more important was how these were distributed over the city. In Tehran, around 1880, there were at least 37 druggists.²⁰⁸ In 1925, there were 615 drugstores. However, to many people such stores were not accessible. It depended on where you lived in town. If you lived, for example, in Shahr-e Now then you were out of luck, because there were only four shops (see Table 3). This is an indication that in this new city quarter the service infrastructure developed only slowly. This was partly due to the relative poverty of the population in the new quarters, partly due to the unwillingness of the established service providers to move their operations beyond their local area.

As a result there also were many street side druggists, although they did not show up in the statistics.²⁰⁹ These were found all over the town; behind stores or in front of a mosque with their wares spread out on a piece of cloth. They sold a wide variety of remedies and they cried their wares that ranged from specialties for women (to get fat, for women's pains, pregnancy), when women passed by, or for men (potency) when men passed by, to generics such as purgatives for pain in the hands or foot. These traders were not only sellers of drugs and herbs but also healers who sold their service to anyone who was willing to pay for it.

---

[207] Javadi, *Tabriz*, p. 227.
[208] Sheikh-Reza'i and Azari, *Gozareshha-ye Nazmiyeh*, Index q.v. `attar`.
[209] For a picture of an itinerant druggist see Rosen, *Persien*, p. 148.

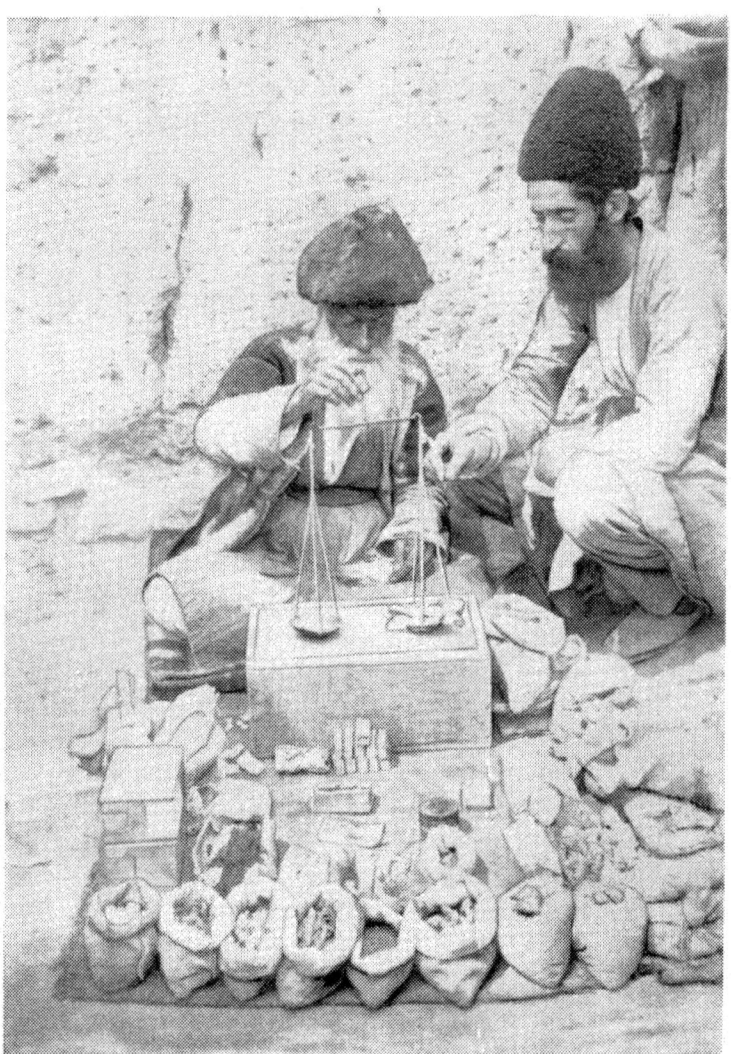

Figure 7: Traditional street side drug seller.

There was not a disease that they were not willing to treat, for they had a remedy for all from the top of the head to the nails of the feet and anything in between, both the inside and the outside of the body. Generally, the patients would whisper their complaint into the ear of the healer-drug seller. Thus, they were even more trusted than regular physicians, because the drug seller did not know his patient, and women, of course, were unrecognizable anyway due to their all-encompassing shroud. Some of them would be specialized in certain diseases such as hemorrhoids (*bavasir*), venereal diseases, female diseases, or male diseases. In addition to those drugs that were spread out for sale, these drug sellers also kept special medications in bottles in boxes. These were for men's diseases such as "medicines to increase the length of the penis, pills to improve sexual performance and the length of ejaculation, etc.; for women, to change the timing of periods (to shorten or lengthen it), for making the vulva smaller and the return of virginity, etc." Some of these street healers had more customers and made more money than regular doctors, particularly those whose specialized in women's medicine.[210]

Table 3: Number of drugstores, their staff and their distribution over Tehran (1925)

Name quarter	# Shops	# Masters	# Workers	# Helpers
Ark	9	9	-.-	2
Dowlat	77	73	45	15
Hasanabad	54	52	37	3
Sangalaj	103	89	26	13
Qanatabad	58	52	20	3
Mohammadiyeh	86	74	55	6
Sharq	32	24	7	6
Bazaar	95	87	71	12
`Owdlajan	97	93	37	22
Shahr-e Now	4	4	1	1
Total	615	557	299	83

Source: Baladiyeh, pp. 78-79.

EYE DOCTORS

There also were eye-surgeons (*jarrah-e cheshm*; *kahhal*) to treat eye problems.[211] They enjoyed enormous fame even beyond the borders. Persian eye powder, consisting of a combination of copper sulfate and myrabolan, also was much sought after and was exported as well. The eye doctors performed a range of operations including entropium, trichiasis, pannus, trachoma, pterygium, and catharact using a variety of techniques. Despite the fame that Persian ophthalmologists enjoyed the number of people suffering from eye diseases or who were blind was high, and thus were a living denial of their efficacy.[212] According to Dr. Häntzsche there were many eye doctors in Qajar Persia. Many of them were itinerant and were not above misleading their patients. However, in Tabriz there were only five of them (*cheshm pezeshk*) in 1869. Häntzsche may have included the many women and other folk medicine practitioners who also operated in the ophthalmological field.[213] Not much is known about the diagnostic and therapeutic practice of Persian eye doctors (*kahhal*). There were, of course, medical texts, but these need not necessarily have had any relationship with actual medical practice. Mostowfi characterized this brand of medicine as follows:

> The field of ophthalmology had always been separate from the rest. Eye doctors carried their own medicine with them in special leather pouches (*quloq*) to drop them with their thumb and the index finger into the sick eye. They also did such operations as couching (*mil zadan*) and catheterization (*ab gereftan*), at which they excelled the European-trained doctors.[214]

---

[210] Shahri, *Tarikh*, vol. 4, pp. 327-31 (with a description of some of the remedies).

[211] Basir al-Molk, *Ruznameh*, p. 421.

[212] Polak, *Persien*, vol. 2, p. 205.

[213] Javadi, *Tabriz*, p. 277; Häntzsche, "Specialstatistik von Persien," p. 442; Ibid., "Physikalisch-medicinische Skizze," p. 561; Collins, *In the Kingdom*, p. 169 ("Besides the regular Hakims, there are numerous old women who are said to remedies of such a marvelous character that they will effect a cure when everything else has failed.").

[214] Mostowfi, *Sharh*, vol. 1, p. 528; see also Safari, *Ardabil*, vol. 3, p. 480. According to `Eyn al-Saltaneh, *Ruznameh*, vol. 2, p. 1249, Nur Mohammad Hakim-e Jadid al-Eslam (possibly a former

The most experienced *qeynaris* (cornea specialists) were from Saveh, who were exceptionally outstanding in couching, according to Mostowfi. They challenged the European-educated doctors in competitions and often won. They did not drain liquid that had collected in the eye, but re-channeled it and it naturally went away. They also operated on trachoma patients who suffered from thick eyelids, by scraping it with a lump of sugar. Salve and bandage was their final touch.[215]

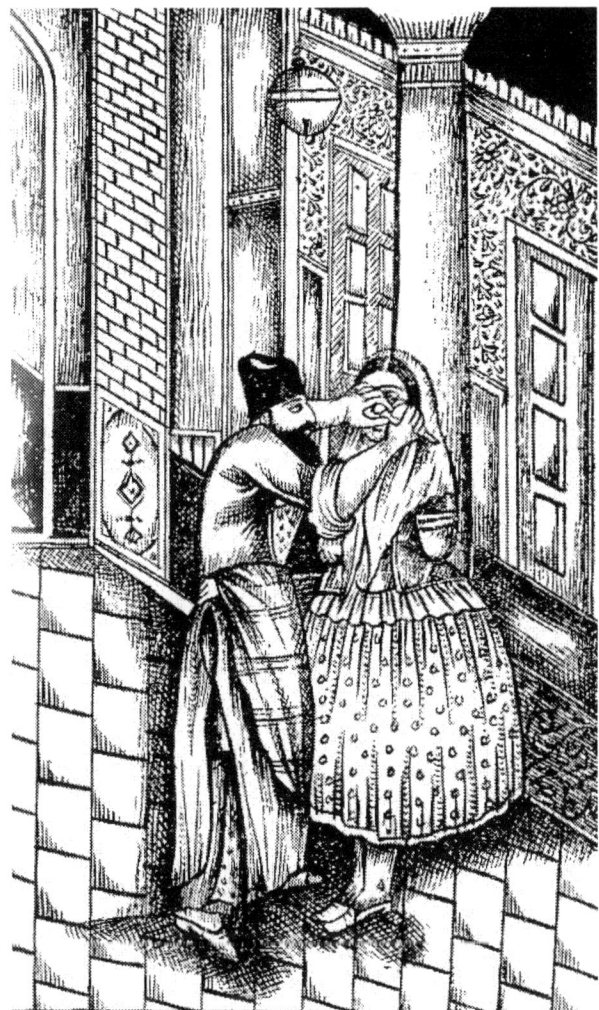

Figure 8: Persian woodcut of an eye doctor and a patient.

Jewish physician) was better in treating eye diseases than Muller, the German physician, the doctor of the American hospital, and other Western doctors. Nur Mohammad did not know Western medicine, only Islamic medicine. In the case mentioned (*lakeh* or spots) he used medicines that he prepared himself that cured the problem (*ghobaresh rafteh* or the mistiness disappeared).

[215] Mostowfi, *Sharh*, vol. 1, p. 529; see also Safari, *Ardabil*, vol. 3, p. 480.

Forbes-Leith experienced that in particular the eye situation of babies was pitiful. They were covered with filth and scabies or suffering from all sorts of congenital disease. Most from "some form of virulent trachoma, and often their inflamed and blind eyes were past treatment." He advised the parents to frequently use soap and water, but this advice fell on deaf ears. He therefore gave the parents colored water with salt or something else to wash them and they loved it, "as medicine of any kind is a fetish with the Persian villager."[216] This simple approach was not always followed. A Yezidi wandering medicine man, for example, examined a Kurdish chief who suffered from trachoma and "diagnosed the watering of the eyes as due to an excess of moisture behind the eye-balls, and had proposed running a red-hot skewer through the Sheikh's head from temple to temple, in order to dry up the 'superfluous moisture' at the fountain of the head!"[217]

The Persian cure for ophthalmia was quite different. "They cover their diseased eyes with a small piece of blue cotton cloth, often very dirty, and scarcely ever change it; thus rendering the remedy worse than the disease; but even experience does not correct them, and of a hundred inhabitants of a town, nearly one half are met with similar rags suspended from their caps."[218] Not all cases were that bad. Browne related the discussion of the Sanitation Council in 1888 about the presentation of a case of acute ophthalmia that had been "successfully treated by inoculation, the merits of which plan of treatment were then compared with the results obtained by the use of jequirity, called in Persian *chashm-i-khurus*, and in Arabic `*aynu'd-dik*, both of which terms signify 'cock's eye'"[219]

Persian ophthalmologists considered white dog's dung (*Album graecum*) or *goh-e sag-e safid* the best remedy for spots on the cornea. To produce this remedy the ophthalmologists believed that the dogs needed to be fed bones only during 40 days, and to use only the product of the 40th day, that was pulverized.[220] According to Dr. Collins, a favorite treatment of inflammations of the eye was fumigations with the smoke of burning donkey's dung. "A form of counter irritation is resorted to in obstinate cases, small issues being kept constantly open on the outer side of the arm by the insertion into them of grains of Indian wheat. I saw one man who had had issues kept open in this way for twenty years, and though he had patiently submitted to this prolonged course of treatment, he expected me to effect a cure in a few days."[221] Ella Sykes reported that sore eyes were even "cured by an application of powdered glass!"[222] According to Dr. Cochran, an American missionary physician, inflammatory diseases of the eye were "treated with powerful caustics, freely applied. Couching for cataract is practiced in places."[223] His British colleague, Dr. Hume-Griffith was not impressed at all with the surgical qualities of Persian ophthalmologists.

---

[216] Forbes-Leith, *Checkmate*, p. 94.
[217] Wigram, *The Cradle*, p. 146.
[218] Tancoigne, *A Narrative*, p. 245.
[219] Browne, *A Year*, p. 107.
[220] Schlimmer, *Terminologie*, p. 24.
[221] Collins, *In the Kingdom*, p. 169.
[222] Sykes, *Persia and its People*, p. 337.
[223] Cochran, "Treatment of the Sick," pp. 105-06. Shabaz, *Land of the Lion*, p. 21, wrote, "I could

> The Persian surgeons also operate for this disease [cataract], using the old Eastern operation known as 'couching.' An incision is made into the white of the eyeball (without any aneasthetic), then a thick, blunt probe is worked into the interior of the eye, directed so as to dislocate the lens. If successful, the lens drops back into the posterior chamber of the eye, and the patient 'sees,' but alas, the vision obtained is, in ninety-eight cases out of a hundred, only temporary! Twenty-four hours later, inflammation of the eye supervenes, and the sight is gone, and the eye lost. Needless to say, the operator obtains his fee either before the operation is done, or during the few hours that this patient is rejoicing in his newly found vision; that if he is wise he disappears from town, and resumes his practice elsewhere.[224]

In all the thousands of cases Hume-Griffith had seen only two cases of couching ever were permanent, in all the other cases there was inflammation and the eye was lost.[225] Dr. Collins, an ophthalmologist, also saw many cases of couching, "a few quite successfully, but a very large number with disastrous results."[226] Mostowfi held a different opinion. He reported that the Persian eye doctors were so good that they had a success ratio of 90-100%! Mostowfi further maintained that Western-educated Persian doctors did not have their experience and sometimes would blind the patient.[227] It is also possible that these eye-surgeons not only extracted cataract, but also practiced non-ophthalmologic medicine such as cutting for stone.[228] For the surgeons (*jarrah*), who would be expected to do this, whom I discuss in the section of traditional healers, do not appear to have had the instruments or the technical finesse to do so.

In Urumiyeh, a town of 30,000 people around 1900 had only two eye doctors. However, during a warm dry season at least 10% of the population would suffer from eye disease. One of the two eye doctors in that town was a woman, Mashadi Zabar Khanom, who practiced her profession at home. Her courtyard was filled with up to 100 patients every day and each had to wait his or her turn.

> Mashady-Zabar-Khanum is seated near the fountain on a nice soft cushion, and each patient in turn lies down and puts his or her head on the doctor's left knee. The doctor has several folded papers containing a variety of medicines of her own make; she takes a little pinch of

---

see no more, and the only remedy was nicotine which they took from their pipes and applied to my eyes." This was a rural folk remedy.

[224] Hume-Griffith, *Behind the Veil*, pp. 153-54. His view was shared by Stuart, *Doctors in Persia*, p. 7.

[225] Hume-Griffith, *Behind the Veil*, p. 154. The success rate of the couching technique was much higher in India around 1900 (50% blind; 50% some vision) and in Senegal around 1950 (81% blind), see Savage-Smith, "The Practice," p. 318.

[226] Collins, *In the Kingdom*, pp. 168-69 ("the old operation of couching for hard cataract, in which the opaque lens is displaced from the axis of vision, but still left in the eye and not removed, as is the custom in Europe at the present day, is the only one resorted to by Persian surgeons.").

[227] Mostowfi, *Sharh*, vol. 1, p. 529.

[228] Neligan, "Public Health," part III, p. 742 (Although cataract was not extracted, but rather pushed down, Neligan explicitly used the word 'extract,' reason why I have also used it).

medicine and sprinkles the eyelids and in a few seconds he is up and another down.

Next is a lady with granulated eyelids. The doctor will put the lid between two round sticks of her own make also, and will roll them over and over until the desired effect is produced. Again, you will see a lady with inverted lids. The doctor will take hold of a portion of the loose skin of the lid and ties a section, 1-6 to 1-8 of an inch, between two sticks; the part becomes withered, and in a few days the shortness of the lid is produced.[229]

Dr. Collins described the same cure for "the exceedingly common affection, namely, a turning in of the margin of the eyelids, so that the eyelashes rubbed against and irritated the eye," which he qualified as "mechanically ingenious, though not very effectual." The operation was also carried out by an old lady, who "had enclosed a fold of the skin of the lid between two pieces of wood, each the size of half a Lucifer match, which were bound tightly together. Each end of the pieces of wood were then connected by strings to a band passing round the patient's head in front of her ears; in this way the lid was drawn away from the eyes, but, needless to say, the patient found the remedy worse than the disease."[230]

Mashadi Zabar Khanom was not the only female eye doctor, but one of many. A very well-known female colleague was *Khanom* Dr. Kahhal, the publisher of the weekly periodical *Danesh*, whose main target audience was women. Dr. Kahhal continued to practice her profession right in her editorial office.[231]

Persian doctors operated without anesthesia. Dr. Collins was astonished at the "considerable fortitude and patience" of Persian patients. He used in most cases cocaine as a local anesthetic. When this was not possible he used chloroform, without having the trouble of the British doctor in Bushire, who had almost been killed because of this. Where patients drew the line, however, was the removal of an eye, even when not removing it was painful or unsightly. Even when they ran the risk of losing the sight to the other eye, patients adamantly refused to have the sick eye removed.[232] As I will discuss later in the section of surgery, Persian patients, generally, refused any kind of amputation.

---

[229] Sargis, "Persia and Her Doctors," p. 584 (this author claims 100,000 inhabitants for Urumiyeh, which is contradicted by other sources such as Aubin, *La Perse*, p. 66).
[230] Collins, *In the Kingdom*, pp. 169-70. E`temad al-Saltaneh apparently also underwent this or a similar treatment, because he mentions that "Mirza Zeyn al-`Abedin Khan, who is healing my eye, came. He put briefly a lancet into my eyelid." E`temad al-Saltaneh, *Ruznameh*, p. 794.
[231] *Shekufeh beh enzemam-e Danesh. Nakhostin nashriyehha-ye zanan-e Iran* (Tehran: Ketabkhaneh-ye Melli, 1377/1998). (advertisement in nr. 2, September 29, 1910 as well in some later issues).
[232] Collins, *In the Kingdom*, p. 170.

TRADITIONAL HEALERS

In 1925, Tehran had "a doctor for every thousand inhabitants. There are, on the other hand, country districts, hundreds of square miles in extent, where there are no doctors at all."[1] But even if a village had access to a Persian doctor, "few can afford to consult him."[2] Those who could afford the money sometimes traveled hundreds of miles distance to seek professional medical help. Many died en route and were buried by the wayside.[3] Because most of the population had no access whatsoever to physicians, they had to fall back on persons, generally old men and women, who because of their experience had more knowledge about medical matters than ordinary people. As a result, "the number of irregular practitioners is legion."[4] These practitioners consisted of female healers, midwives, barbers, bonesetters, and surgeons.

Female healers
Mainly old women, called *mama* or *qabeleh*, dealt with childbirth and with diseases of young children. Women either delivered, while squatting, without assistance, or with the help of traditional midwives. According to Dr. Wills, in urban areas, "Midwifery is in the hands of the Jewesses and old women."[5] These midwives "make internal examinations and introduce strange substances to hasten labour."[6] According to Dr. Lichtwardt these strange substances were "some harmless decoctions of carrot-seeds, sage-tea, or bitter-sweets."[7] However, among the nomadic population "There are no *sages femmes*. Every woman is supposed to be able to help her neighbour in her hour of need. Maternity is easy. The mother is often at work the day after the birth of her child, and in less than a week regains her usual strength."[8] After birth, "The umbilicus of children, here, too, as in Western Persia, is tied at birth in two or three places with a common string, and the remainder cut with a pair of scissors or a knife. A midwife, called *daya*, is requested to perform this operation."[9] Because of the 'magicking' involved with childbirth, in

---

[1] Neligan, "Public Health," part III, p. 742; Häntzsche, "Specialstatistik," p. 442; Saad, *Sechzehn Jahre*, p. 182.
[2] Rice, *Persian Women*, p. 62.
[3] Sargis, "Persia and Her Doctors," p. 588.
[4] Neligan, "Public Health," part III, p. 742; Häntzsche, J.C. "Specialstatistik von Persien," *Zeitschrift der Gesellschaft für Erdkunde zu Berlin* 1869, p. 442; Amir Hoseyni, Karim Nikzad. *Shenakht-e Sarzamin-e Char Mahall* (Isfahan, 1357/1979), p. 38; Ts., "Persidskie Doktora," p. 157.
[5] Wills, *Persia*, p. 89; Polak, *Persien*, vol. 1, pp. 219-20; vol. 2, p. 205; Häntzsche, "Physikalisch-medicinische Skizze," p. 561 ("there are midwives in name only"). The Jewish midwives, called *mama*, while aiding the delivery would utter Persian or Persian/Hebrew prayers, see Loeb, *Outcaste*, p. 220; Saad, *Sechzehn Jahre*, p. 188; Safari, *Ardabil*, vol. 3, p. 480 (*mama*; after the Russian revolution two trained midwives settled in Ardabil); Lichtwardt, "Western Medicine," p. 237 ("enthusiastic but ignorant mid-wives.').
[6] Neligan, "Public Health," part III, p. 742.
[7] Lichtwardt, "Ancient Medicine," p. 83.
[8] Bird, *Journeys*, vol. 2, p. 75; Lichtwardt, "Ancient Medicine," p. 83 gives a less optimistic view on childbirth in Persia.
[9] Landor, *Across*, vol. 2, p. 182.

particular towards the end of the pregnancy and the first 40 days after birth, the midwives were believed to have magical powers.[10]

According to Dr. Neligan, "Every woman is an authority on medicine and uses remedies such castor oil, cassia, manna, infusions of violets and decoctions of various herbs, and opium."[11] Women, mostly midwives, were the primary health care givers for the majority of the rural and urban population, in particular of women and children. These women not only treated children's diseases, but also those of adults, in particular women. The latter, as was discussed above, had no access to male doctors. The female healers also treated *salek*, also called 'date boils,' which were a nuisance and because of possible disfigurement people wanted to be rid of them. Mrs. Bishop reported that, "Various remedies, including cauterization, have been tried, but without success."[12] One of these remedies was *Anacardii longifolii semen* or the cashew nut (*balador*). It was a caustic used by Persian matrons against the *salek*. They heated the nut with a candle by concentrating towards its point the acid oil it contains. "This causes quite an intense cauterization, which I cannot recommend, [commented Schlimmer] because even a light superficial cauterization has no effect whatsoever. Moreover, the penetration of this oil into the ulceration sometimes causes excessive deformed and hideous scars."[13]

There were even women who specialized in certain diseases, such a class of female healers in Jolfa, the Armenian suburb of Isfahan, who were known as *makhmalu'i*s, i.e., healers of scarlet fever, in which illness they specialized,[14] while others specialized in the treatment of syphilis.[15] Brugsch further remarked that it was odd that many women in Persia were exclusively engaged in the treatment of eye-disease, "which often have positive results, European doctors assured us."[16] Basir al-Molk also used such female eye specialists, one of whom he referred to as Mirza's wife, to treat his son's eyes.[17]

For the nomadic population access to medical care was even more difficult. They had, therefore, developed their own 'health-care system,' which in the case of the Bakhtiyaris was composed of experienced old women, who often carried out this hereditary function. Isabelle Bird, the intrepid British traveler, characterized the situation as follows:

> I have often wondered that the Moslem contempt for women does not prevent
> even the highest chiefs from seeking a woman's medical help, but their own
> *Hakims* of whom there are a few, though I have never seen any, are mostly
> women, and the profession is hereditary. The men, they say, are too unsettled to

---

[10] On the role of women as healer and witch in pre-industrial society, see Heiler, *Erscheinungsformen*, p. 412.

[11] Neligan, "Public Health," part III, p. 742; Ts., "Persidskie Doktora," pp. 157-58.

[12] Bird, *Journeys*, vol. 1, p. 39. For other Persian remedies see Jozani, *La beauté*, pp. 184-85.

[13] Schlimmer, *Terminologie*, p. 37; also Ibid., pp. 12 (q.v. acetas cupri or *zengar*), 117 (q.v. caustiques). *Zengar* or verdigris was used just like copper sulfate as a caustic for the *salek* or Baghdad boil.

[14] Schlimmer, *Terminologie*, p. 503 (q.v. scarlatine).

[15] Neligan, "Public Health," part III, p. 742.

[16] Brugsch, *Reise*, vol. 2, p. 17.

[17] Basir al-Molk, *Ruznameh*, pp. 211, 285 (*zan-e mirza*).

be *Hakims*. Some of these women are renowned for their skill as bullet extractors. If a father happens to have any medical knowledge he communicates it to his daughter rather than to his son. Aziz's grandmother learned medicine from a native Indian doctor in Fars, and his mother had a repute as a bullet extractor. A woman extracted the three bullets by which he had been wounded. The 'fees' are very high, but depend entirely on the cure. A poor man pays for the extraction of a bullet and the cure of the wound from fifteen to twenty *tumans* (from £5 to £6:10s.), a rich man from forty to sixty. In all cases they only give medicine so long as they think there is hope of recovery, and have no knowledge of any treatment which can alleviate the sufferings of the dying. When death seems inevitable they stuff the nose with a paste made of aromatic herbs.[18]

Dr. Ross reported that the Bakhtiyaris Bibis, i.e., the head wives of the Bakthiyari chiefs were great doctors, who treated their own families and their villagers and dependants. Around 1910, they had French medicine chests with all kind of European drugs.

> They weigh and measure out powders most accurately and I must say seldom make any mistake as to the therapeutic properties of the drugs employed. It proves rather embarrassing to the doctor sometimes, when everything he suggests has been tried. "Sore eyes! I have used boracic lotion, zinc lotion, yellow ointment, etc. etc. Have you nothing fresh to suggest?" "I have a headache. I have taken phnacetin, caffeine, antipyrin, calomel, quinine; I want something new."[19]

John Malcolm and most of the rest of his mission suffered from snow blindness in 1800. Although he knew with time the effect would pass, he was delighted when the wife of the chief of a nomadic group he was staying was told him that she knew a speedy remedy. When he agreed to the remedy, "a large vessel, full of snow, was put before me, and I was desired to place my face near it: a red hot stone was then thrown into the vessel, and the sudden dissolution of the snow caused a very great perspiration, which was increased by a cloack being pulled at the same moment over my head. This remedy, (which was administered twice,) though very disagreeable, proved efficacious, and my sight was completely restored."[20] John Malcolm reported another folk remedy in Kurdistan in 1810, where the tribe concerned, according to its chief, had but one remedy, "a purgative, in which the chief ingredient was the fat of a sheep's tail. 'This was boiled,' he said, 'and given, sometimes in small, and at others in large doses. It answered very well,' he added, 'in all complaints; and it saves us a great deal of trouble, and the expense of doctors.'"[21]

Isabella Bird also related the case of the Bakhtiyari khan's son, who suffered from various things. "He had been sewn up in raw sheepskins, his ears had been filled with fresh clotted blood, and he had been compelled to drink blood while warm, taken from behind the ear of a mare, and also water which had washed off a verse of the Koran from

---

[18] Bird, *Journeys*, vol. 2, p. 74. Even in the twentieth century, medical care continued to be practice by old women, see Roney Jr., "The Occurrence of Trephining," p. 491.
[19] Ross, *A Lady Doctor*, pp. 94-95.
[20] Malcolm, *The History*, vol. 2, p. 533, note *
[21] Malcolm, *The History*, vol. 2, pp. 533-34, note *

the inside of the bowl. It transpired that the Khan, who is a devout Moslem and a *mollah*, could not allow his son to take my medicine unless a piece of paper with a verse of the Koran upon it were soaked in the decoction."[22] Given the fact that the boy was sewed in sheepskins he may have suffered from pneumonia, for a remedy for it "is to wrap the sick person up in a raw hide."[23] Percy Sykes reported that the sewing up of a patient in a sheepskin freshly flayed from the body of the animal was in high repute, in general, and not only among the Bakhtiyaris.[24]

Gun wounds were very common in rural areas, in particular where nomadic groups operated. These needed to be taken care of, because "necrosis and caries are very common troubles following accident of gunshot."[25] It is interesting to note that the Bakhtiyari method to treat gun wounds was different from that of the Baluchis. According to Schlimmer, who spent some time in Baluchistan:

> Surgeons in Baluchistan and the Gamsir in case of gunshot wounds rarely attempt to extract the bullet. They prefer to pour every six hours virgin honey (which has been liquefied over a fire or in the sun) into the wound during the first seven days and to position the body part in such a way that the honey be maintained as best as possible. After the seventh day, the position is reversed, to favor the ejection of the foreign element. Also from the very beginning, if the condition of the wounded person allowed it, they surround him from top to bottom, until very close to the wound, with a more or less compressive bandage, but not too tight. For they believe that this would prevent the pus to make its way by fistulous paths. The wounded observed absolute rest and I have witnessed that an entire nomadic tribe pitched their armed and entrenched camp around a wounded chief, rather than oblige him to be transported over a great distance.[26]

The Bakhtiyaris treatment of wounds was indeed different from that of the Baluchis. "They dress wounds with an astringent paste made from a very small gall-nut found on one species of oak."[27] In general, and especially in compound fractures and bullet wounds, according to Cochran, "water is considered dangerous, the pus being simply wiped off daily. In the earlier course of the trouble, a fresh warm skin of a kid tied over the part is considered the best treatment, as is proven by the profuse and malodorous pus which "it extracts from the seat of the trouble.'!"[28] According to Ella Sykes, probably referring to the practice in Kerman, "if anyone was badly burnt the wounds would be smeared with soot from the bottom of the cooking vessels, and pomegranate juice would be taken internally.[29]

---

[22] Bird, *Journeys*, vol. 2, p. 7.
[23] Sykes, *Persia and its People*, p. 337; Saad, *Sechzehn Jahre*, p. 186.
[24] Wills, *Persia*, pp. 90-91.
[25] Cochran, "Letter," p. 85.
[26] Schlimmer, *Terminologie*, p. 210, note 1.
[27] Bird, *Journeys*, vol. 2, p. 74. For a discussion of the treatment of the various kinds of wounds see Jozani, *La beauté*, pp.170-74.
[28] Cochran, "Treatment," pp. 105-06. According to Rice, *Mary Bird*, p. 111, "a wound may be filled with peas to keep it open."
[29] Sykes, *Persia and its People*, p. 337; Ibid., *Through Persia*, pp. 111-112. According to Rice,

BARBER

The barber (*salmani, dallak*) enjoyed "the monopoly of dentistry, shampooing, phlebotomy, and the actual cautery; he also cups and performs the operation of circumcision, and often is a bone-setter, while he generally pretends to a special knowledge of diseases of the eye."[30] Phlebotomy (*rak zadan, fasad*) also included dry cupping (*badkesh*), scarification (*hejamat-e ferangi*), and the application of leeches (*zalu* or *`alaq*). The barber also took care of the pulling of teeth and shampooing which included taking care of patrons in the bathhouse as masseur, shaving of head hair and trimmer beards and mustachios, and applying henna and indigo (*rang*).[31] Finally, depending on market conditions, the barber also practiced as bonesetter and surgeon. In short, the barber was a hands-on healer.

There were two kinds of barbers: (i) those that had a fixed shop with a large array of accessories, and (ii) those who had a small handbag with their basic necessaries and were ambulatory and did their work in the streets, shops, and coffeehouses. You could easily recognize these ambulatory barbers by their implements.[32] Some barbers had no regular shop, but nevertheless had a kind of fixed location. In Tehran during the first decade of the nineteenth century, for example, at the Meydan, in front of the principal royal palace, in the form of a parallelogram, "a small rivulet crosses the square in its whole length, and the public barbers have established themselves on its borders. Here it is that they shave the heads of passengers, bleed, and perform operations; for they are the only surgeons in this country."[33] Others just operated wherever clients asked them to, which usually was right in the street.

Mary Bird, p. 111, "for a burn, the ashes of a piece of calico dyed with indigo, or an ointment composed of pomegranate juice, white of egg, and gunpowder, are applied on a piece of rag, or brown paper, which need not be clean."

[30] Wills, *Persia*, p. 90; Neligan, "Public Health," part III, p. 742. Old women also did cupping, for the female clientele, Lichtwardt, "Western Medicine," p. 237. Ther barber also dealt with other disorders such as venereal diseases, see Shahri, *Tarikh*, vol. 2, pp. 696-97.

[31] Polak, *Persien*, vol. 2, p. 203; Shahri, Ja`far. *Tarikh-e ejtema`i -Tehran dar qarn-e sizdahom*, 6 vols. (Tehran: Farhang-Rasa, 1368/1989), vol. 2, pp. 684-716; Landor, *Across*, vol. 1, p. 309; Benjamin, S.G.W. "Farm Life and Irrigation in Persia," *The Cosmopolitan* 9/June (1890), pp. 139; Schlimmer, *Terminologie*, pp. 315, 495.

[32] Shahri, *Tarikh*, vol. 2, pp. 708-11, 717-20 (pictures); Polak, *Persien*, vol. 1, p. 201; vol. 2, p. 203.

[33] Tancoigne, J. M. *A Narrative of a Journey into Persia* (London: William Wright, 1820), p. 99. In Kermanshah, barbers operated in the *meydan-e `allaf*, according to Soltani, *Joghrafiya*, vol. 1, p. 534.

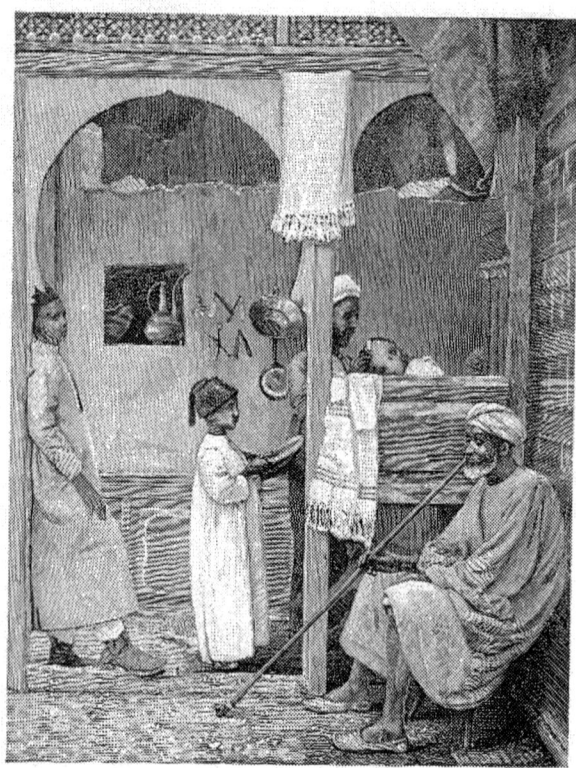

Figure 9: A village barber.

Barbers catering to the needs of the wealthy elite were, of course, a category apart. This held in particular for the royal barber. "Their skill in shaving the heads and trimming the beards of kings and nobles, though highly prized, is subordinate to that which they display as attendants at the warm bath. It is on their superior address in rubbing, pinching, joint-cracking, and cleansing the human frame at the hummums that their fame in established." Fath `Ali Shah's barber had made so much money that he had built a splendid villa not far from the royal bath. Just like Shah `Abbas I's barber had built the Pol-e Dallak, or the main bridge on the road from Tehran to Qom.[34]

Prior to the Russian conquest of Eastern Armenia (Erevan khanate) in 1828, there were 64 barbers in Erevan itself (50 Moslems, 14 Armenians) and 78 barbers in the so-called *mahall*s (16 Moslem, 62 Armenians).[35] According to Höltzer, there were 25 barbers (*dallak*) in Isfahan around 1890, and 6 in Jolfa. However, there were many more, because Höltzer did not count those working in the 72 bathhouses of Isfahan. Around 1920, there were 50 master barbers (*salmani*) in Isfahan.[36] In Qazvin, in the Meydan-e Gosfand quarter,

---

[34] Anonymous, *Sketches*, vol. 2, pp. 72-73.
[35] Bournoutian, *Eastern Armenia*, pp. 204-05.
[36] Höltzer, *Persien*, pp. 23, 82; Tahvildar, *Joghrafiya*, p. 121; Janab, *Ketab*, p. 78.

there were 31 barbers (*salmani*) unequally divided over the seven neighborhoods.[37] In 1925, in Tehran, there were 232 barber (*salmani*) shops, employing 224 masters, 122 workers (*kargar*), and 106 boys (*padu*), as shown in table 4.[38] Barbers, according to one source, were even obliged to have one apprentice, if they had no son, to ensure that his trade would be continued.[39]

From Table 4 it is clear why there was a need for ambulatory barbers. For apart from a difference in cost, the new city quarters had very few barbers shops compared with the older ones. Shahr-e Now and Sharq, for example, were relatively under serviced. This situation was the market niche for the itinerant barbers, who made their service more accessible to their clients, both in geographic and income terms.

Table 4: Number and distribution of barbershops and staff over Tehran city quarters (1922)

Name quarter	# Shops	# Masters	# Workers	# Helpers
Ark	23	19	20	14
Dowlatabad	43	40	26	14
Hasanabad	26	26	11	14
Sangalaj	24	38	17	21
Qanatabad	14	15	5	5
Mohammadiyeh	13	15	5	9
Sharq	6	6	1	3
Bazaar	38	38	29	16
`Owdlajan	26	26	7	9
Shahr-e Now	1	1	1	1
Total	232	224	122	106

Source: Baladiyeh, pp. 74-75.

Barbers were not only an urban phenomenon. Because of the need for a regular haircut and the medical services provided by barbers they were also found in all the larger villages. The Persian village barber, according to Benjamin, was "only next to the mollah and the ketkhoda [village chief] in importance, and doubtless in his own opinion, the biggest man in the village is the barber. Well does he know his value as the fulcrum around which everything turns in his little world." [He was] "a personage of the first rural magnitude, and his shop, whether in a wayside booth or under a spreading chenar [plane-tree] in the heart of the village, naturally becomes a sort of resort or club where idlers meet and the gossip of the neighborhood is discussed with all the gravity of which your village bumpkin is capable."[40] In the villages, barbers usually also had other economic interests. For example, Mostowfi reported that in his family's village, Nayeh, Rahman, the village barber, also kept some heads of cattle.[41]

---

[37] Sadvandian, "The Inhabitants of Meydan-Gusfand," p. 52. (two quarters with 9 barbers, three with one, one with 6, and one with no barber at all).

[38] See also Sheikh-Reza'i and Azari, *Gozareshha-ye Nazmiyeh*, Index q.v. *Salmani*. As to the requirements for an apprentice see Shahri, *Tarikh*, vol. 2, pp. 712-13.

[39] Anonymous, "Ärtze und Arzneiwissenschaft," p. 97.

[40] Benjamin, "Farm Life," pp. 138-39; Lichtwardt, "Ancient Medicine," p. 82.

[41] Mostowfi, *Sharh*, vol. 1, p. 529. For the payment of barbers in the village context see Lambton, *Landlord*, pp. 346-48. See also Money, *Journal*, p. 76.

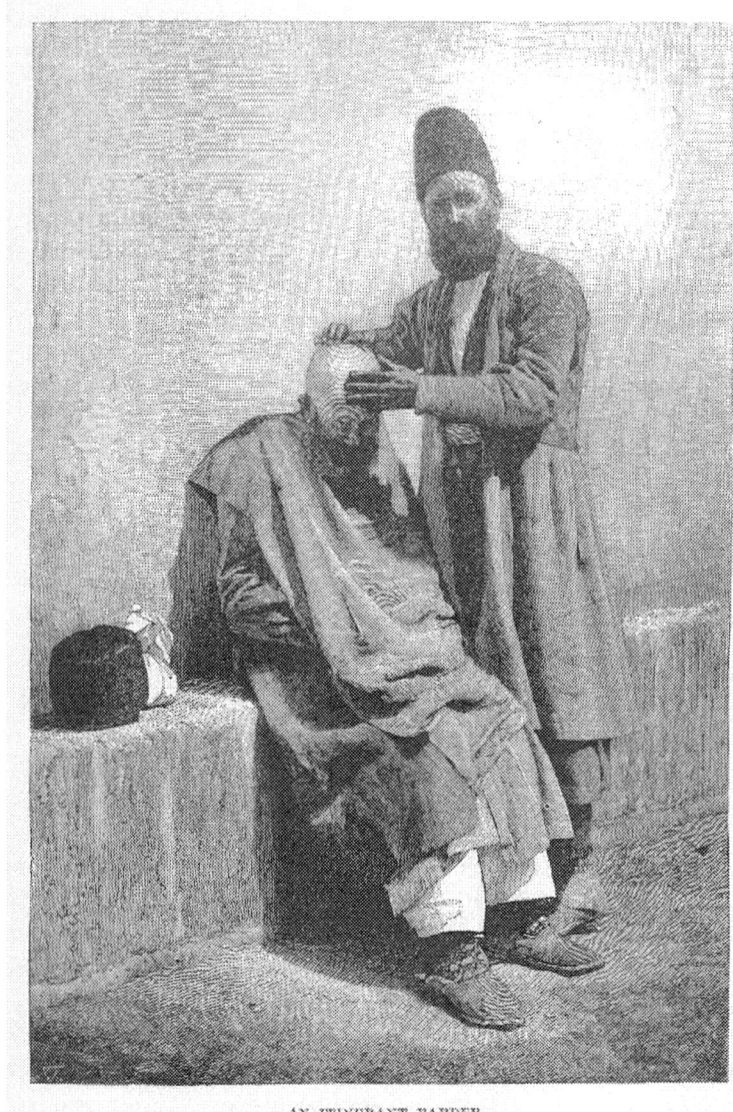

Figure 10: An itinerant barber.

Those barbers who had fixed shops were to be found both in the main bazaar as well as in the smaller bazaar in the city quarters. There also were such shops in the small towns and larger villagers. They were small, like other shops in the bazaar. They were swept and garnished, and very clean. It basically was small square room, one side open to the street, with whitewashed walls and a brick floor. Later in the twentieth century they had a wooden door with small square glass pieces. "Up to some five feet along the walls is nailed a cloth, usually red, against which the customers rest their heads while being shaved." […] "In the centre was a tiny bed of common flowers sunk in the floor some two feet square; from the middle of this rose an octagonal stone column some yard high, the capital of which formed a receptacle for the water in which the barber dipped his hand ever and anon, as he shaved his customers."[42]

Hung upon the walls, or placed in the *taqcheh*s or recesses, were the various instruments of the barber's art. Scissors (*meqraz*) of all sizes, razors, the fleams and lancets (*tigh*) for bleeding, the hand-mirrors, square and circular, "the *one* pair of huge pincers with which all the teeth are extracted, the small clamp and knife used for certain operations on the youthful male Persians [circumcision]; the branding-irons used for the actual cautery- favourite remedy in Persia- a variety of well-made native wooden combs, [preferably] of ebony- absolutely no brushes, these being unused by Persians." Further, copper mirror-frames (*a'ineh-ye qab*) of 60 x 90 that were hanging from a rope or hook. Some barbers even had a number of glasses with flowers in their shop. Finally, there usually was a small carpet for the more opulent customers. The barber himself was properly equipped to deal with his clients. "From his girdle, a yard or two of white calico, hung the round copper water-bottle, the needful utensil of the peripatetic barber in a country where water is scarce; also his strap on which he sharpens his razors; and a small leathern pouch, which holds a handy stock of implements of his trade. In his bosom is a small mirror, the presentation of which to his customer is the sign that his functions are completed. On his head the tall shub-kolah (or night-cap)." An apprentice or two shaved the heads of villagers unworthy of the master's skills, usually at the street side. They also looked after the water pipe for the important customers.[43] Towards the end of the Qajar dynasty the barber was already becoming modernized. His necessaries included a narrow painted table of about one meter in length and height. He further had a soapbox, a shaving brush (*fercheh*) and other items, all of which had not been used traditionally, but now had become part and parcel of his trade. There also was a wooden chair for clients to sit on, rather than on the floor, that was a bit higher than normal chairs.[44]

BLEEDING

"Our barber also acts as venesector,"[45] although there also were women (*abji*) specialized in this art.[46] In fact, "nearly every village has its official bleeder, usually a toothless, wrinkled old woman, who possesses as instruments only an old rusty knife and the hollow horn of a goat or a cow."[47] Purging (*tanqiyeh kardan*) and bleeding were the almost universal start of medical treatment.[48] However, it was "not only in sickness bleeding and leeching [are] practiced in Persia, but it is also the custom, as a supposed

---

[42] Wills, *Persia*, p. 131; Shahri, *Tarikh*, vol. 2, pp. 684f.; Landor, *Across*, vol. 1, p. 309. For an illustration of a village barbershop see Benjamin, "Farm Life," p. 142.
[43] Wills, *Persia*, pp. 133-36; Landor, *Across*, vol. 1, p. 309.
[44] Shahri, *Tarikh*, vol. 2, pp. 684-85.
[45] Benjamin, "Farm Life," pp. 139; Wills, *Persia*, p. 129. According to Saad, *Sechzehn Jahre*, p. 185, some barbers used a sharp flint rather than a knife. Phlebotomy also was done under the tongue.
[46] N.N. "Esfand Mah va Abji Kuchek," *Ettela`at-e Mahaneh* 107 (Bahman 1335/1956), pp. 34-35 (these women also pierced earlobes and made tattoos or *khal kubidan*).
[47] Lichtwardt, "Ancient Medicine," p. 83.
[48] De Windt, *A Ride*, p. 178 ("purging and bleeding are the two remedies most resorted to by the native hakim."); Anonymous, "Ärtze und Arzneiwissenschaft," p. 97.

preventive of ill-health in a warm climate, for every one to be bled at least once a month; the horses are also lanced during the warm season every four or five weeks."[49]

There were three techniques of bloodletting: (i) phlebotomy or venesection (*rag zadan, fasd kardan*); (ii) cupping (*hejamat kardan*); and (iii) leeching (*zalu andakhtan, ersal-e `alaq*). In case of phlebotomy, "the patient squatted on the ground and a small hole was dug in the earth beside him. The operator put a ligature around his arm, massaged the desired vein, and finally plunged in the tip of the lancet. The filling of the hole in the ground showed when enough blood had been let. When this moment arrived or when the patient fainted, the barber took a little soil, rubbed it on the vein, and applied some strands of cotton, and to keep them in place tied up the arm with the patient's own handkerchief."[50] The lancet that the barber used was long as a poniard, but, according Drouville, the barber expertly opened the vein without ever maiming the patient.[51] Although Elgood reported that bleeding was usually done in a garden or courtyard, and that it was forbidden to do so in public, phlebotomy was often just done in the streets and the blood was dropped wherever the patient was sitting. The British visitor Rees related with some surprise, "Apropos of bleeding, it is very odd to see four or five men squatting contentedly by a barber's shop, each holding one forearm, from which the blood drips, over the gutter. I don't think the operation is so much resorted to in the villages. At any rate it only came under my notice in big towns."[52] The barber was an equal opportunity venesector, for both "male and female, were bled into the gutter."[53]

Cupping was often done when phlebotomy was contra-indicated. In that case the use of wet or dry cups was preferred, which removed the rarified rather than the more viscid blood. In case of wet cupping, known as *hejamat-e ferangi*, the cupper made several parallel incisions or scratches in the dry skin, without any preliminary cleansing, with a bad razor until blood flowed, and then the cup (the large end of a cow or sheep's horn or horn-shaped glass), which had a hole in the tip of the horn, was placed over the wound. The barber or the old woman, who performed the cupping, then sucked vigorously at the small end of the horn to create a vacuum, so that the horns filled with blood rapidly. The horn was emptied on the ground, "more sucking, more blood, and the treatment is continued until the patient falls over in a faint from weakness." An attached piece of leather allowed the cupper to close the hole in the horn after removing the cup. Usually one to three horns of blood were taken. Usually the blood was taken from between the shoulders. The wound did not heal normally by suppuration. All Persians kept the scar for the rest of their life, as a kind of mark of nationality, which looked like welts from the lash. In case of small children the

---

[49] Benjamin, "Farm Life," pp. 139; Wills, *Persia*, p. 129; Shahri, *Tarikh*, vol. 2, p. 689-93 (with picture); Lichtwardt, "Ancient Medicine," p. 83. According to Dieulafoy, *La Perse*, p. 121, even babies of three days old were bled to rid them of their mother's bad blood. See also, Willem Floor, "Bloodletting," *Encyclopedia Iranica*, vol. IV, pp. 315-16.
[50] Elgood, *Medical History*, p. 300; Polak, *Persien*, vol. 2, p. 238.
[51] Drouville, Gaspard. *Voyage en Perse pendant les années 1812 et 1813*. 2 vols. (Paris, 1819 [reprint Tehran: Imp. Org. f. Social Services, 1976], vol. 2, p. 165.
[52] Rees, J.D. *Notes of a Journey from Kasveen to Hamadan across the Karaghan Country* (Madras, 1885), p. 3; Elgood, *Medical History*, p. 300.
[53] Landor, *Across*, vol. 1, p. 309; Wishard, *Twenty Years*, p. 211 ("usually in front of their door").

monthly bleeding was replaced by scarification between the shoulders, one time at least each spring.[54] According to Polak, in the nineteenth century dry cupping (*hejamat-e badi* or *kuzeh*) was mainly done. The cup was applied to the unbroken skin (*badkesh kardan*) and was not meant to draw blood. Paste was spread on the infected part of the body; a burning candle or piece of cotton was used to heat the cups; a jar (*kuzeh*) with a mouth of three to four inches wide was then placed over that area. The resulting vacuum, due to cooling caused the skin under the jar to swell and burst. The discomfort was supposed to reduce pain in another place.[55] The barber did not only do bleeding in his shop, or in the street, but often people went to the bathhouse to have it done. Basir al-Molk did so, he reported that "the phlebotomist (*hajjam*) came for the cupping; I took five horns (*shakh*) of blood."[56]

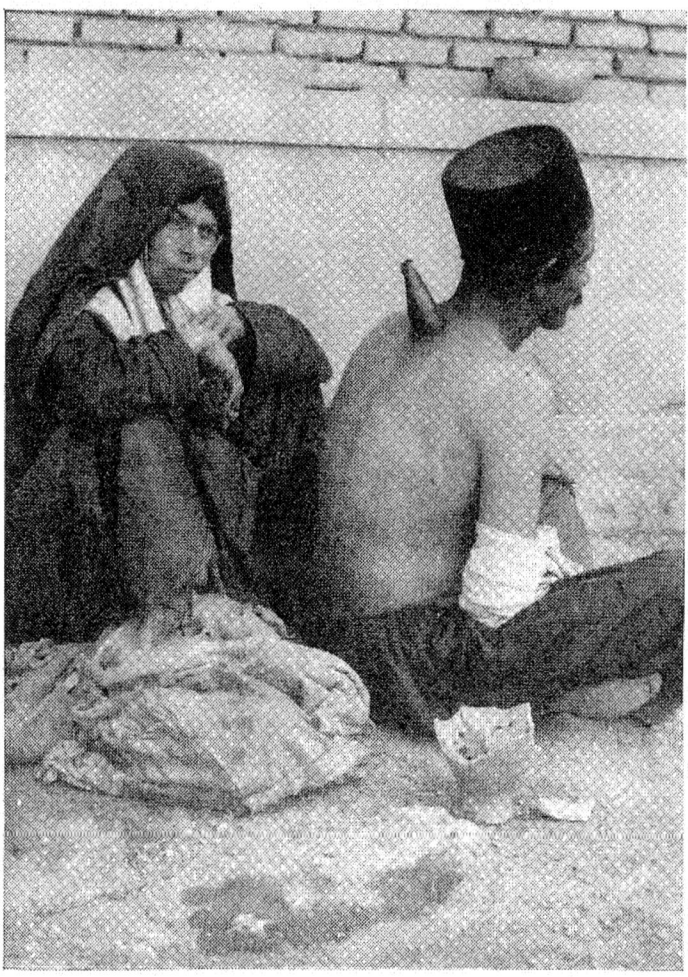

Figure 11: Cupping in the street.

---

[54] Schlimmer, *Terminologie*, pp. 495, 549; Elgood, *Medical History*, p. 300 (the best time for cupping is the middle of the month, when the humours are in a state of agitation, and when the moonlight is increasing); Lichtwadt, "Western Medicine," p. 237; Ibid., "Ancient Medicine," p. 83.
[55] Floor, "Bloodletting," p. 316; Polak, *Persien*, vol. 2, pp. 239-40.
[56] Basir al-Molk, *Ruznameh*, p. 379.

The third method was leeching in which leeches were allowed to suck blood. They were applied on or near to the alleged diseased spot. For example, in case of eye sore they were placed on the temples. The leeches were mainly procured from the Caspian Sea littoral and the Lake Urumiyeh region. There was also export of leeches to Europe. In Tehran, there were hawkers (*zalu-forush*) who cried their leeches in the streets and found a ready market for them.[57]

As a result of the national habit to have oneself bled without any objective medical need, every month, or at least at the change of each season, or at least once a year, and that before March 20, anemia or *qellet-e dom* was quite widespread in Persia. It was believed this would renew the old blood. Among young women the sedentary lifestyle predisposed them to plethora. To re-establish equilibrium they had themselves cupped once or twice a month by leeches on the thighs. This diluted their remaining blood too much. Their courses became quite voluminous and that further weakened them. Schlimmer prescribed with success quinine peel, cod-liver oil or stearine.[58] "Even the lepers, barely existing on their allowance of thirty cents a month, will spend a cent or two each spring and fall to have their unclean blood sucked out!"[59]

Bleeding was thus more of a problem than a remedy. Everyone had him or herself bled without the intervention of a physician or without objective need, just because they believed they had too much blood. All kinds of unfortunate results were the outcome of this activity. Often Persians were preferably bled once per month, and for reasons unknown, on Thursday afternoon. According to Schlimmer, the repeated bleeding resulted in early aging and three-fourth of the suppressed menstruations that he and his colleagues often observed in Persia.[60]

According to Arnold, the Persian physician had:

> a decided tendency to blood-letting, and a delight in strong medicines. In a morning's walk through the streets of Ispahan, we have often seen the snow blood-stained, as if slaughter had been done in these public places. Sometimes we saw, in passing, the actual operation, a patient extending his bare arm in the street for the barber's lancet. We inquired of several why they were thus bled?

---

[57] Shahri, *Tarikh*, vol. 6, pp. 170-75; Blau, Otto *Die commerzielle Zustände Persiens* (Wien: Decker, 1858), p. 76; Polak, *Persien*, vol. 2, p. 239; Lichtwardt, "Ancient Medicine," p. 82; Elgood, *Medical History*, p. 301. For pictures of leeching see Hasanbeygi, *Tehran-e Qadim*, p. 208. There also were many leeches near Kushkzar (at the border of Fars and Isfahan), but these probably were too big for medicinal purposes. Pirzadeh, *Safarnameh*, vol. 1, p. 20, described them to be as big as small snakes.

[58] Schlimmer, *Terminologie*, pp. 40 (q.v. anemie), 495 (q.v. saignée). How to prepare yourself for the annual bleeding is related by Polak, *Persien*, vol. 2, pp. 222-23, 238.

[59] Lichtwardt, "Ancient Medicine," p. 83.

[60] Schlimmer, *Terminologie*, pp. 495, 549; Lichtwardt, "Ancient Medicine," p. 83 ("for the poor, anemic, under-nourished folks, who submit to it, it is often disastrous."); Elgood, *Medical History*, p. 300 (after the morning meal and movement of the bowels, but before noon); see also Ibn Qayyim, *Natutral Healing*, pp. 36-42.

One replied that he had a clod; another that he had a pain in the stomach; a third that his head ached, and so on. Perhaps it may be said without error, that such drastic treatment, whether purgative or phlebotomic, will remove, in ninety-nine cases out of a hundred, the particular sensation which led the patient to the doctor. It is not for us to assess the amount of subsequent injury or physical deterioration.[61]

If people did not have recourse to bleeding they had the option of cupping. The reasons for cupping were various and do not seem to have followed a certain objective logic or theory. According to Elgood, it was because cupping removed the rarified rather than the more viscid blood.[62] O'Donovan related that when he had a sprained ankle, "the hakim suggested a dozen leeches. To get out of the subject I agreed with him, but was not getting off that easy. "I presume you are an astronomer? I presume you can foretell a favourable conjunction for the application of the leeches, and drawing the blood of His Excellency?"[63] When Naser al-Din Shah said that, all of a sudden, he had had vertigo, his physicians recommended to put leeches on the box of his ear or on his belly. The shah took an omen (*estekhareh*) that indicated that putting the leeches on the belly was good. Because the shah was afraid of leeches he wanted to put them on E'temad al-Saltaneh, who demurred. Finally, Hajji Heydar put the leeches on the shah, where they were left for one hour.[64] Leeches were also used to alleviate a condition of general indisposition. Basir al-Molk did so a number of times. He usually applied about 10 leeches, one time explicitly on his face. He reported that two leeches cost five copper coins (*pul*).[65] After having applied leeches, people who could afford to usually went to the bathhouse to wash off the marks left by the leeches.[66]

Leeching, like all other operations carried out by the barber, also was done in the open air by the wayside.[67] "These leeches are kept in great jars in the shops of the barbers."[68] Leeches were in great demand and there was even export of Persian leeches to Europe.[69] But they were not available everywhere. The American journalist Weston reported that a peasant from Yazdekhvast had joined his caravan. The man was walking 180 miles and back, "to get some leeches for a rich and prominent citizen of his town who was desperately ill."[70]

---

[61] Arnold, *Through Persia*, p. 261.
[62] Elgood, *A Medical History*, p. 300.
[63] O'Donovan, *Merv Oasis*, vol. 1, p. 196.
[64] E'temad al-Saltaneh, *Ruznameh*, pp. 248, 922 (shah put on leeches again).
[65] Basir al-Molk, *Ruznameh*, pp. 421, 442.
[66] Basir al-Molk, *Ruznameh*, p. 368.
[67] For a picture see Weston, Harold F. "Persian Caravan Sketches," *National Geographic Magazine* 39/4 (1921), pp. 462. According to Drouville, *Voyage*, vol. 2, p. 165, the barber never did "enemas, leeching, visicatories, cautery, and no exterior applications, which often have such a powerful effect," which is contradicted by the facts as reported by other contemporary authors.
[68] Wishard, *Twenty Years*, p. 211.
[69] Blau, Otto *Die commerzielle Zustände Persiens* (Wien: Decker, 1858), p. 76.
[70] Weston, "Persian Caravan Sketches," pp. 465.

British doctors also sometimes recommended the application of leeches, as Arnold found out when he was ill.[71] To do so the services of a professional Persian leecher were retained. He "prescribed a hot bran mash to be used as a vapor-bath, and before applying the leeches, provided himself with a quantity of the tinder of burned linen, in which he placed the utmost faith for stopping undue bleeding from the leech bites. He did his work well; and came on three consecutive days to see how his work was progressing; and when asked to name his own remuneration, mentioned three krans."[72]

Insects were not always looked upon as a pest; in fact, they were sometimes considered to be medically beneficial. Rees related that when he was washing himself in the village in which he was staying, Persians saw him covered with bites and stings. He complained to them about the torment of bugs that the traveler was exposed to in Persia. His Persian hosts explained to him that he did not understand. "These insects are as good as daily bleeding. No man can be bled daily. Praise be to God who has devised this substitute."[73]

CIRCUMCISION

Only males were circumcised (*khotneh*; *sonnet*) in Qajar Persia, although among the Lurs apparently girls also were "circumcised." This took place during the first 40 days after birth (*chelleh*), often, in the second week. The barber was usually called to do the operation, which was a festive occasion. At that time the baby-boy also received his name.[74]

DENTISTRY

The Persian barber was not just a bleeder, a circumciser and a shampooer. "Besides bleeding and setting dislocated limbs, he is the village dentist. He uses no anaesthetics, his weapons of torture are of the simplest description; but if there are any aching teeth in the village, he is the man to extract them, and he does it vi et armis!"[75] Indeed, the barber was an expert at tooth extraction, although he often had to ask a bystander to help him by sitting on the patient's knees and keep him from moving and make the operation more painful.[76] Many people, including children, suffered from bad and rotten teeth.[77] Doctors

---

[71] Arnold, *Through Persia*, p. 260; Lichtwardt, "Ancient Medicine," p. 82 ("the modern doctor, who has never used or even seen a leech, would marvel at the splendid results achieced with it in certain cases.')
[72] Arnold, *Through Persia*, p. 262.
[73] Rees, *Notes of a Journey*, p. 3.
[74] Yonan, *Persian Women*, p. 25; Wills, *Persia*, p. 90; Shahri, *Tarikh*, vol. 2, pp. 695-96; Sheikh-Reza'i and Azari, *Gozareshha-ye Nazmiyeh*, Index q.v. *khotneh-suran*, and *majles-e namgodhari* (*shab-e shesh*); Feilberg, *Les Papis*, p. 133 (the circumcision was done by so-called *luti*s, a gypsy tribe, who, under different names such as *qereshmal*, performed similar 'medical' functions elsewhere in Persia). For various customs associated with the circumcision ceremony see Massé, *Croyances*, vol. 1, pp. 51-53.
[75] Benjamin, "Farm Life," pp. 139; Hasanbeygi, *Tehran-e Qadim*, pp. 205-06. There were also other people, such as a molla, who was famous for both his tooth extraction as well as leeching skills. E`temad al-Saltaneh, *Ruznameh*, p. 663.
[76] Wills, *Persia*, p. 136; Soltani, *Joghrafiya*, vol. 1, p. 534; Hasanbeygi, *Tehran-e Qadim*, p. 205; Shahri, *Tarikh*, vol. 2, p. 694.
[77] Hasanbeygi, *Tehran-e Qadim*, p. 203.

treated gum disease; if a tooth had to be drawn they recommended a barber. When Mostowfi was staying at his farm at Savojbolagh around 1912, he had problems with his wisdom teeth. "Rahman, the village barber, came to see me with his forceps. I hesitated, but he convinced me that it was nothing. Wisdom teeth were weak ones with two roots, and indeed, in 30 seconds they were out."[78] Barbers pulled teeth with forceps and pincers (*kalbateyn*; *gazonbor*) made in Isfahan, and did not use any anesthetic. False teeth were not known in Persia.[79]

Here as in case of bodily illness, Persian took an omen to decide what to do. Malcolm related the case of "a woman with raging toothache got permission from the beads to send for a European lady to extract the tooth, but on taking the beads for the extraction after her arrival they were unfavourable, so arrangements were at once made for divining with the Quran at a mosque, which would of course overrule any result with the beads."[80] There were no modern dentists in Persia until Naser al-Din Shah brought a dentist back from Europe, but even the wealthy aristocracy did not avail themselves much of his services.[81]

---

[78] Mostowfi, *Sharh*, p. 529. For a photograph of a Persian barber extracting teeth photo, see Sykes, Ella. *Persia and its People* (London: MacMillan, 1910), p. 336. For the same photo see also Rosen, *Persien*, p. 149.
[79] Mostowfi, *Sharh*, vol. 1, p. 529.
[80] Malcolm, *Five Years*, p. 120.
[81] Mostowfi, *Sharh*, vol. 1, p. 529; E`temad al-Saltaneh, *Ruznameh*, p. 663.

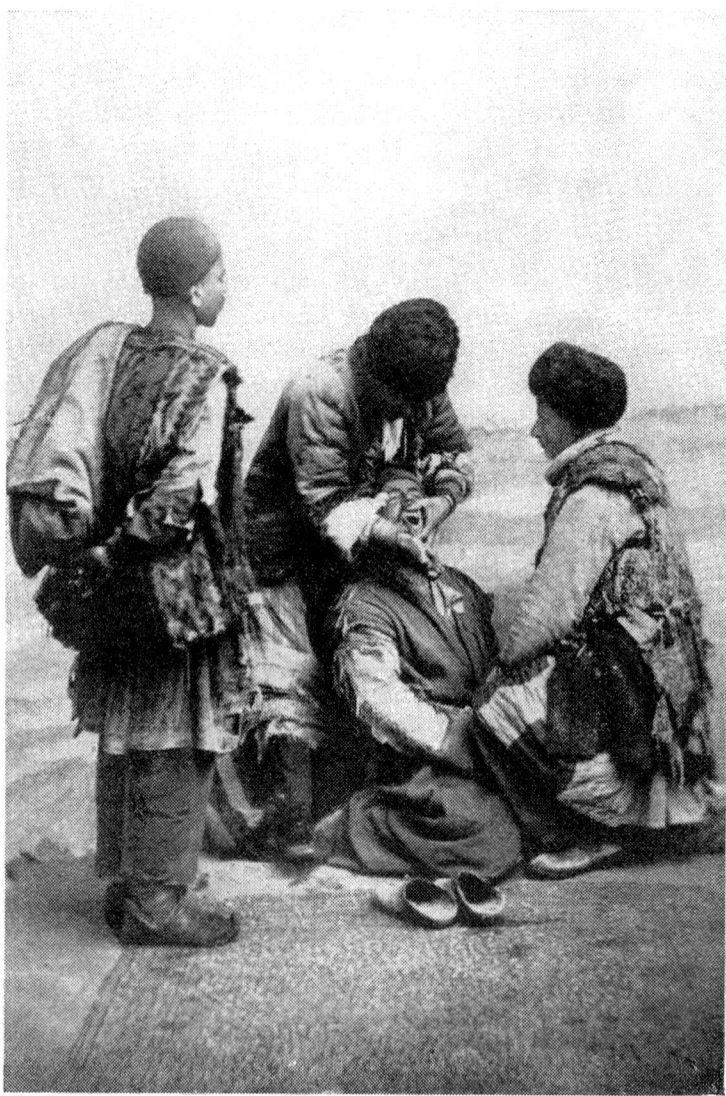

Figure 12: Street side teeth drawing.

HAIR CUTTING

"Consider for a moment that an ordinance of Mahometism commands all Mussulmans of the male sex to shave their heads, beginning the practice in boyhood. A man may be able to shave his face, but the crown of the head can only be razored by a barber. A Persian village, therefore, can no more exist without its barber than without its mollah or ketkhoda. While it is true that in the chief cities a few of the prominent dignitaries are now venturing to leave the hair on their heads like Europeans, yet this innovation has not yet reached the lower-classes nor the people in the rural districts, who are invariably the last to break away from the strict observance of religious ordinances. Every male in our village must therefore come under the hands of the barber several times a month. He knows them all, their foibles, their weaknesses, their peculiarities, the secrets of their lives, which, with his insinuating palaver, he well understands how to draw from them."[82]

"Shaving is a serious matter in Persia. To get shaved does not merely mean to get rid of superfluous beard: it signifies among the Persians to shave the entire scalp in most cases. Among the young, often a kharkul or tuft is left in the centre of the top of the scalp; this little patch of hair has probably never known the razor, and is often a foot or even two in length; it is carefully tied in a knot, and hidden from view by the wearer's skull-cap of white embroidered linen. Mahommedans think that it has a use, for after death the Prophet by it will draw up the true believer into paradise. As a rule, too, among the younger men, the whole temporal bone is left covered with hair, and this hair is allowed to grow long, and forms the zulf, or love-lock, which the boys and beaux of Persia allow to hang down behind each ear. But the rest of the scalp is shaven certainly once a week."[83] ... "The lower orders generally have the hair over the temporal bone long, and this is brought in two long locks, turning backwards behind the ear; the are termed 'Zulf;' the beaux and youths are constantly twisting and combining them. The rest of the head is shaven. Long hair, however, is going out of fashion in Persia, and the more civilized affect the cropped hair worn by Europeans, and even have a parting in it. The chin is never shaved, save by 'beauty men,' or 'Kashangs,' though often clipped, while the moustache is usually left long. At forty, a man generally lets his beard grow its full length, and cherishes it very much; part of Persian's religious exercises is the combing of his beard."[84]

"The middle-aged, on the contrary, generally shave the entire scalp, and allow the beard to grow long. Beards in Persia are generally worn long, and often attain a portentous growth." "To pluck a man by the beard is the greatest insult that can be offered. It is dyed black or red, by means of henna or indigo, or both." The cheaper clients were served on an earthen platform outside the shop.[85] A de luxe treatment was to have one's hair washed "with the clay of Shiraz, so celebrated throughout the east, and afterwards to trim it, much in the severe style in use among our regimental and ship's barbers."[86]

Persian barbers used no soap. They had a bowl of water at their side, and regularly dipped a finger in the bowl with which they would wet the client's chin or face, his skull and neck, which were all clean shaved. They further held the client's nose when going under the chin and the Adam's apple. Their short razor was stuck in a straight wooden handle, and was

---

[82] Benjamin, "Farm Life" pp. 139. On the importance of the treatment of hair, moustache and eyebrow, how they should look like, related disorders and treatments see Jozani, *La beauté*, pp. 111-31; Shahri, *Tarikh*, vol. 2, pp. 697-99 (head), 702-04 (hair and lock), 714-16 (moustache).
[83] Wills, *Persia*, pp. 131-32.
[84] Wills, *In the Land*, pp. 321, 323 (regarding women's faces); Landor, *Across*, vol. 1, pp. 309-10; Buckingham, J.S. *Travels in Assyria, Media and Persia* (London, 1829 [Westmead: Gregg Int., 1971]), p. 108. In addition to the hair-pulling device, "Persians say that this custom of shaving the head is out of compliment to Ali, who was bald and who dyed his long beard." Sykes, *Persia and its People*, p. 73.
[85] Wills, *Persia*, p. 132.
[86] Wills, *Persia*, p. 127.

stropped on the barber's arm, or occasionally leg, and was quite sharp.[87] The male lip, however, was always covered. "All men cultivate a moustache, a hairless upper lip being looked upon as effeminate, and at about thirty a short clipped beard is grown, which after the age of forty is never cut."[88]

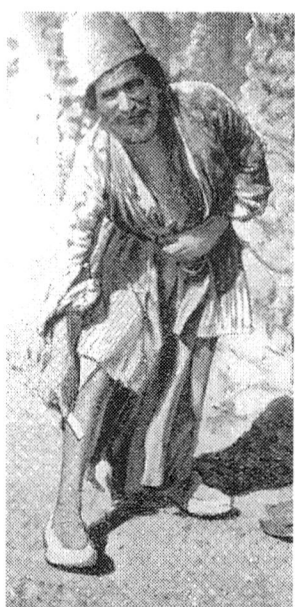

Figure 13: Village barber stropping a razor on his leg.

"The hair is dyed a glossy blue-black with indigo and henna, and the nails and finger-tips of the middle classes are tinted with the juice of the latter plant."[89] To that end the Persians used a very fine powder made from dried indigo (*rang*). They let it absorb water till it required the consistency of a paste. Before applying it the barbers washed your hair with soapy water to rid it of fatty substances. Then they washed the hair to get rid of the soap. Then the paste was applied to the hair so that none remained uncovered. Afterwards, you would be massaged for one to two hours. The paste was then removed with warm water and a fine comb. If this was done for the first time the process had to be repeated two days later. At first, the hairs looked a bit green, but later acquired a perfect black gloss. It then had to be renewed six weeks later. It was even better to first apply henna, which dyes the hairs red, and then black dye (*rang*), because the black became darker.[90] If a person's hair was dark, henna was first put on, which turned the hair red. When dry it was washed off, indigo was substituted, and a jet black was produced. "As my hair was light, the indigo only was used."[91]

---

[87] Wills, *Persia*, pp. 128; Landor, *Across*, vol. 1, pp. 309-10.
[88] Sykes, *Persia and its People*, p. 73.
[89] Sykes, *Persia and its People*, p. 72-73.
[90] Drouville, Gaspard. *Voyage en Perse pendant les années 1812 et 1813*. 2 vols. (Paris, 1819 [reprint Tehran: Imp. Org. f. Social Services, 1976), vol. 1, pp. 43-44.
[91] Keppel, George. *Personal Narrative of a Journey from India to England*. 2 vols. (London: Henry Colburn, 1827), vol. 2, pp. 128, 146 ("the eyelids of the king, stained with surmeh.")

The barbershop also served as an exchange of gossip, and consequently, the barber knew all the scandal of the town. In his shop also the water pipe was served.[92] "While the individual fees are small, yet this steady demand keeps the barber and his chagird, or apprentice, busy a good part of the time and makes him one of the most substantial members of our village."[93]

BONESETTER
"Most accidents are caused by fire-arms, by falls from horses, or trees or roofs, by burns."[94] Such persons were in need of the bonesetter or the surgeon, if family intervention had not produced the desired result. This type of work was usually also taken care of by the barber, but also often by healers specialized in this art. In Ardabil such bonesetters were known as *senekhchi* and they were known for their ability.[95] For the barber did more than cupping, bleeding, extracting teeth and cutting hair, in his shop. He also reduced dislocations and fractures, and took care of 'ricked' necks. The barber that Wills employed for his shave and haircut "had 'nafas' [breath of soul] and inherited it from his father."[96] According to Neligan, bonesetters (*shekasteh-band*; *jabbar*) were mainly "butchers, who adjust displaced bones and produce disastrous effects in the case of fracture," while Lichtwardt opined that they "made up in power what they lacked in science," and "ignorant of anatomy or physiology, and knowing even less of asepsis, are in a position to do much good, or much harm, to their patient."[97] Dr. Carr recounted the case of a woman who had broken her arm above the elbow and went to the bonesetter for treatment. He "took money from her and tied up her arm. This he did with such success that the circulation in the arm was stopped. The unfortunate woman, suffering much pain, went again to the bone-setter, who after a few days took off the splints, only to find that the fingers had mortified. Seeing what he had done, he thought the best he could do was to try to bring the fingers to life again. To accomplish this he applied some strong caustic remedies to the arm so effectually that the skin peeled off the whole arm from the fingers to the shoulder. He then proceeded to take more money, and apply remedies to cure the results of his last treatment. He applied some filthy black compound, and then, finding that his victim's slender stock of money was exhausted, he told her he could do no more, but was afraid she would die." She then went to the CMS hospital in Jolfa, where after a long treatment she recovered.[98]

Dr. Wills gave the following description the bonesetter's operations, which bears out the above characterization of the bonesetter's art.

---

[92] Landor, *Across*, vol. 1, p. 310; Wills, *Persia*, pp. 127-28.
[93] Benjamin, "Farm Life," p. 139.
[94] Rice, *Persian Women*, p. 259; Häntzsche, "Physikalisch-medicinische Skizze," p. 569.
[95] Safari, *Ardabil*, vol. 3, p. 485.
[96] Wills, *Persia*, pp. 129; Knanishu, *About Persia*, p. 186 ("When you have a blister on your tongue rub your hand upon the head of a first born child. That will cure the blister.").
[97] Neligan, "Public Health," part III, p. 743; Lichtwardt, "Western Medicine," p. 237; Ibid, "Ancient Medicine," p. 82; Polak, *Persien*, vol. 1, p. 201.
[98] Stileman, *The Subjects*, pp. 47-48; for similar cases see Malcolm, *Children*, p. 89; Rice, *Persian Women*, p. 254; Speer, *Hakim Sahib*, p. 282; Lichtwardt, "Ancient Medicine," p. 82.

> The bone-setter is in better repute than the surgeon, and enjoys considerable popularity. He always informs the patient that his limb is either fractured or dislocated; and even should the injury be merely a bruise or sprain, he wraps it up in bandages smeared with yolk of egg; or, should he have diagnosed a fracture, with bitumen (mum yai), which latter is supposed to possess almost miraculous properties; and he keeps the limb in a state of perfect rest so long as the patient will pay for his visits. The results of this are limbs of various degrees of shortness and curvature, ankyloses, etc.; but, by this mode of treatment, the bone-setter has the credit with the simple of working extraordinary cures, and I have been gravely shown supposed united fractures of the femur and humerus while compound fractures generally result in gangrene and death, though at time they are brought to what is considered a successful termination by the spontaneous separation by mortification of the distral extremity of the limb, leaving a useless stump.[99]

Stack confirmed Will's report on the use of egg yolk in bandaging limbs. "From various kinds of mint, elixirs (araq) are extracted; the large white anemone is beaten up with eggs and used to bind up broken bones."[100] The use of white of egg "actually may have kept germs out and protected the wound as collodion does."[101]

In this connection Pirzadeh's accident is also of interest, as it shows what happened in case of an accident. Also, that some surgeons were also called *hakim*, and probably were therefore of a higher professional standing than the barber-surgeon. Pirzadeh had wounded his shinbone en route to Bushire. He bandaged it with a kerchief till he arrived in the next halting place where a poultice of egg yolk was applied. When he finally arrived in Rishahr a surgeon (*jarrah*) was called named Hakim `Ali Mohammad. He prepared and applied a wax-cloth (*moshamma`*) on the wound, which reduced the pain. The next day, after Pirzadeh had taken a bath, the surgeon renewed the wax-cloth. He later had it treated again in the bathhouse of Bushire. When he arrived in Bandar `Abbas, Pirzadeh had the surgeon again attend to the wound. Six days later an English doctor looked at his leg. The latter applied an ointment consisting of oil and fat, which did not improve his condition at all. Then Pirzadeh asked the captain of the British vessel that took him to India for help. The ship's doctor took some oil that he rubbed on Pirzadeh's foot and then bandaged it; he kept it this way during two days. This was quite an improvement. After two days the bandage was removed, the foot was washed with soap, and once again the oil was applied and the foot bandaged, and the shinbone healed.[102]

Chirikov reported that Persians believed that if they had a piece of *mumiya* (bitumen) with them they would not fall off a horse; it would stop tooth pain and would counter any

---

[99] Wills, *Persia*, pp. 88-89; also A Friend of Iran, *"Dawdson," The Doctor. G.E. Dodson of Iran* (London: Highway Press, 1940), p. 6; Linton, *Persian Sketches*, p. 79.

[100] Stack, Edward. *Six Months in Persia*. 2 vols. (New York: G.P. Putnams, 1882), vol. 2, p. 58; Rice, *Persian Women*, p. 255; A Friend of Iran, *"Dawdson," The Doctor*, p. 2 ("much yolk of egg and saffron"); Polak, *Persien*, vol. 1, p. 201.

[101] Morton, *A Doctor's Holiday*, p. 214. If handled properly, the inside of the egss is sterile and if the egg yolk film on the wound was not touched and penetrated it would indeed provide some protection.

[102] Pirzadeh, *Safarnameh*, vol. 1, pp. 114-15.

disorder. They dissolved it in olive oil and would rub it over the broken or painful limb. It was sold for gold at a high price. Many kept it in a silver box, as if it were a person's eye. The best were kept in the shah's treasury.[103] But not only Persians had a strong belief in the healing properties of *mumiya*, so did de Bode, Chirikov's compatriot. De Bode wrote, "The author of these pages has himself experienced the efficacy of the Persian mumia, on applying it to a bruised side occasioned by a fall down some rocky cliff. A piece of the hard black substance of which it consists is mixed with melted sheep's fat, and, while hot, the bruised part of the body is well rubbed with it."[104] *Mumiya* also had other uses. The Bakhtiyaris, for example, ate it when they suffered from dyspeptic pains and 'bad blood.'[105]

Mumiya (*qir, zaft-e rumi*) was a kind of bitumen that was only found in small quantities at certain locations. It was exuded from the mountains at Behbahan, Darab, Jahrom and other localities in Fars province as well in certain locations near Shushtar and Dezful. Schlimmer had never been able to verify any of the claims of miraculous healing by mumiya despite his endeavors to do so. He further reported that the druggists were unable to tell what the qualities of real mumiya were so as to be able to distinguish it from fake mumiya. Schlimmer knew in fact a druggist who had grown rich by selling fake mumiya. In particular, the naphtha at Daleki was used to apply as an ointment for sores and bruises. Its healing properties were celebrated, and it was used widely, with great efficiency on man and beast.[106]

Despite the general negative opinion about Persian bonesetters, Dr. Lichtwardt commented that, "Some, with surprising intelligence, have, by observation and practice, developed quite a commendable technique in the reduction of simple fractures of the long bones, and we occasionally see healed fractures, the end results of which would be approved by the most critical surgeon."[107]

SURGEON

The surgeon (*jarrah*) was generally of the same as, if not lower in position than, the barber. In fact, it often was the barber or farrier who acted as surgeon.[108] Around 1800, Olivier described, in fact, the role of the barber when he wrote that Persian surgeons were engaged in bleeding, plastering wounds, cupping, applying moxa on hurting parts, cautery, reduce luxation, open an abscess. He wondered, however, how they could do all this

---

[103] Chirikov, *Siyahatnameh*, p. 101; Polak, *Persien*, vol. 1, p. 201-02.
[104] De Bode, *Travels*, vol. 1, p. 324. Babin and Houssay, "A Travers," p. 98 who were at the bitumen source at Jeyzun commented that it must have been of a very bad quality indeed, judging by the number of sick people that sought gratis medical care from them.
[105] Bird, *Journeys*, vol. 2, p. 74.
[106] Schlimmer, *Terminologie*, p. 62 (q.v. asphaltum); Ballantine, Henry. *Midnight Marches Through Persia* (Boston: Lee & Shepard, 1879), p. 78. On the use of naphtha for medical purposes see Floor, *The Traditional Crafts*, p. 145, n. 129; see also A. Dietrich, "Mumiya," *Encyclopedia of Islam²*.
[107] Lichtwardt, "Ancient Medicine," p. 82.
[108] Wills, *Persia*, p. 90; Polak, *Persien*, vol. 1, p. 199; Safari, *Ardabil*, vol. 3, p. 485 (there usually were one or two per quarter). In the Meydan-e Gosfand quarter of Qazvin there was only one *jarrah*. Sadvandian, "The Inhabitants, p. 51.

without having any knowledge of anatomy.[109] According to John Malcolm, "in cases of surgery the treatment is very rude," while according to Hume-Griffith, a British missionary doctor, "the Persian surgeon is a man to be avoided at all costs,"[110] and opinion shared by Dr. Wishard who qualified the barbers' methods as "most cruel, foul, and objectionable."[111] Drouville shared that opinion, because he considered surgery in Persia worse than anything. He wrote that "in most of Persia a few Jews practiced surgery, and they were as ignorant as they were miserable." Their knowledge consisted in the application of rancid unguents, the secret of which was passed from father to son. The unguent was a passe-partout for it was applied in case of an ulcer as well as a gunshot wound. Those unfortunate enough to be administered by them owed their healing to Mother Nature rather than the remedy, as he knew from his own experience. He had received a gun wound and the Jewish surgeon was the only help available. Drouville had lost much blood and he marveled that he had survived the cure of the rancid balsam. At first, he had gangrene that disappeared after two days due to applications of vinegar. "After three months of suffering the Jewish butcher declared him healed," but Drouville maintained that his own constitution and care had hauled him through. He firmly believed that if he had continued with the unguent that he would have died of gangrene.[112]

> These people do not know the abatement of fractures, and if somebody is so unlucky to have one, they let him just like that on his back, to the mercy of God, without stretching the broken limb that will in truth attach itself again, but remaining crooked and much shorter than the other. A limb that has been broken by a gunshot is practically always a mortal wound. These ignorant practitioners abandon those that have been wounded in this manner, and maintain that this accident is without remedy. At the end of the Oslanduz affair, about 50 unfortunate soldiers were in such a condition as well as a colonel, named Jaffer-Kouli-Khan, son of one of Persia's magnates. They were treated by Dr. Cornik [sic; Cormick], the meritorious English doctor. Because not a single one of them was maimed, his Persian colleagues became so furious, that they spread about that he had concluded a pact with the devil. However, this did not prevent the sick and wounded to come to him. His reputation even reached that of the Prince's [`Abbas Mirza] harem, where he was called each time whenever there was a real malady or an imaginary one such as migraine, vapors, hysteria, etc.[113]

---

[109] Olivier, *Voyage*, vol. 5, p. 112; Polak, *Persien*, vol. 1, p. 199. Moxa is a soft woolly mass prepared from the young leaves of *Artemisia Chinensis*, and used as a cautery by burning it on the skin; hence, any substance used in a like manner, as cotton impregnated with niter, amadou.

[110] Malcolm, *The History*, vol. 2, p. 534; Hume-Griffith, *Behind the Veil*, p. 160.

[111] Wishard, *Twenty Years*, p. 211; Saad, *Sechzehn Jahre*, p. 186 ("the barber's method of treatment is like that of our shepherds").

[112] Drouville, *Voyage*, vol. 2, pp. 165-66. It may be that Drouville was wrong. Saad, *Sechzehn Jahre*, p. 187 describes the case of a man with a deep wound that had been filled with donkey fat by a local healer. To Saad's surprise, who had told the man's relatives that this treatment would kill him, the man had healed rather well two weeks later. The balsam may have been a composition of "yolk of eggs, flour, and some other ingredients not quite so wholesome." Linton, *Persian Sketches*, p. 77 (by 1900 it was applied "with a piece of blue paper from a sugar bag" and "tied round with some old and very dirty rags.")

[113] Drouville, *Voyage*, vol. 2, p. 166-67.

There were also non-Jewish army surgeons such as Avakimeh, who was an Armenian surgeon and whom 'Abbas Mirza granted tax exemption (*mo'af va mosallam*) as a reward for his services to his troops.[114] Common Persians were not so negative either about their traditional surgeons, as Drouville was, and remembered them for their good deeds, even of treating fractures caused by gunshots.[115]

The barber-surgeon usually did not treat the moneyed class; the latter only needed him for bleeding.[116] A few female surgeons also performed minor non-invasive operations on women, and they enjoyed a good reputation.[117] There were also some surgeons, who occupied a more elevated status, such as the *jarrahbashi* in Zenjan, who was an army-surgeon, and the one who treated Pirzadeh's wound bore the title of *hakim* or doctor.[118] In 1869, there were four surgeons (*zakhm-band, jarrah*) in Tabriz.[119] Whether these were any better than the barber is not clear. Wishard related the visit he received from a Persian surgeon who had just been at the royal palace of Dushan Tepe. When he saw Wishard's operation room he said that all these instruments that he had seen there "were quite unnecessary, that when he wished to perform a surgical operation he did not need sterilizers, gowns, and assistants, but simply rolled up his sleeves, called to the prophets for aid, and before the spectators had realized what had been done, the operation was finished. 'Do the patients get well?' I asked. 'That rests with God,' was the fatalistic answer; 'my work is done when the operation is finished!'"[120]

Open wounds were not cleaned with cold water, but allowed to fester. Contact with water had to be avoided, reason why the patient was not allowed to drink water or sherbet during three days. The surgeons maintained that if the wound came into contact with water, then a serious skin infection (*erysipelas*) would occur (*zakhm sim mikashad*). Therefore puss in the wound would be cleaned with some cotton.[121] According to Dr. Malcom, "it is in surgery that one sees the Persian doctor as his worst." They would plaster a broken skull and a large wound with mud; "burns are smeared with sticky white of eggs covered over with leaves; it will take days of proper dressing to get the wounds clean" or the wounds were treated with camphorated oil that the patients would be so inflamed that s/he would cry all the time. They treated scalding with Indian ink.[122] The burns were mostly caused by children falling into fire placed under the *korsi* as well as by people upsetting lamps and

---

[114] Todua, Magali A. and Shams Esma'il K, *Tiflisskaia Kollektsia Persidskix Firmanov* 2 vols. (Tiflis, 1989), vol. 1, p. 348.
[115] Homayuni, *Molk-e 'Anbar-amiz*, pp. 92-93; Ghani, *Yaddashtha*, vol. 1, pp. 68-69, 192 (the famous Dr. Rajab 'Ali was an illiterate man, who had learned simple surgery on-the-job as an assistant to a Polish doctor, who had practiced in Sabzavar and Nishapur). This kind of on-the-job training also occurred in the case of mission hospitals, see, for example, A Friend of Iran, *"Dawdson" The Doctor*, pp. 34, 58.
[116] Wishard, *Twenty Years*, p. 211.
[117] Polak, *Persien*, vol. 1, p. 202.
[118] 'Eyn al-Saltaneh, *Ruznameh*, vol. 2, p. 1564; Pirzadeh, *Safarnameh*, vol. 1, p. 114.
[119] Javadi, *Tabriz*, p. 277.
[120] Wishard, *Twenty Years*, p. 210.
[121] Polak, *Persien*, vol. 1, p. 199.
[122] Malcolm, *Children*, pp. 88-89; Rice, *Persian Women*, p. 255.

pots with hot water.¹²³ "Wound, ulcers and open sores are dressed with green leaves some of which may have some definite therapeutic value." These leaves included those of mirabilis jalapa, of waterlilies, and of the marigold. "These various leaves are probably less harmful and surely much cleaner than the pieces of dirty paper which they often stick over their wounds, often the first piece of old paper they can pick up in the street, sometimes a carefully written paper. With the arrival of products of western civilization these too are used, and when a man came in with his ulcers covered with a thick black mass, and was asked what it was, he proudly replied 'mobiloil.'"¹²⁴

In Urumiyeh, doctor Harun was a well-known surgeon and physician. Every day, up to 300 people mobbed his house, so that many had to wait for days before he could see them, unless it was an emergency. "He has only three or four home-made knives, and uses no needles, does not make any difference how large the wound may be, not a stitch is taken, so all his wounds are healed by second intention (granulation). Now there comes a fellow with a large cut on his arm and suffering great pain. Doctor will tell him to go to the fountain and wash it clean, then he puts some medicine on it and then bandages it with a handkerchief, and tells him to call to-morrow. When next day he returns there may be pus formation, and as to treatment that will be the same. The result is, a large per cent die."¹²⁵

The fear of surgery on part of the patient, or his friends and relatives, and the ignorance of Persian doctors led to often unnecessary consequences.

> Jahangir Khan's leg had become severely infected and needed treatment. Dr. Tholozan, one of Naser al-Din Shah's personal physicians, had suggested that surgery be performed on the infected area. The women in the harem objected to this, and as a result the operation was cancelled. Instead, a traditional physician, Mirza Hasan was called, who claimed that he could cure the infection in a few days. Mirza Hasan used leeches to suck out the infected blood, but it was not long before the infection spread and the entire leg had to be amputated.¹²⁶

Generally speaking, surgery was accorded a low social ranking partly due to the inferior status of the surgeon, "and partly to the great objection that the Persian has to all operations which result in mutilation; for amputation of the arms, feet, or hands is the common punishment of theft, and the mutilated person is considered infamous. Hence it is rare that a Persian of the lower class will consent to them, while the upper ranks of society are, of course, less liable to require these operations."¹²⁷ Even if it would save their life most Persians refused amputation. The reason was that they could not appear

---

¹²³ Rice, *Persian Women*, p. 259.
¹²⁴ Lichtwardt, "Ancient Medicine," p. 84.
¹²⁵ Sargis, "Persia and Her Doctors," p. 585; Polak, *Persien*, vol. 1, p. 199. It does not seem likely that 300 patients mobbed the doctor's office every day. Assuming 200 working days per year that would mean 60,000 patients, or twice the number of inhabitants of Urumiyeh. It is more likely that the 300 people were an inflated number and were patients and accompanying family and that the number of patients was much lower.
¹²⁶ Hedayat, Mehdi Qoli Khan, *Khaterat va Khatarat* (Tehran: Zavvar, 1344/1965), p. 36; for another case of a botched tumor operation see Polak, *Persien*, vol. 2, p. 200.
¹²⁷ Wills, *Persia*, p. 88.

before Allah "short of limb, or in any other than complete state, it would incur his wrath and ridicule to such a degree that they would be refused admission to Paradise."[128]

The low esteem that surgeons were held in by Europeans was an understandable attitude, given the fact that "the surgeons are absolutely ignorant of anatomy, and the knife is scarcely used for anything but superficial abscesses. When some deep affection must be reached, as caries or necrosis of the bone, the part involved is denuded, gradually, by caustics."[129]

When amputation was done, no anesthesia was used. Chloroform or ether (*qiluruform* or *keloruform*) was unknown; its use was also dangerous, because relatives or friends of the patient might think that you had put the person to death, of which Wills gave a concrete example. "The medical officer to the Residency of Bushire having narrowly escaped a pistol-shot from a tribesman on seeing his relative apparently put to death by the unknown drug."[130] The operation itself was rather one that resembled that of a butcher shop. "The primitive methods observed in Europe before the invention of the ligature are in use. The limb is struck off by repeated blows of a mallet on a chopper or short sword, or, in case of a finger or toe, a razor, and then dipped into pitch or oil which is boiling. Lithotomy is frequently performed above the pubes, and is always fatal."[131] To make it possible for the patient to be whole again, the amputated limbs were given to the relatives for burial.[132]

Refusing amputation was often indeed a death penalty for the patient concerned. Hume-Griffith reported on a case of a man who came with a swelling of the leg that prevented him from straightening it. Hume-Griffith's diagnosis was that of a malignant cancer of the thighbone that needed amputation. The man refused, and later died because he went to a Persian surgeon, who said that, unlike the European doctor, he saw no problem in straightening the leg. The man's father and some other people held the man down, while others held his leg, "then seizing a huge slab of stone in both hands, he brought it down

---

[128] Forbes-Leith, *Checkmate* p. 92; Hume-Griffith, *Behind the Veil*, p. 142; A Friend of Iran, "*Dawdson,*" *The Doctor*, p. 2; Cochran, J.P. "Letter from Persia," *Medical Press of western New York* 2 (1887), p. 84 ("The Persian would sooner die than have his arm or leg amputated"). Cochran also details in this letter the conservative methods he applied to save the affected limbs. In some cases, however, amputation took place to save the patient, or toes, in case of frostbite. Ibid., p. 85 and Speer, *Hakim Sahib*, pp. 218, 282.

[129] Cochran, "Treatment ," pp. 105-06.

[130] Wills, *Persia*, p. 88. Its existence was known, however, because in 1854 an article appeared in Government of Iran, *Vaqaye`-ye Ettefaqiyeh*, vol. 2, pp. 1115 (nr. 173, 7 Sha`ban 1270/25 May, 1854), 1181 (8 Dhu'l-Qa`deh 1270/2 August, 1854), explaining its use and benefits. Invasive operation were dangerous, because patients were already on death's doorstep when they arrived, and the relatives often did not understand what was going on. Polak had to save himself by flight one day, after a hernia operation. Polak, "Medicinische Briefe," p. 175. Around 1870, the prince-governor of Shiraz initially refused to have his carbuncle on his back removed with the help of chloroform, see Waters, *Travel Reminiscences*, p. 23.

[131] Cochran, "Treatment," pp. 105-06 ("Median lithotomy is practiced some"); De Windt, *A Ride*, p. 178.

[132] Hume-Griffith, *Behind the Veil*, p. 142.

with all his force on the bent knee. The leg was straightened ... and needless to add, the poor patient only survived a few days."¹³³

According to Schlimmer, the Persian executioners who were accustomed to cut off limbs drenched the mutilated limb in boiling ricinus oil to stop hemorrhaging. Hemorrhaging or gangrene seldom occurred after these amputations (*boridan-e alat* or *qat`-e `ozv*), if the limb was not interfered with.¹³⁴ Sargis, who concurs with Schlimmer as to the method applied, adds that if hemorrhage was small, they "cover the part with either spider web or fine dust."¹³⁵ Forbes-Leith was less positive than Schlimmer, may be because he did not refer to simple amputations, while the number of more complicated operations also had increased by his time, which was some 50 years later. One of the problems in case of surgery that Forbes-Leith encountered was sepsis. This occurred because the family of the patient opened the bandages to see what had been done. He forbade it, and to be sure that his ban was respected he, in the case of his own patients, put a lead seal on the bandages. How unfortunate this family inquisitiveness could be was clear from as case in Hamadan after a successful operation of a double cataract. The patient's female relatives took off the bandages and opened the blinds of the room where the patient lay; the result was perpetual blindness.¹³⁶

Surgeons, male and female, also treated syphilis and other venereal diseases. They treated syphilis with inhalation, mercury fumigation, and mercury pills. The most common treatment was inhalation.¹³⁷

---

¹³³ Hume-Griffith, *Behind the Veil*, pp. 160-61.
¹³⁴ Schlimmer, *Terminologie*, pp. 35-36 (q.v. amputer).
¹³⁵ Sargis, "Persia and Her Doctors," p. 586 ("hemorrhage, if large, dip the part in boiling water or oil"). By 1920, criminals with amputated limbs were taken to the nearest mission hospital for treatment. Linton, *Persian Sketches*, p. 61.
¹³⁶ Forbes-Leith, *Checkmate*, pp. 92-93.
¹³⁷ Polak, J.E., "Ueber den Gebrauch des Quecksilbers in Persien," *Wiener Medizinische Wochenschrift* 10 (1860), pp. 566-67 with a detailed description of the prescriptions; Polak, *Persien*, vol. 2, p. 223-24.

THE PROGRESS OF MODERN MEDICINE

In the preceding pages I have shown that people in Qajar Persia suffered from a broad range of diseases against which the existing traditional medical infrastructure had little to offer in terms of effective treatments. The reasons for this enduring medical affliction of the population were the prevailing unsanitary and unhygienic public and private conditions in which people lived, behaved, and dressed. The other reason was that the prevailing medical systems that were available to the Persian population were not able to explain scientifically why disease occurred, and therefore also unable to recommend effective methods how to prevent it; and if you fell ill, in spite of preventive efforts, how to treat it. Theurgic folk medicine and prophetic medicine that both ascribed everything to divine and supernatural causes (both the illness and the treatment) Islamic-Galenic medicine that ascribed disease to system imbalance of the humors offered insufficient, let alone effective, explanation or treatment for the wide range of disease patterns. The arrival of modern Western medicine offered an alternative to the existing medical system, and one that increasingly proved to be more effective than the prevailing traditional Persian medical systems.

The introduction of modern, Western medicine started with the arrival of the French and British embassies during the first decade of the nineteenth century. The physicians who accompanied these embassies extended their services to the public in general and also tried to initiate a program of smallpox vaccination. One of them, Dr. John McNeil treated Fath `Ali Shah at several occasions, the first time, at the recommendation of one his favorite wives, Taj al-Dowleh, whom McNeil had treated with success in 1826. He continued to treat the shah and members of his harem in the years thereafter, even when he had become the British Minister in Tehran.[1] Modern medical assistance became somewhat more permanent with the appointment of Dr. John Cormick in 1812, or thereabouts, as the personal physician of `Abbas Mirza, the heir presumptive. In addition to treating his royal patron, Cormick also extended his services to the small European community, as well as those Persians who were interested. One of his main accomplishments was the authorship of a book on smallpox vaccination that was one of the first books printed in Qajar Persia. Another of his contributions was the introduction of Artemisia absinthium Linn. (*qurt-e udi*, *kharagush* in Gilak), or common wormwood, as a vermifuge, which afterwards was widely used. He is also credited to have introduced the use of calomel or mercurous chloride.[2] In addition to Dr. Cormick, there also were the physicians at the British Legation at Tehran, who treated the sick in Tehran.[3] Even if there were confidence in European medicine, which was not always the case, Persian patients and doctors often would refuse to follow a European doctor's advice if it was contrary to their hot-cold system. Dr. Jukes observed cases in which people died, because

---

[1] Elgood, *Medical History*, pp. 455-56. On McNeil's activities see Ebrahim-Nejad, "La médecine européenne," p. 73; Wright, *The English*, pp. 123-24.
[2] Schlimmer, *Terminologie*, p. 9; Polak, *Persien*, vol. 2, p. 221; Elgood, *Medical History*, p. 467 (Cormack died in November 1833, three weeks before `Abbas Mirza); Ebrahim-Nejad, "La médecine européenne," p. 74.
[3] Wilbraham, Richard. *Travels in the Transcaucasian Provinces of Russia* (London: John Murray, 1839), p. 69; Wright, *The English*, p. 124.

the Persian physician had decided that a disease (ulcerated sore throat) was a hot one. The patients were bled and received cooling remedies and many died. Likewise, in case of dysentery, a hot disease, Juke's proposed treatment (mercury) was also a hot one and thus not acceptable. The patients were treated with cooling draughts and ice, and several died.[4]

The reason that `Abbas Mirza, the heir presumptive, hired Dr. Cormick was that he wanted to promote the use of European medical knowledge with a view to maintain a healthy army. To that end he had sent five students to Great Britain for training. Two of them studied medicine. Hajji Baba Afshar obtained his medical degree and became later Mohammad Shah's personal physician. Mirza Ja`far Tabib, although he stayed longer in Great Britain than his fellow students to finish his studies did not do so. He was finally forced to return, but there is no information available on his later vicissitudes and employment.[5] `Abbas Mirza also ordered the translation of European medical textbooks. To overcome opposition to the introduction of modern Western medicine by the medical and religious profession, `Abbas Mirza commissioned the writing of a text that justified the European approach of medical practice, one that included surgery. This text further argued that Persian medicine was as valuable as European medicine.[6] Also, the Persian government, allowed the establishment of an American missionary mission in 1835 in Urumiyeh to work among the Nestorian Christians and provide them, amongst other things, with medical assistance.[7]

At first, Western medicine did not meet with much opposition. This was due to the fact that there were very few Western medical practitioners in Persia during the first half of the nineteenth century. Also, most of them either worked for the court (royal or princely), for a foreign diplomatic mission, or for an isolated minority group (Christians in Urumiyeh). Most Moslems had no contact with them, and the pious ones did not even want to have anything to do with them, because Christians could not heal Moslems, or so they believed. Only the desperate ones among the rural population afflicted with many diseases or alleged barrenness for which they had found no help, appealed for help and treatment on a regular basis to any European who passed by. Even the institutionalization of the appointment of a European doctor as one of the personal physicians to the shah hardly upset anybody. After all, the shah had always employed and consulted more than one physician, who were accustomed to compete with one another for the royal favor. One or two more, even if they were experienced and effective European doctors, did not

---

[4] Malcolm, *The History*, vol. 2, pp. 531-32, note; Ts., "Persidskie Doktora," p. 167. On Jukes activities see Ebrahim-Nejad, "La médecine européenne," pp. 72-73. Kurdish healers often prescribed to put the afflicted person on a fabric drenched in petroleum, according to Saad, *Sechzehn Jahre*, p. 187.

[5] Elgood, *Medical History*, pp. 465, 474; Ebrahimnejad, "La médecine européenne," pp. 74, 76; Wright, *The Persians*, pp. 71-73, 75, 77, 80-82 and plate 6 for Mirza Ja`far Tabib's portrait. Hajji Baba, who had been for nine years in England did not like it in Persia and wanted to return to England. "On returning to Persia he was attached to Abbas Mirza's person, but, seeing that fatal consequences would ensue from that Prince's folly and mode of living, left him, and followed his [eldest] son as physician." Money, Journal, pp. 191-92, 189.

[6] Ebrahimnejad, "La medicine," p. 70 (the text was by Mohammad b. `Abd al-Sabbar, *Jame` al-Hekmatayn va Majma` al-Tibbayn*).

[7] Perkins, *A Residence*, p. 134; Elgood, *Medical History*, pp. 533-35.

make that much of a difference. Persian physicians were able to hold their own against their colleagues and, in fact, tended to have more effective access to the royal ear and favor.

The example given by 'Abbas Mirza, *i.e.*, to employ a European physician, in addition to a number of Persian physicians, was followed by his son Mohammad Shah and other Qajar royalty, and became an established practiced thereafter. His brother and rival, Mohammad 'Ali Mirza, employed the French doctor Labat, while his other brother, Malek Hasan Mirza, employed doctor Bertoni, an Italian, as his personal physician. He also was Judge of the Christians (*Qadi al-Masihun*) in the prince's jurisdiction (Urumiyeh).[8] 'Abbas Mirza's son, Mohammad Shah, did not use a European personal physician until 1844, when he first employed William Cormick, the son of Dr. John Cormick.[9] The French Dr. Labat soon replaced the latter in that same year. His compatriot Dr. Cloquet succeeded him in 1846 and continued to serve Mohammad Shah's son, Naser al-Din Shah,[10] as personal physician or *hakim-e hozur*, which was the official designation for court physicians. After Cloquet's death in 1855, Dr. Jacob Polak succeeded him and, when he left Persia in 1860, was temporarily replaced by the Dutchman Dr. Johan Schlimmer. The Frenchman Dr. Barthelemey succeeded him in that same year, and was replaced by his compatriot Dr. Tholozan in 1864, who served in that function until 1893, with an absence of two years from 1889-91.[11] After Tholozan followed Dr. Schneider (1891-1907), Dr. Coppin (1907-10), and Dr. Georges (1910-11).[12]

Despite the employment of European physicians the shahs also continued to use a number of Persian physicians at court, one of whom was the chief royal court physician. The latter retained the title of *hakim-bashi*. The title of *hakim-bashi* was also conferred on the leading physician of each major provincial town, and later, due to the depreciation of the value of titles in general, to the leading physician of a city quarter. Also, in popular parlance, the title was conferred upon any well-known leading physician. To distinguish between the royal physician and the other doctors who also were known as *hakim-bashi*

---

[8] A.D. "Chronique," *Revue de l'Orient*, p. 112; Piemontese, Angelo Michele. "Gli Ufficiali Italini al servizio della Persia nel XIX secolo," in G. Borsa, P. Beonino Brocchieri, *Garibaldi, Mazzini et il Risorgimento nel resveglio dell'Asia et dell'Africa* (Milano: Franco Angeli, 1984), p. 103.

[9] On his further activities see Wright, *The English*, p. 124.

[10] Dr. Cloquet, who was paid 35,000 francs per year by Mohammad Shah, probably was asked to remain as personal physician because he had been able to cure the mother and sister of the later Naser al-Din Shah from cholera in 1846. Mohammad Shah out of recognition gave Cloquet a diamond studded medallion, see Dequevaullier, "Notice," pp. 5, 17, 23.

[11] Elgood, *Medical History*, pp. 488, 494-96 (Tholozan had arrived in Persia during the winter of 1858-59); Hassendorfer, Colonel. "Les médecins militaries français fondateurs et organisateurs de l'Enseignement Médical et de la Santé Publique en Iran," *Histoire de la médicine* 4/7 (1954), 58; Ekhtiar, Maryam Dorreh. *The Dar al-Funun: Educational Reform and Cultural Development in Qajar Iran* (thesis, New York University 1994), pp. 156, 159; Ghaffari, *Khaterat va Asnad*, p. 329; Najmabadi, Mahmud. "Hakim Shelimer Felamanki, *Rahnama-ye Ketab* 13 (1349/1970), pp. 574-80.

[12] Hassendorfer, "Les médecins," pp. 60-62.

the former was sometimes referred to as *hakim-bashi-ye koll*.¹³ The title *tabib-bashi* also occurs, although it is not clear whether it conferred a special responsibility on its holder. However, one text explicitly states that the Mirza Ebrahim Khan received the title of *hakim al-molk* and the presidency of all physicians in Persia, which seems to indicate that neither the *hakim-bashi* nor the *tabib-bashi* were chiefs of all physicians.¹⁴

The fact of employing physicians representing two different medical schools and traditions reflects the adherence of the Persian population in general to the traditional medical system. The rivalry between these representatives of two medical systems was more than just medical; it also, and more so, was about one's standing in society, power, influence, and 'face.' An event that E`temad al-Saltaneh noted in his Diary is telling in this connection. "Dickson, the physician of the English Legation, who is one of the world's devils, and the reason why the English are very hostile to me, had told Tholozan that 'So-and-So has written your name in the Government Yearbook (*Salnameh*) after that of Mirza Nasrollah.' Three days earlier when I was in Tholozan's house he had drawn my attention to this. I soothingly told him that he must have been mistaken, because he could not read Persian. European physicians were listed separately, like Persian physicians were written separately. This has been customary for 12 years. Yesterday, I gave him one copy of the Yearbook to prove my statement." Tholozan was and remained furious despite the explanation and even complained to the shah about this, who told E`temad al-Saltaneh to satisfy Tholozan. That did not happen for a number of weeks and E`temad al-Saltaneh and Tholozan who had been very close avoided one another for a long time until they made up.¹⁵ Tholozan also used his position of trust to obtain various concessions for himself and interested financial parties in France. Whereas everybody in Persia was upset about the 1872 Reuters concession, the concession that Naser al-Din Shah granted to Tholozan in 1875 very much resembled that of Reuter's without upsetting those who had protested against the Reuter's concession. The British government was the only one that protested and engineered its annulment.¹⁶ Tholozan was not the only doctor who wanted to enrich himself; he was only less adept at doing so. Much more successful was Hakim al-Molk, the Persian physician of Mozaffar al-Din Shah. The Russian diplomat Kalmykov recalled: "I had met in Tabriz, a Persian doctor, Hakim ol-Molk. He looked very humble and obsequious at that time. Upon the succession to the throne of Mozaffar ed-Din, Hakim ol-Molk followed the new shah to Tehran and soon accumulated a hundred thousand dollars in bribes and opposed the grand vizier Amin os-Soltan. I saw Hakim ol-Molk in Tehran, driving in state in a fine carriage and surrounded by mounted servants."¹⁷

---

¹³ Sheykh-Reza'i and Azari, *Gozareshha-ye Nazmiyeh*, Index q.v. *Hakim*; Sykes, *The Glory*, p. 103.
¹⁴ Nezam al-Saltaneh Mafi, *Khaterat va Asnad*, vol. 1, p. 278 (Mirza Abu'l-Qasem Khan Tabib-Bashi Soltan al-Hokama), vol. 2, p. 295.
¹⁵ E`temad al-Saltaneh, *Ruznameh*, pp. 388-89 (*shanbeh* 26), 403 (*yekshanbeh* 17), 437 (*sehshanbeh* 19).
¹⁶ Kazemzadeh, Firuz. *Russia and Britain in Persia 1864-1914* (New Haven: Yale UP, 1968), pp. 156-58. Tholozan was also involved in obtaining other concessions and schemes, see Nezam al-Saltaneh Mafi, *Khaterat va Asnad*, vol. 1, pp. 121,148, 170, 174.
¹⁷ Kalmykov, Andrew D. *Memoirs of a Russian Diplomat. Outposts of the Empire, 1893-1917* (New Haven, Yale UP, 1971), p. 80.

Treatment of the royal patient by these physicians of different disciplines was consecutive, concurrent, or sometimes even joint.[18] This was nothing new, because it also applied to Persian physicians. For example, in 1858, in case of the illness of Amir Qasem Mirza, Naser al-Din Shah's first heir-apparent, half a dozen Moslem and two Jewish doctors were called in. The British Minister Murray ascribed the six-year old child's death to the conflicting therapy recommended by these doctors. At the last moment, Polak also was asked to offer his views, which he did, albeit reluctantly. Apart from professional differences of opinion, the Jewish doctors had a close relationship with the shah's mother, while the main Moslem doctor was a confidant of the grand vizier, a political opponent of the shah's mother. Thus, their political affiliation may have influenced their professional opinion, and it certainly had great influence on the aftermath of the heir-apparent's death. The fall of the prime minister resulted in the arrest of 'his' physician.[19]

There was a daily medical royal audience. Dr. Feuvrier remarked that he had the impression that his service consisted mainly in being present at the Naser al-Din Shah's breakfast. For all the royal physicians would present themselves prior to the moment that the shah ate his breakfast, standing according to their rank, with the European doctor at their head. Other physicians present were: Feylosuf al-Dowleh, Loqman al-Molk, Malek al-Atebba, Fakhr al-Atebba, Sheikh al-Atebba, Hakim Shams al-Ma'ali and others. Sheikh al-Atebba was their spokesperson. When the shah had sat down to eat his breakfast he would stretch out his arm to the *hakim-bashi* who then respectfully would take the royal pulse and feel it. Then the others would follow and each in their turn, after having kissed the shah's hand, would feel his pulse. During breakfast the shah would ask one of the doctors what the characteristics were of the particular food item he then was eating. The doctor then replied by elaborating on the influence the food item had on the various parts of the body.[20]

This also shows that there was not just one European and one Persian royal physician. There were more, both of the European and Persian persuasion. Ebrahimnejad, therefore, makes too much of the French hold on the position of the shah's European personal physician. Naser al-Din Shah and his successors always used more than one physician, whether European or Persian. For example, Naser al-Din Shah also consulted Dr. Joseph Dickson, physician to the British Legation in Tehran (1848-1887), regularly. Naser al-Din Shah also asked Dr. Dickson to join him on his first European tour in 1873.

---

[18] Feuvrier, J.B. *Trois ans à la Cour de Perse*. (Paris: F. Juven, 1900), pp. 70-71; Ebrahim-Nejad, "La médecine européenne," p. 72; E'temad al-Saltaneh, *Ruznameh*, p. 389.

[19] Elgood, *Medical History*, p. 508; Amanat, Abbas. *Pivot of the Universe. Nasir al-Din Shah Qajar and the Iranian Monarchy, 1831-1896* (Berkeley: UCP, 1997), pp. 336-37; Polak, *Persien*, vol. 2, pp. 33-34.

[20] Mo'ayyer al-Mamalek, Dust'Ali. *Yaddashta'i az Zendegani-ye Khosusi-ye Naser al-Din Shah* (Tehran: 'Elmi, 1351/1972), p. 124; Polak, *Persien*, vol. 2, pp. 207-08 (the royal physicians also had to be present at official audiences and the royal hunt); Feuvrier, *Trois Ans*, pp. 55, for the shah's treatment by the four physicians (one European, three Persian) including the taking of his pulse and the prescription of different remedies, see pp. 66-80.

Similarly, Mozaffar al-Din Shah retained Dr. Hugh Adcock, who had been his personal physician when he was still heir-apparent in Tabriz, as consulting doctor-in-chief, in addition to his French and Persian personal physicians. Dr. Adcock also accompanied Mozaffar al-Din Shah on his visit to Great Britain in 1902.[21] Moreover, Mozaffar al-Din Shah also used the skills of the German Dr. Damsch, who has been credited to have kept the shah alive until the heir-apparent, Mohammad `Ali Mirza, arrived in Tehran and thus ensured his smooth succession to the throne.[22] Another British physician, Dr. Lennox Lindley, had been assistant court physician as of 1900 and continued to serve all future Qajar shahs, including Ahmad Shah.[23]

In short, a French physician may have been regularly appointed as *hakim-e hozur*, but it did not mean that he had an exclusive claim on who the shah consulted in medical matters. In fact, Nafisi related an interesting story about his father, Nazem al-Atebba, who had been called urgently to court during the night to treat Mozaffar al-Din Shah. When he had arrived there he found a number of young courtiers hovering near the shah. One of them, a recent medical graduate from Europe already had given the shah a drug, which Nazem al-Atebba found was too high a dosage that risked killing the shah. Due to his intervention the shah survived. This event clearly shows that nobody had the monopoly of medical access to the shah or his treatment.[24] Moreover, even if a French physician had optimal access it did not matter than much. Afzal al-Molk wrote in 1896 about Mirza Mohammad Khan Hakim-Bashi, the personal physician of Mozaffar al-Din Shah that, "expect for him, none of the other government doctors, be they European or Persian, had the place of trust and confidence in taking care of H.M. health and the blessed pulse was in his hands."[25] It was also for this reason that Dr. Schneider, who clearly resented the Persian doctors' influence with the shah, started to verify whether his colleagues had really studied medicine in France as they had claimed. Another reason was that British physicians scoffed at the very idea of medical training for Persians in France, where, they claimed, it was so easy to obtain a diploma.[26]

---

[21] Wright, *The English*, pp. 124-25; Ebrahimnejad, "Introduction," pp. 77-81; Nafisi, "Doktor `Ali Akbar Khan," pp. 58-59; Nezam al-Saltaneh Mafi, *Khaterat va Asnad*, vol. 1, p. 149. The same is also clear from the shah's Diary where not only Tholozan is mentioned, but so is Dickson and Begmez Hakim, a convert to Islam, who was Mo`tamed al-Haram, and thus may have had even more influence due to his contact with the harem inmates. Badi`i, Parviz ed. *Yaddashtha-ye Ruzaneh-ye Naser al-Din Shah (1300-13003 qamari)* (Tehran: Sazman-e Asnad-e Melli, 1378/1998), Index q.v. Begmez Hakim, Dikson Hakim, Tuluzan, Hakim (several), Sheykh al-Atebba, Fakhr al-Atebba. For the location of the Begmez's house see Sa`dvandiyan, Sirus and Ettehadiyeh (Nezam-Mafi), Mansureh. *Amar-e Dar al-Khelafeh* (Tehran: Nashr-e Tarikh, 1368/1989), p. 375.

[22] Litten, Wilhelm. *Persische Flitterwochen* (Berlin: Georg Stilke, 1925), p. 171.

[23] Wright, *The English*, p. 125.

[24] Nafisi, "Doktor `Ali Akbar Khan," pp. 59-60.

[25] Afzal al-Molk, Gholam Hoseyn. *Afzal al-Tavarikh*. ed. Mansureh Ettehadiyeh (Nezam-Mafi) and Sirus Sa`dvandiyan (Tehran: Tarikh-e Iran, 1361/1882), p. 56 (the shah did not deny him anything); Ghaffari, Mohammad `Ali. *Khaterat va Asnad-e Mohammad `Ali Ghaffari Na'eb-e Avval Pishkhedmat-Bashi*. eds. Mansureh Ettehadiyeh (Nezam-Mafi) and Sirus Sa`dvandiyan (Tehran: Tarikh-e Iran, 1361/1982), p. 172.

[26] Nategh, Homa. "Les Persans à Lyon," in Balaÿ, C. Kappler, C. and _. Vesel eds. *Pand-o Sokhan*

The physician who may have had more influence on the development of political and economic affairs in Persia than any other European physician was Dr. M. Y. Young. He was employed by the Anglo-Persian Oil Company (APOC), but also treated the Bakhtiyari khans and their families. The APOC used him to negotiate various matters with the Bakhtiyari khans and the sheikh of Mohammerah. Wilson credited him to have seen to it that there was no trouble in the oil fields in 1914, when there was no communications with the coast due to Arab insurgency fomented by the Ottomans.[27]

TEACHING OF MODERN WESTERN MEDICINE

Thus, it would seem that there was no opposition to the introduction of Western medicine into Persia through the presence of one or two European doctors at court or to the small number present in the country itself, or even to the printing of some outdated Western medical text books, but there was some opposition against its formal teaching in Persia.

Although there was a presence of a very small number of European and American physicians in Persia, there was as yet no formal training of Persians in modern Western medicine before 1850. Naser al-Din Shah had instructed his personal physician, Dr. Cloquet, to educate a number of Persians in European medicine. Amir Kabir, the grand vizier (1848-52), was convinced that Persia needed to be strong militarily and economically, and that an institution of higher learning within its own borders was key to achieve that objective. In 1851, with the establishment of the *Dar al-Fonun*, the teaching of modern Western medical science became a permanent and institutionalized fact in Persia. It was a major step forward in the propagation of modern Western medicine. For one of the subjects taught at the school was medicine.[28]

Initially the teachers at the *Dar al-Fonun* were Austrian. However, in the medical field the teachers were multi-national after 1860. The medical teaching staff began with the Austrian Jacob Polak and the Italian Fochetti, who together shared the teaching load during the first decade of the *Dar al-Fonun*'s existence. At the end of the 1850s, the Dutchman Johan Schlimmer joined them, while in the 1860s the Frenchman Joseph Tholozan (part-time) and in the 1880s the German Albo also joined the teaching staff.

(Paris-Tehran: IFRI, 1995), pp. 192-93. A review of all the dissertations written by Persian graduates at French universities until that time may or may not confirm the British derision. The sons of the Jewish doctor Rabbi Nahurai "spent six weeks in Paris, studying medicine as they told me, though the one was in bed nearly all the time, and his brother was overawed by the asphalt and the gas around him." Adler, *Jews in Many Lands*, p. 189.

[27] Wright, *The English*, pp. 126-27; Williamson, J.W. *In A Persian Oil Field. A Study in Scientific and Industrial Development* (London: Ernest Benn, 1927), p. 123.

[28] On the establishment of development of the *Dar al-Fonun* see Ekhtiar, *The Dar al-Funun*. Dr. Cloquet gave medical courses to familiarize courtiers with the principles of Western scientific medicine, see Government of Iran, *Vaqaye'-ye Ettefaqiyeh*, vol. 1, p. 277, nr. 52 (Rabi` al-Thani 1267/February 9, 1851). Already in 1845, Mirza Sadeq (not a student of Dr. Cloquet, as Wright wrongly has it) had been sent to Great Britain to study medicine, about whose later career in Persia nothing is known. Wright, *The Persians*, pp. 141-42

The European teachers realized that their Persian students lacked the necessary background (no knowledge of the basic sciences) and time (four years) to become fully trained physicians. According to Schlimmer, the objective of the training of students in medical science was therefore the following:

> To better understand the reasons which have made me always prefer with regards to my Oriental students, the narrative genre that combines that which is instructive with that which is amusing, I have to say that these students are too little accustomed to serious study and that the only requirement for their admission as medical students is the knowledge of the Persian language (read and write fluently) and of Arabic, sufficient to understand the derivations and the grammatical roots. In general, they have no preliminary idea of science at all, and may, with much effort on their part and of that of their teachers, become what were Health Officers in Europe at the beginning of the [nineteenth] century. Nevertheless, let's not despair. It would be impractical for the Persian government, with its limited means and the limited number of teachers of diverse nationalities that it found to be available at the moment of the creation of the School to dictate study plans such as are current in Europe. It was therefore necessary to be content and train practical Persian physicians, who would know to diagnose diseases in an encyclopedic manner based on pathognomic symptoms, which European science have established in an unequivocal manner, and to treat these maladies with remedies that have been accepted by the most famous professors. In all civilized countries one demands in addition that one makes the students recognize at the same time the different modifications that the nature of the country and the way of life of its inhabitants make necessary. As to surgeons, we require just enough knowledge of topographical anatomy that is required to be able to generally perform non-mortal [i.e., non-invasive] operations, dress wounds and the necessary routine capacities to be able to prepare themselves in the field the required drugs.[29]

Thus, the idea was to provide the students with a good basis of medical science that would allow them to deal with the most common diseases and to do simple surgery as well as to continue their studies abroad after graduation and then become a real physician. Polak, for example, gave his students training in anatomy, "a course which normally takes a year, in three months." He also took at least two of them to attend him when he did surgery, so that they might see surgical procedures up-close.[30] During the 1852, cholera epidemic in Tehran, Polak took three of his students with him when he made house calls.[31] Polak himself wrote that, "I would like to teach my students how to perform small operations. Then, they would be able to come with me to visit patients and assist me in important operations, and in this way they became familiar with how to stop bleeding and the treatment of other cases. After some time, I allowed them to perform small operations in my presence and later alone; even in case of some amputations I could let them work independently. One of my students, who presently resides in Tabriz,

---

[29] Schlimmer, *Terminologie*, pp. 228-29.
[30] Government of Iran, *Vaqaye`-ye Ettefaqiyeh*, vol. 1, p. 583 nr. 98 (5 Rabi` al-Avval/February 2, 1854).
[31] Government of Iran, *Vaqaye`-ye Ettefaqiyeh*, vol. 2, p. 997, nr. 157 (4 Jomadi al-Avval/February 2, 1852).

Mirza Abd-al Ali, has become famous in the field of surgery. On numerous occasions he performed lithotomies."[32] Polak himself also performed many lithotomies; according to his own count he performed the operations 158 times during his ten-year stay in Persia.[33]

Apart from acquainting the students of the *Dar al-Fonun* with Western medical science and its latest developments mainly through oral teaching, some of the professors also wrote textbooks for the school, most of which remained in manuscript form. Apart from the fact that there were no textbooks on modern Western medicine in Persian, the European professors realized the need for the creation of a body of medical knowledge in Persian to modernize Persian medical practice as well as to facilitate the transition from Islamic-Galenic to Western medical methods. Schlimmer wrote: "In the beginning of the teaching the absence of a scientific nomenclature in Persian was a great handicap."[34]

Polak and Schlimmer taught most of their classes in French, and also wrote their course materials in French, which were translated by students or translators working at the *Dar al-Fonun*.[35] Polak soon noticed, when he had picked up enough Persian to do so, that the interpreters translated what he said in Galenic terms and thus taught Islamic-Galenic medicine rather than Western medicine. He therefore realized that he had to learn Persian fast, and even 40 years later a Persian minister noted that Polak's Persian was pretty good.[36]

Between 1854-1875, four professors wrote most of the available books and manuscripts for use as teaching material at the *Dar al-Fonun*. The Dutchman Schlimmer wrote the largest number (14) of manuscripts on various subjects, such as pharmacology, pathology, ophthalmology, and pediatrics. The Austrian Polak wrote 10 manuscripts, mainly on anatomy, cholera, ophthalmology, surgery and internal medicine. The German Albo, who joined the *Dar al-Fonun* only in the 1888s, produced six manuscripts, mostly on surgery, physiology and general medicine, while the Frenchman Tholozan, contributed two manuscripts, one on smallpox vaccination and the other general medicine. In addition, there were Abu'l-Hasan Khan who wrote on therapeutics and 'Ali Ra'is al-Atebba on anatomy.[37] The Italian Fochetti taught chemistry, physics and

---

[32] Polak, *Persien*, vol. 1, pp. 305-06. The newspaper *Danesh* also highlighted a surgical operation done by a former student of the *Dar al-Fonun*, see, for example, Qasemi, *Danesh*, p. 20 (nr. 5, Shavval, 1299/16 August, 1882) reporting on the successful excision of a large tumor from a thigh of an old man at the request of the Imam Jom'eh of Qom.

[33] Polak, *Persien*, vol. 2, p. 318; see also E'temad al-Saltaneh, Mirza Hasan Khan. *Mer'at al-Boldan* 4 vols in 3. ed. 'Abd al-Hoseyn Nava'i and Mir Hashem Mohaddeth (Tehran: Daneshgah, 1368/1989), vol. 2, p. 1165, according to whom Polak performed 23 lithotomies in 1852-53 (20 males, three females) of which only one died.

[34] Schlimmer, *Terminologie*, p. 229.

[35] Government of Iran, *Vaqaye'-ye Ettefaqiyeh*, vol. 1, p. 997 (nr. 157, 4 Jomadi al-Avval/February 2, 1852); vol. 2, p. 1738 (nr. 271, 4 Sha'ban 1272/10 April, 1856).

[36] Polak, *Persien*, vol. 1, pp. 303-06.

[37] Arjah, *Ketabshenasi* (index); Elgood, *Medical History*, p. 502. Two of Schlimmer's texts were published. Shteglova, O.P. *Katalog Litografovannyx Knig na persidskom yazykev sobranii Leningradskovo otdelelniya instituta vostokovedeniya AN SSSR* 2 vols. (Moscow: Nauka, 1975), vol. 1, pp. 307-08 (*Ketab-e Serr al-Hekmeh* in 1862; *Ketab-e Zeynat al-Abdan* in 1862).

pharmacology at the *Dar al-Fonun*.³⁸ Some of these texts were printed by the *Dar al-Fonun* Press,³⁹ most remained, however, in manuscript form. The students were also encouraged to distribute their lecture notes on cholera among doctors and laymen alike to be used in the case of an outbreak of cholera.⁴⁰ Fochetti together with Polak introduced the use of ether as a general anesthetic in 1852, when Polak performed his first lithotomy in Persia.⁴¹

Prior to the publication of Polak's book on anatomy (*Tashrih*) in 1852,⁴² Persian physicians only had `Ali b. al-`Abbas `Ala al-Din al-Majusi's *Kamel al-Sena`ah* (from 994 CE) and Avicenna's *Qanun fi'l-Tebb* (from 1037 CE) to guide them in matters anatomic." There also was an earlier European-type study on anatomy, published in Arabic by the Abu Zabel School. Mullah Mohammad Ghobuli published a Persian translation in lithographic form around 1854. However, according to Schlimmer, this Persian translation was filled with mistakes and mysterious formulations, which he ascribed to the ignorance of the translator. Finally, this book's main function was to serve as packing material for the druggists.⁴³ Polak also had his students handle real skeletons. After initial reluctance to perform such a ritually unclean act, they soon overcame this attitude. Thereafter, they made haste to get skulls from gravesites to be used as study objects.⁴⁴ There was further the treatise that Mirza Mohammad *Hakim-bashi-ye koll* had written. It was a study on medicine entitled *Anvar-e Naseriyeh* in three volumes. The first volume was on anatomy with 56 plates and an index. The second volume was on surgery, and the third volume on general medicine.⁴⁵

Tholozan's book on the plague was printed in Tehran in 1876, see Ibid., vol. 1. p. 309 (*Resaleh dar keyfiyat-e marz-e ta`un*). It is therefore highly questionable whether Tholozan initiated the *réforme litéraire*, as Ebrahimnejad, "Theory and Practice," p. 171 has it.

³⁸ Piemontese, "Gli Ufficali Italini," pp. 102-03; Ekhtiar, *The Dar al-Funun*, pp. 158-59.

³⁹ Government of Iran, *Vaqaye`-ye Ettefaqiyeh*, p. (4 Jomadi al-Avval/December 17, 1852) ("Books and treatises written by the teaching staf at the school were often translated by the students and printed by the *Dar al-Fonun* Press. This Press is operated by the students, thus facilitating the rapid printing of books. The first medical book to be printed by the *Dar al-Fonun* Press was The Anatomy of the Human Body by Dr. Polak.").

⁴⁰ Ebrahimnejad, "Theory and Practice," p. 173.

⁴¹ Government of Iran, *Vaqaye`-ye Ettefaqiyeh*, p. (12 Rabi` al-Avval, 1269/December 24, 1852); Piemontese, "Gli Ufficali Italini," p. 101..

⁴² Polak's *Tashrih-e Badan* (Anatomy of the [Human] Body) was printed at the *Dar al-Fonun* Press and sold at a price of 6,000 dinars. Government of Iran, *Vaqaye`-ye Ettefaqiyeh*, pp. 1115 (nr. 173, 7 Sha`ban 1270/25 May, 1854)

⁴³ Schlimmer, *Terminologie*, pp. 38-39; Government of Iran, *Vaqaye`-ye Ettefaqiyeh*, pp. 1105 (Polak's anatomy), 1115 (Polak's anatomy), 1121(Polak's anatomy in Persian, 6,000 dinars), 1988 (*Anvar-e Naseriyeh*). For the earlier period see, e.g., Newman, A. "Tashrih-e Mansuri: Human Anatomy Between the Galenic and Prophetic Medical Traditions," in *La Science dans le Monde Iranien*, ed. Z. Vesel, et. al. (Tehran: Institut Francais de Recherche en Iran, 1998), pp. 253-72 and Savage-Smith, E. "Tashrih, *Enyclopedia of Islam*², vol. 10, pp. 354-56.

⁴⁴ Polak, *Persien*, vol. 1, p. 304.

⁴⁵ Government of Iran, *Vaqaye`-ye Ettefaqiyeh*, vol. 2, p. 1988 (nr. 305, 4 Rabi` II 1273/2 December, 1856). Not having seen this treatise it is not possible to form an opinion about its value added.

The Persian physicians' anatomical knowledge remained, however, still very theoretical despite their improved sources of information. Autopsy was not allowed according to the interpretation of Islamic law at that time, because it was believed that a post-mortem dissection was disrespectful to the deceased.[46] The only case that ever occurred was an autopsy done by Dr. Polak on the corpse of his compatriot Zatti, (who had taught mathematics and engineering at the *Dar al-Fonun*) to determine whether foul play had been involved.[47] Dr. Tholozan, who joined the teaching staff on a part-time basis as of 1864, gave lessons concerning descriptive and microscopic anatomy of the nervous system as well as a special course on the dissection of the sanguinary system using sheep as subjects in the late 1860s. The course was followed with great interest by the students and even by some practicing traditional doctors, who had never studied at the school.[48]

Tholozan further introduced aegophonia or auscultation (*sowt-e bozi*) in the *Dar al-Fonun* to which end he wrote an Auscultation and Percussion Treatise that clearly demonstrated its workings in its lithographed version. He further wrote a Quinology (the science which treats of the cultivation of the cinchona, and of its use in medicine) in Persian, dealing with pharmacological and therapeutic applications as well as the most recent European developments in the field. Tholozan finally wrote a textbook, *Badaye` al-Hekmat*, which was published in lithographed version in Tehran in 1277/1861, while some of the interpreters of the European professors at the school translated various medical texts into Persian.[49] Schlimmer published his very important *Terminologie Medico-Pharmaceutique* in 1874. It had started as a small dictionary of Persian equivalents for the common French terms, but had grown into a major pharmacopoeia. According to Elgood, "it was indeed a gigantic attempt to make the transition from Avicenna to Harvey least abrupt, to fit the old nomenclature to the new ideas, and to standardize the technical terms of the new university."[50] In this way, these pioneering teachers and translators created much of the medical terminology used in Persia to-day.

---

[46] Autopsy is allowed, according to Moslem law, if it serves a purpose that advances human knowledge. Savage-Smith, E. "Tashrih," *Encyclopedia of Islam*², vol. 10, p. 354-56, and Ibid., "Attitudes towards Dissection in Medieval Islam," *Journal of the History of Medicine and Allied Sciences* 50/1 (1994), pp. 67-100. However, socially and religiously it was a practice that was not accepted during the Qajar period. Anybody touching corpses was considered to be of a ghoulish disposition. Clarke, "Sketches," p. 708 ("A man to be seen dissecting would be taken for a ghoal, and he would be shunned as a degraded being"). Even the washers of the dead, for example, were only allowed inside the towns during the day. Gilmour, *Rapport*, p. 61.

[47] Schlimmer, *Terminologie*, p. 69 (q.v. autopsy or *fath*); Government of Iran, *Vaqaye`-ye Ettefaqiyeh*, vol. 2, (nr. 138, Dhu'l-Hejjah 1269), p. 1029 (no. 161, 10 Jomadi II 1270/October 3, 1854); Polak, *Persien*, vol. 1, p. 313 wrote that he died of coal dust suffocation, but Slaby, H. *Bindenschild und Sonnenlöwe* (Graz: Akademische Druck, 1982), p. 73 reported that he had been strangled by an infuriated Persian officer;

[48] Schlimmer, *Terminologie*, p. 229.

[49] Schlimmer, *Terminologie*, pp. 17, 229; Arjah, *Ketabshenasi*, p. xi.

[50] Elgood, *Medical History*, p. 502. For an analysis of these treatises written by the European teachers of the *Dar al-Fonun* see M. Najmabadi, "Tebb-e Dar al-Fonun va Kotub-e Darsi-ye An," in Iraj Afshar ed. *Amir Kabir va Dar al-Fonun*, pp. 202-37, and Ibid., *A Bibliography of Printed Books in Persian on Medicine and Allied Subjects* (Tehran, 1364).

Schlimmer further published in Persian a treatise on Animal Chemistry, a Treatise on skin diseases, and a first edition, without notes, of the *Terminologie*. "My course on pathology and special therapy together with a large pharmacopoeia of about 700 pages remains in manuscript and half done on lithographic stone due to lack of funds; my Treatise of medical ophthalmology with illustrations after Beer and others is ready to be lithographed. I also have dictated a Treatise of Pharmacodynamics, a Medical Primer, a course on pathology and general therapy, and a course on semeiotics (the cenoscopic science of signs), all of them in manuscript with my students, and even some traditional doctors have made haste to obtain copies of them."[51]

There also was a polytechnic school in Tabriz, with one director, one artillery instructor, one medical instructor, one mathematics teacher, one French instructor, and one Arabic teacher. It had been established in 1876. In 1880, there were 25 boarding (*dakheleh*) students and 25 gratis (*majani*) students, and eight support staff.[52]

The number of European physicians was still limited around 1860. There usually were one or two at the British and Russian legations, as well as the British residency at Bushire and the British consulate in Tabriz. Russia had two doctors at Ashuradeh Island as well as a small hospital, and a physician at its consulate in Tabriz. One of the two Russian doctors, each year, spent a couple of weeks in Astarabad and Mazandaran. In addition there had been one American doctor at the mission of Urumiyeh, while there were usually one or two European doctors at the *Dar al-Fonun*. In Shiraz, there was a Swedish physician (Fagergrin) as chief army-surgeon of Fars, while in the 1850s there had been a German doctor in Resht. Finally, there was the personal physician of the shah. This added up to about 12 European doctors present in Persia.[53] In 1864, there further was a Maltese British subject, Stagno, who was surgeon-in-chief to the Persian army, while, in 1855, de Gobineau met a Polish doctor, who was surgeon-in-chief of the army of the province of Fars. De Gobineau was unable to ascertain his medical qualities and qualifications. As of the early 1860s, a British adventurer and veterinarian, Dr. Dolmage, also taught at the *Dar al-Fonun*, but he was soon let go for incompetence.[54] The Italian doctors Castaldi and Cabuzzi came from Istanbul in 1871 to help with the plague epidemic in Persia and, on behalf of the Ottoman government, to monitor Persian activities to prevent the spread of cholera and other epidemics.[55]

---

[51] Schlimmer, *Terminologie*, p. 230.
[52] E'temad al-Saltaneh, *al-Ma'ather*, p. 405. For the publication of the Tabriz school's newspaper called *Madraseh-ye Mobarakeh-ye Dar al-Fonun-e Tabriz* see Qasemi, Sayyed Farid ed. *Danesh* (Tehran: Markaz-e Gostaresh-e Amuzesh-e Resanehha, 1374/1995) to which it has been appended. The last page of the introduction to this newspaper publication also provides additional information on the vicissitudes of this school.
[53] Häntzsche, "Specialstatistik," p. 442, note 1; Polak, "Lepra," p. 177 (Dr. Bock, physician of the Russian mission in Tehran); de Gobineau, *Trois Ans*, vol. 1, pp. 194-95 (Fagergrin); Polak, *Persien*, vol. 2, p. 206 (only seven). The German doctor in Resht probably was the Dutchman Dr. Schlimmer.
[54] Elgood, *Medical History*, p. 511 (Dolmage later showed up in charge of the arsenal in Mashad); de Gobineau, *Trois Ans*, vol. 1, pp. 136, 138, 244 (short presence of a French pharmacist).
[55] Piemontese, "Gli Ufficiali," p. 103; G.D. "Sanitätsreformen," pp. 299-300.

By 1858, 18 students who had majored in medicine graduated, and their number continued to grow thereafter. For medical science remained a pillar of the *Dar al-Fonun*. Students were also sent to France to be trained in medicine and surgery, and by 1859 some 18 students (in three waves) to study medicine and four students to study chemistry (*davasazi*) had been sent.[56]

SOME OPPOSITION AGAINST WESTERN MEDICINE
Thus, by 1860 there were less than 35 doctors trained in modern Western medical science in Persia, half of them Persian students who had just graduated from the *Dar al-Fonun*, and who, properly speaking, were not really physicians. Despite this small number of Western trained doctors, there was some opposition against the penetration of modern Western medicine in the second half of the nineteenth century. Before dealing with that opposition I first want to discuss who was this opposition by?

As has been detailed in the preceding chapter medical assistance in Qajar Persia was provided by: (i) the dead, (ii) the spirits, and (iii) the living. It was and is difficult to compete with the dead, especially when, if they spoke up, it was through their spokesmen, members of the clergy. However, Western medicine did not even try to compete with the dead providers of solace and cures. After all, if Western trained doctors had treated a person successfully that person would still go on pilgrimage, not so much for a cure, as he might have done before, but to give thanks for his cure. Thus business for the dead did not necessarily drop off. In effect, it may even have increased, because more people had reason to give thanks due to Western medical science. Consequently, there was no opposition from this segment of the medical establishment as far as the introduction of Western medical science was concerned. The clergy would sometimes speak about it, but because of other, although related, reasons.

The benevolent spirits also had no reason to complain because doctors trained in Western medical science did not try to compete with them either. Doctors only made people's efforts to combat the bad spirits, such as divs, jinns, etc. more effective by giving them modern tools to prevent diseases that were ascribed to supernatural causes. If you had ran afoul of the jinns and you had broken, burnt, or chafed something the modern doctors also here provided effective cures. The evil spirits may have had cause to complain about their own less effective means to defend themselves against human encroachments on their way of life, but this was not new and had been accepted for centuries. Also, apart from causing disease and ill-luck, spirits had no other means to express their opposition, which therefore became over time less relevant.

If it were not the dead or the spirits opposition had to come from the living, the only group left. However, even here we have to make a distinction between the various sub-categories of healers. For example, opposition did not come from the large majority of traditional healers such as bonesetters, surgeons, midwives, wise women and other general practitioners. Even if they felt that Western medicine was reducing their

---

[56] Ardakani, Hosein Mahbubi, *Tarikh-e Mo'assesat-e Tamaddon-e Jadid dar Iran* 3 vols. (Tehran: Daneshgah, 1368/1989), vol. 1, p. 303. For an overview of the graduates and their careers see Ekhtiar, *Dar al-Funun*, pp. 178-82, 184-85, 188-91, 195-99.

importance there was little that they could do about it. They were for the most part illiterate, unorganized, and without political contacts to channel their grievances, if they had them. Part of this apparent lack of manifested opposition was also due to the fact that if business dropped, it did so gradually, and that only towards the end of the nineteenth century and in certain towns. For practitioners of Western medicine, even in the early twentieth century, still only served part of the total population. Also, if there was a drop in demand it was partly compensated by the increase in population. However, because Persians tended to go first to traditional healers before asking help from Western doctors, it seems unlikely that there was a drop in the demand of their services. Finally, a few traditional practitioners had adopted some of the Western medical techniques such as in the treatment of wounds. Thus they had found it profitable to go "west.' When Western medicine had become dominant, it was too late to complain, because everybody (government, population, and religious and political forces) had already gone over to the other side.

The only group that remained then was that of the Islamic-Galenic healers. Even here there was no universal opposition. It did not come from the eye-doctors, who seem to have embraced Western medical science and made it their own. This is clear from the publication by Dr. Kahhal and her periodical *Danesh*, and although I cannot claim that she represented all her colleagues it is an important indication of the sentiment among that group of doctors. Opposition also does not seem to have come from the druggists (`attar`), although they must have suffered from the fast growth of their new competitors, the chemists (*davasaz*). However, there does not seem to have been a major problem. This is probably due to the fact that druggists were mainly found in towns, and towns were growing fast after 1880. Thus, loss of business to the chemists, most of which were established after that date and then in large towns only, was partly compensated by population growth. Also, this situation, combined with a low literacy rate, lack of organization and political contacts made any opposition quite unlikely and ineffective.

This means that the only ones left were the doctors of internal medicine (*hakim*). They were the heirs and bearers of the flagship of ancient medicine, the Islamic-Galenic system. They were literate, many of them even well educated, and of a studious bent of mind. Although they were not organized, their leading proponents had excellent contacts at the highest level of government and the religious establishment; in fact some of them were religious persons.

Having dealt with the question who felt threatened, I now discuss the nature of the threat. Was it the size of the threat? By 1860 there were less than 35 doctors trained in modern Western medical science, half of them Persian students who had just graduated, and who were not really physicians. It cannot have been this small, but growing, number of physicians trained in Western medicine that caused trepidation amongst some of their colleagues trained in Islamic-Galenic medical science.

So what was the real nature of the threat; what exactly was found to be objectionable in Western medicine? Much of the sphere of intervention of Western trained doctors was in the hands-on (*yadi*) part of medicine. Small and large surgery interventions were areas in which the *hakim*s were not interested.⁵⁷ But it was in this area that Western doctors established a reputation of enormous effectiveness. Galenic medicine was a hands-off method. Doctors rarely touched their patients; it sufficed to listen to their complaints and on that basis make a diagnosis and prescribe proper treatment and medicine. Polak reports that in the 1850s, when European doctors operated upon patients, Persian doctors (*hakim*) to denigrate their work would tell people that the European doctor was but a surgeon (*jarrah*), i.e., the doctor had no knowledge whatsoever about medicine.⁵⁸ I do not think, as Ringer has suggested, that the ban on autopsies was of particular importance between the two schools of thought. Although the European teachers, of course, wanted their students to be trained in that branch of medicine as well, no Persian at that time was really willing to learn or to do autopsy because of Islamic and culture prejudice. Even, as late as 1926, Neligan noted that, "Persian practice is largely medical. There are very few surgeons."⁵⁹

Thus, the field of internal medicine, the domain par excellence of the *hakim*, was the real battlefield. But here also, what was the problem? I do not think that the reason was that Western medical science had a different, if not diametrically opposed, approach to both diagnostic and therapeutic methodology and that most of its practitioners considered Islamic-Galenic medicine hocus-pocus. For there was a growing openness to new ideas among the Persian medical class in the second half of the nineteenth century. Morier poked fun at the traditional physician, whom he characterized as being steeped in ancient tradition and driven by self-interest. The royal physician told Hajji Baba, Morier's fictional hero, that he opposed the European doctor, because: "He makes no distinction between hot and cold diseases, and hot and cold remedies, but gives mercury by way of cooling medicine; stabs the belly with a sharp instrument for wind in the stomach; and what is worse than all, pretends to do away with the small-pox."⁶⁰

Persian physicians on their own accord had 'discovered' Paracelsus, one of whose books had been translated into Persian three times (in 1810, 1820s, and 1836), although only one of which was published in lithographed form in 1829 in Tabriz. Although no Western trained doctor would have introduced Persian doctors to Paracelsus, whose theories had been abandoned, it nevertheless demonstrated the readiness of some Persian doctors to question the foundation of humoral theories.⁶¹ This is also clear from the work of some of the more independent thinking Persian physicians such as Mohammad Taqi Shirazi, an opponent of Western medicine. In one of his works he broke with Galenic medical tradition in his treatise on cholera.⁶² The same open attitude to explore, if not accept new

---

⁵⁷ "The native *hakims* were utterly ignorant of surgery." Stuart, *Doctors in Persia*, p. 7.
⁵⁸ Polak, *Persien*, vol. 2, p. 199.
⁵⁹ Neligan, "Public Health," part III, p. 742. Lichtwardt, "Western Medicine," p. 239 ("at one time … the medical missionaries were the only trained surgeons and physicians.")
⁶⁰ Morier, James. *The Adventures of Hajji Baba*, chapter XIX.
⁶¹ For the titles of the translations and their location see Ebrahimnejad, "Religion and Medicine," p. 100. According to Ts., "Persidskie Doktora," p. 162, Persian doctors were not willing to question the tenets of the Galenic system at all; in fact, he maintains they were forbidden to do so.
⁶² Ebrahimnejad, "La médecine d'observation," and Ibid., "Un traité d'épidémologie." Islamic-Galenic doctors had not yet embraced the notion that there was a link between the plague and 'contagion' although a few had made such a link. They, as many of the Western doctors (*supra*) thought that it was caused by supernatural phenomena and the will of God, see Dols, Michael W.,

medical ideas, was also demonstrated by the publication of the new modern anatomy book, as has already been discussed. However, I do not think that the few Persian Islamic-Galenic physicians who were in an evolutionary process of change were representative of their profession. Ebrahimnejad's thesis that it was "the internal evolution of traditional medicine which paved the way for anatomical-clinical [=Western] medicine," in my view is not supported by the facts. I agree with him that it was an internal Persian evolution that paved the way for Western medicine, but it was a socio-political evolution, not a medical one that was instrumental in making this happen. For the acceptance of Western medicine was the result of the Persian power elite's objective to modernize, which meant adopting Western technology lock-stock-and barrel.[63]

I do not think either that the opposition was due to a bread-and-butter issue. The newly trained doctors certainly began to compete for the same influential and remunerative posts, such as that of court physician or physician to the high and mighty, that traditional doctors coveted. But they would also have done this if they had remained pure Islamic-Galenic professionals. Also, the selection of physicians by the high and mighty was not solely based on whether the doctor concerned had studied in Europe or not. Other, social and cultural reasons played a much more important role.

But even though most of the Persian *hakim*s did not oppose Western medicine, some did, and for a variety of reasons. First there was *amour-propre*. It takes a strong personality to be able to admit that much, if not all, that you have believed in is no longer relevant. The more so, if you strongly believed that these ancient truths should not be questioned at all. Those that accepted this fact made it easier for themselves by gradually going over to the 'competition.' Having a foot in both systems and slowly withdrawing from the Galenic system made the transition easier for them. For example, the *hakim*s who traditionally did not examine their patients, under influence of the practice of Western doctors, also began to look at the patients' tongue and feel their pulse.[64] Those Persians who had studied medicine in Europe (mostly France), such as Mirza Sheikh Jalal, still remained tradition-bound doctors.[65]

For those who found it difficult to accept Western medicine, there were other reasons to oppose it. Not only did Western medical science originate from a suspicious, even infidel,

---

The Black Death in the Middle East (Princeton, 1977, 1979), pp. 74-142, in particular 93-98, 110 and Ibn Qayyim, *Natural Healing*, pp. 32-34 (quoting the Tradition that "If you hear of a plague in a land, do not go there, but if it occurs in a land where you are, do not flee from it."), 106-07 (avoid contact with leprosy)..

[63] The modernization process in Qajar Persia developed in three stages, each one being stronger and having more societal support than the previous one. For a discussion of the modernization process see Floor, *Traditional Crafts*, chapter one, and with regards to the medical sector in particular see Richter-Bernburg, "Avicenna gegen Pockenimpfung," pp. 73-87.

[64] Lichtwardt, "Western Medicine," p. 236; Ts., "Persidskie Doktora," pp. 162-63; Morier, *Hajji Baba*, chapter XXI.

[65] Lycklama, *Voyage*, vol. 2, p. 166; `Eyn al-Saltaneh, *Ruznameh*, vol. 1, p. 795 (Dr. Ehya al-Molk Sheykh Morad had studied in Paris); Polak, *Persien*, vol. 1, p. 311 (Dr. Mirza Hoseyn, Dr. Mirza Reza b. Moqim and Dr. Mirza `Ali Naqi); Dieulefoy, *La Perse*, p. 453; Ebrahimnejad, "Religion and Medicine," pp. 100-07.

source, but it was part of the same Western onslaught that was also trying to take over the country politically, economically, morally, and now also medically. Standing up against Western medicine was therefore the moral thing to do; it was patriotic and would strengthen the country's so far feeble resistance in the political and economic field against Western domination. Also, some religious and secular leaders looked with suspicion on the nature of Western medicine and thus provided moral cover for an oppositional stand. Polak mentioned that until Mirza Agha Khan Nuri, the grand vizier (1852-58) had been dismissed he could not do much to improve matters in preventive health, because Agha Khan Nuri was against all new ideas and reforms.[66] But these were 'socio-religious and political' reasons, not medical scientific ones. Similar types of anti-modernity and reform expressions occurred when electricity, the railway, and other modern innovations were introduced into Persia. These were branded as un-Islamic, and as capitulation to Christendom.[67]

The most outspoken and vociferous opponent of European medicine was Hajji Mirza Baba Shirazi, Malek al-Atebba, who wrote a treatise refuting European medicine. It is of interest to note that the medical arguments from the Persian opposition were not against the nature of the scientific method, but rather against the nature of the medicines used. Western medicine not only offered an alternative approach, it also used a different delivery mechanism, *i.e.*, chemical instead of herbs. The new European drugs were based on the essence (*jowhar*) of simple or compound herbal drugs. Instead of plants and herbs, its medical representatives prescribed chemical products. Medical pills or powders contained elements that were poisonous. This was, of course, a misleading argument, because Persian doctors also prescribed medicines that contained poisonous substances in non-lethal dosage to their patients. Mercury and arsenic were examples of two substances often prescribed by Persian doctors, which, according to Häntzsche, was the reason why mercury poisoning occurred so frequently in Persia.[68] Nevertheless, this was one of the main arguments used in Mirza Mohammad Taqi Shirazi's Arabic treatise against the introduction and use of Western drugs, entitled *Resaleh-ye Jowhariyeh* (Treatise on Essences). The alleged use of so-called poisons and essences by European doctors was a refrain that was parroted by many a Persian doctor, and as a result, many Persians were reluctant to have recourse to Western doctors for matters of internal medicine.[69]

The following story is instructive in this context. One of the well-known and leading Persian physicians, Fakhr al-Atebba, argued during a social gathering that European drugs were all bad and had nothing special to recommend them. He maintained that anyone who used them was mad, and would never properly heal. It would seem that European doctors

---

[66] Polak, "Medicinische Briefe," p. 140.
[67] Richter-Bernburg, "Avicenna gegen Pockenimpfung," pp. 73-87.
[68] Dieulefoy, *La Perse*, pp. 456-57; Häntzsche, "Physikalisch-medicinische Skizze," pp. 565-66 (the sale of mercury had been banned in Tehran, due to a failed poisoning attempt on the shah, but at Resht it was freely available); Ts., "Persidskie Doktora," p. 170.
[69] Polak, *Persien*, vol. 2, p. 206. Rice, *Mary Bird*, p. 98 reported that "the wife of the high priest came with bad rheumatism the other day, but she could only have liniment, as she has never been permitted to defile herself with medicine not prepared by her own people; the other Parsis were most surprised at her coming at all."

gave iodide potassium (*yodurudupatas*) for all disorders, argued Fakhr al-Atebba. This had negative consequences. It made women's breasts and men's testicles smaller, for example. To remain hale and sound it was better to eat a vegetable soup (*ash-e reshteh*) and vinegar juice (*sarkeh-ye shireh*) each night and then to vomit (*qey kardan*). Alternatively, after dinner you had to take a glass of oxymel (*sekanjebin*), and then smoke two strong water pipes that had to be drawn deeply. That also would result in vomiting. Never in your life would your temper (*mazaj*; *atesh-e mezaj*) be so sound. Fakhr al-Atebba said: "You should do that every evening." All those present laughed at him. He then said. "In the [traditional Persian] medical books it is written: each year you should bleed and each day you should vomit."[70]

Astarabadi, one of Mirza Mohammad Taqi Shirazi's pupils, also argued that Western drugs were harmful, "because they were altered through their transformation from their natural state to their essence; secondly because they were produced in a different climate from that of Iran and consequently they did not fit the temperaments of the local population."[71] These arguments had nothing to do with medical issues and more with ritualistic or financial matters. For many of these drugs and their ingredients had already been used since the beginning of the nineteenth century. For example, Astarabadi opposed the use of quinine imported from Europe, but not of that, which had been locally processed.[72]

Another more likely reason for the opposition against European drugs was that they were efficacious and undoubtedly created a feeling of uncertainty, if not jealousy among Persian doctors. Morier has an interesting tale about the royal physician telling Hajji Baba to steal the wonder drug from the European physician that cured the shah.[73] But not only in court circles was the efficacy of European drugs well-known. Mme Dieulafoy, for example, mentioned meeting some road-guards en route, who asked for a medicine given by a European traveler in the past that had been so effective.[74] Although a very small minority opposed Western medicine, the majority of the population could not care less about what Persian Islamic-Galenic physicians felt about European doctors and drugs. The former were not accessible to them, while the latter were, despite their limited number. Therefore, whenever a European passed a village he was mobbed by the sick. For in Qajar Persia, all Europeans were supposed to be deeply versed in the art of healing, and "'Feringhi medicine' is all they care for, and in their eyes every Feringhi is a Hakim."[75] Persians

---

[70] 'Eyn al-Saltaneh, *Ruznameh*, vol. 1, p. 795; see also Safari, *Ardabil*, vol. 3, p. 484; Polak, *Persien*, vol. 2, p. 233.
[71] Ebrahimnejad, "Religion and Medicine," pp. 100-101; Government of Iran, *Vaqaye'-ye Ettefaqiyeh*, vol. 1, pp. 194 (nr. 37, 20 Dhu'l-Hejjah 1267/16 October, 1851) quotes a price of 8,000 dinars, 382 (same price).
[72] Ebrahimnejad, "Religion and Medicine," p. 105.
[73] Morier, *Hajji Baba*, chapters 19 and 20.
[74] Dieulefoy, *La Perse*, p. 436; Linton, *Persian Sketches*, p. 30 (a Persian had been left to die at the road; he was saved by emetine injections and totally recovered).
[75] Bird, *Journeys*, p. 74; Brugsch, *Reise*, vol. 2, p. 17; Arnold, *Through Persia*, p. 261; Bonvalot, Gabriel. *Du Caucase Aux Indes* (Paris: E. Plon, Nourrit & Cie, 1889), pp. 195, 225; Stirling, *The Journals*, pp. 43, 86; Collins, *In the Kingdom*, p. 162 (so many people came to see him at his house, or accosted him in the street, that he had to ask protection to keep the crowd at bay); Forbes-Leith,

also accepted it as quite normal that Western missionary doctors mixed religion with their healing. Mary Bird wrote, "Most patients expect me to pray for and with them, and attribute many cures to this practice, though some repeat their Arabic prayers in a low monotone as an antidote."[76]

The argument against European drugs, therefore, was more of a religious ritualistic nature rather than a medical one. It was similar to those arguments that orthodox Moslems had made, for example, with regards to imported refined sugar.[77] Moreover, Persian physicians as well as patients who could afford them were quick to use European drugs. Calomel or mercurous chloride as well as Epsom salt, Seidlitz salt (both salts were hydrated magnesium sulfate and known in Persian as *gerd-e safid* and *namak-e ferengi*), effervescent powder, and quinine had already been in use since the 1820s. Also, whenever newer products became available in the market, the elite and their Persian physicians were quick to use them.[78] In fact, according to Polak, in the homes of the power elite in Persia there always was at least one ounce of calomel and quinine in storage. In case of slow indigestion, for example, the wealthy Persian would take one small wooden spoon, containing 4-6 grains of calomel in the evening and the following morning a dosage of castor oil or Epsom salt. Such a dosage was considered to be a solvent necessary to liquefy the *Materia peccans*, and then to get rid of it with a purging. Such a purging without a preceding solvent was considered to be dangerous.[79] The Bakhtiyaris preferred pills rather than powders. They believed that pills were more efficacious than *dava-ye ab* (water medicine). Dr. Ross reported that the Bibis insisted powdered medicines and were upset if any water was added.[80] It is therefore not surprising to note that an opponent of Western medicine, such as Eftekhar al-Atebba did not oppose Western pharmaceuticals per se, for he translated a modern English pharmacopoeia into Persian under the title of *Asrar al-Hekmah*, while other Persian physicians also produced similar pharmacological books with a view to propagate Western drugs.[81] Western medicine thus influenced Islamic-Galenic medicine, because traditional Persian physicians gradually adopted its terminology and concepts in their treatises and translations. As discussed above, to facilitate the transmission of European medical science many of the textbooks developed for teaching at the *Dar al-Fonun* were also translated into Persian. These were used by students as well as by opponents to

---

Checkmate, p. 89 (Because he cleaned and stitched a wound of a servant all those ailing in the village came to see the 'hakim.' The next day they came from neighboring villages); Heinrich, *Auf Panthersuche*, pp. 38-39; Linton, *Persian Sketches*, pp. 30, 87.

[76] Rice, *Mary Bird*, p. 127.

[77] Floor, *Traditional Crafts*, pp. 337, 356-59.

[78] Bélanger, *Voyage*, vol. 2, p. 217; Clarke, "Sketches," p. 708, Schlimmer, *Terminologie*, p. 522 (q.v. sulphas magnesiae); `Eyn al-Saltaneh, *Ruznameh*, p. 262. Polak, "Medicinische Briefe," p. 139 reported that he used quinine for those who acould afford to, and for the poor he administered a decoction of cort. salicis fragilis.

[79] Polak, J.E. "Ueber den Gebrauch des Quecksilbers in Persien," *Wiener Medizinische Wochenschrift* 10 (1860), pp. 564.

[80] Ross, *A Lady Doctor*, pp. 94-95 ("I had to get over this difficulty by taking round the water corked and labeled bottles ad telling them it was 'aqua distillata,' which saved my reputation, as the Khans have not yet added Latin to their curriculum.").

[81] Sajjadi, Sadeq. "Drugs," *Encyclopedia Iranica*, vii, p. 559, for other examples and more details.

Western medicine and thus influenced the theoretical framework in which they carried on their discussion.[82]

The opposition against the teaching of only European medicine was sufficiently strong for the government to give in. Naser al-Din Shah's increased lack of interest for the *Dar al-Fonun* at that time facilitated such a change of course. Also, the shah himself continued to employ both Persian as well as European doctors, and thus there was a perfect model for the use of a similar combination of medical systems at the medical school. As a result, the teaching of Islamic-Galenic medicine became part of the *Dar al-Fonun*'s curriculum in January 1860, when the school's director, E'tezad al-Saltaneh announced in the government newspaper *Vaqaye'-ye Ettefaqiyeh*: "Since some of the people of Iran are not yet convinced of European medical practice, in order to inform medical students of the prevailing Persian medical practice, Mirza Mohammad Hakimbashi Kashani, who, both in terms of practice and knowledge is the best of the Iranian doctors, was assigned to teach Persian medicine in the blessed school."[83]

In practice, the teaching of both Western and Islamic-Galenic medicine did not constitute a major problem. The new generation of medical students preferred to study Western medicine. Moreover, some of the European teachers did not reject Islamic-Galenic medicine blindly and totally. Schlimmer made great effort to learn how Persian doctors dealt with their patients so as to better understand how to serve his students by better translating Western medical concepts and methods into Persian practitioners' needs. He also found some of the Persian doctors' practices very useful and even suggested that the Persian prescription system be copied in Europe. Polak, who was very leery of the indiscriminate use of mercury by Persian surgeons, nevertheless made a study of their therapies and its results. Because he saw positive results of the use of mercury in many cases, he adopted some of these methods, even going so far as to refer syphilis patients to Persian surgeons for the inhaling therapy.[84]

Over time the attitude of the olama and the conservative elite changed. Initial opposition to European doctors was usually transformed into acceptance after a while.[85] Even conservative mullahs allowed themselves to be treated by European doctors, despite the fact that some of them also dabbled in healing. On the one hand, European doctors welcomed such a change of mind, but, on the other hand, they also were very careful and circumspect when treating the olama, because of the possible backlash if the treatment did not work. If the patient died his death would be ascribed to the incompetence or worse of the European physician.[86]

---

[82] Ebrahimnejad, "Theory and Practice," p. 176; Ibid., "Religion and Medicine," pp. 104-05.
[83] Government of Iran, *Ettefaqiyeh-ye Vaqaye'*, vol. 4, p. 2990 (no. 406 19 Jomadi 1276/January 13, 1860).
[84] Polak, "Ueber den Gebrauch," p. 567.
[85] Malcolm, *Five Years*, p. 54. In the mid-nineteenth century Ts., "Persidskie Doktora," p. 170 remarked that although Persian patients had faith in European doctors they nevertheless also would secretly consult a Persian one.
[86] Hume-Griffith, *Behind the Veil*, pp. 146-48; Colins, *In the Kingdom*, p. 162 ("I operated on several of them, and have no hesitation in saying that the *seyeds* of Ispahan are, as a rule, the most sour-

Because of Naser al-Din Shah's fear that better education might result in subversive activities, this also diminished his interest in the *Dar al-Fonun*. This translated itself in a cessation of the flow of government–sponsored students to Europe to receive further training and education. It also was shown in the quality of teaching at the *Dar al-Fonun* that left much to be desired after 1880, according to both European and Persian observers. Eyn al-Saltaneh qualified the school in 1892 as a farce (*luti-bazi*), while Dr. Neligan, looking back at the results obtained towards the end of the Qajar era, opined that, "Medical education in Persia, in spite of years of experience and expense, is, it must be candidly stated, of a very low standard."[87]

After 1880, most of the teaching was done by Persian physicians, who were graduates of the *Dar al-Fonun* and of French universities, such as Mirza Sayyed `Ali (Persian, *i.e.*, Islamic-Galenic medicine), Mirza Ahmad Tabib Kashani (Islamic-Galenic medicine; until 1870), Mirza Taqi Khan Ansari (Western medicine), Mirza Reza (Western medicine), Mirza Kazem Mahallati (chemistry), Mirza Abu'l-Qasem Hakim-Bashi (Islamic-Galenic medicine; as of 1877), Mirza `Ali Doktor Mo`tamed al-Atebba (Western medicine; as of 1877), Mirza Hoseyn Doktor (Western medicine; as of 1864), Dr. Abu'l-Hasan Khan Bahrami (Western medicine to second year students; as of 1879), and Mirza Mohammad Doktor Kermanshahi (Western medicine; as of 1881; also head of the public hospital). The drop in quality of the teaching was not necessarily due to the use of Persian teachers. Maybe more important was the lack of interest that Naser al-Din Shah showed in the school in particular and Western education in general.[88] The few students who still went to Europe to study medicine, according to Dr. Schneider, often did not have sufficient educational background, stayed too short a time (two years at most) and did not even formally register with the medical faculty of the university where they were supposed to be studying. Dr. Schneider, who became the shah's personal physician in 1893, was instrumental in establishing a sound medical curriculum, within the *Dar al-Fonun* as well as to send qualified Persian students to the military medical school in Lyon (France). The *Dar a-Fonun* had only two European professors around 1890 (Albo, a German physician, and Basil, an Armenian British-trained physician). The staff was expanded in 1905 to include specialists in gynecology, pharmacology, physics, chemistry, natural history, and veterinary medicine.[89] The French also sent a midwife, Ms Marguenot to train Persian women in modern techniques of obstetrics.[90] It was only in 1918 that the medical school became an independent entity in a separate building, although still within the compound of the *Dar al-Fonun* in the Naser Khosrow Street. It

---

minded, hypocritical, ungrateful individuals that can be met with anywhere.")
[87] Government of Great Britain, *Geographical Handbook*, pp. 408-09; `Eyn al-Saltaneh, *Ruznameh*, pp. 330, 505, 577, 849.
[88] Ekhtiar, *Dar al-Funun*, pp. 171-74 (Persian teachers), 205-10 (changing shah's attitude); for the year 1882 see Qasemi, *Danesh*, p. 7.
[89] Schneider, "La médecine persane," p. 13; Nategh, "Les Persans," pp. 191-99; Ekhtiar, *Dar al-Funun*, pp. 163, 168 (Drs. George and Gaulet [medical], and Roquebrun, Olmer, and Danton later replaced by Drs. Gachet, Duchesne and Maulion [medical] and by LeBlanc and Latess); see also Hassendorfer, "Les médecins français," pp. 61-62.
[90] Hassendorfer, "Les médecins français," p. 61.

was only in July 1924, that the medical school was moved to another location in Razi Street. In 1935 it was integrated into the newly founded University of Tehran.[91] At the end of the Qajar era there also was still a medical school in the *Dar al-Fonun* at Tabriz.[92]

All the good efforts spent to improve the medical school proved to be in vain. According to Dr. Neligan, the medical school at Tehran in the early 1920s was "very poorly equipped and the teaching is largely theoretical. No fees are charged. There is a long list of so-called professors, two (the lecturers on surgery and bacteriology) are French, the others are Persian, some of whom have French diplomas. The two Europeans have no say in the management of the school. The religious law does not permit dissection. Hospital attendance is not compulsory."[93]

WESTERN IMPACT ON MEDICAL INSTITUTIONS AND SERVICES

Although the teaching of modern Western medical science at the *Dar al-Fonun* was very important, equally important was the growing presence of European and American physicians in Persia as well as institutions that they created (hospital, dispensaries) or helped create (government regulations). Most of these physicians were attached to foreign Legations, foreign agencies (Indo-Euro telegraph; Russian Red Cross, etc.), or were missionaries (American; British, French; German, Russian). In addition there were a few physicians attached to the royal court and some to provincial governors.[94] It was in particular the missionary physicians with their hospitals and dispensaries who would introduce the general population to modern Western medicine.

The first, though short-lived, European medical dispensary was established by Dr. Salvatori, the physician of the French diplomatic mission between 1807-09, led by general Gardane.[95] The French dispensary did not last, and therefore it was the American Presbyterian mission that established the first permanent dispensaries in 1835.[96] Towards the end of the nineteenth century, other dispensaries and hospitals were opened, often attached to foreign Legations and Consulates or by missionaries in Tehran, Bushire, Isfahan, Mashad, Kerman and other towns. Two state hospitals also were established, about which more in what follows.

Doctors of foreign legations were at first looked on with suspicion. But the hostile attitude changed over time. Mme. Serena's statement that Persian doctors and mullahs opposed foreign medical aid, because the foreign doctors asked a small sum of one *shahi* from everybody makes sense, if she meant to say that they opposed unfair subsidized

---

[91] Ekhtiyar, *Dar al-Funun*, p. 230; Sadeq, `Isa. *Yadegar-e `Omr – Khaterati az Sargodhasht* 3 vols. (Tehran: Amir Kabir, 1345/1966) vol. 2, p. 183.
[92] Rice, *Persian Women*, p. 252.
[93] Government of Great Britain, *Geographical Handbook*, pp. 408-09.
[94] E`temad al-Saltaneh, *al-Ma'ather*, p. 390 (there were three European court physicians and nine Persian physicians in 1880). By the end of the nineteenth century there were Dr. Coppin (Mozaffar al-Din Mirza), Dr. Sorel (Zell al-Soltan), Dr. Broussière (Customs Service in the Gulf), Dr Bongrand (Na'eb al-Saltaneh) Dr. Roth (Shams al-Saltaneh-Fars) and Dr. Ferte (`Azud al-Saltaneh, Gilan), see Hassendorfer, "Les médecins français," p. 61
[95] Elgood, *Medical History*, p. 441.
[96] Perkins, *A Residence*, p. 134; Elgood, *Medical History*, pp. 533-35.

competition.⁹⁷ Normally, mullahs "expressed surprise that Christians should look after patients who could not pay."⁹⁸ The European doctors in Tehran only treated patients that could pay, with the exception of the British legation doctors, who treated the poor free of charge.⁹⁹ The Indo-European Telegraph Department (IETD), which was established in 1865, employed a number of physicians, who also operated some dispensaries for the poor. Of course, the main task of these physicians was to keep the IETD staff hale and healthy. This was not an easy task, because many, including one of the physicians, died in the course of their service of the same diseases of which the population amongst which they lived died.¹⁰⁰

HOSPITALS AND DISPENSARIES

MILITARY HOSPITAL

In 1810, according to Price, the Persians had no surgeons attached to their military. He made this remark when Russian prisoners-of-war arrived in Tehran whose wounds had not been taken care of since their capture at Qarabagh (Azerbaijan). The two doctors of the Ouseley mission, viz., Cormick and Sharpe, therefore treated them.¹⁰¹ However, Drouville, who served with the army, reported that Jewish and other surgeons were attached to the military.¹⁰² It was clear, however, that the situation of medical care to the military was in need of improvement.¹⁰³ In 1851, Amir Kabir therefore appointed a doctor to each military regiment (*hakem-e fowj*), a decision clearly aimed at improving the quality of medical care and military hygiene available to and practiced by the troops. He further hired a number of Europeans and one Persian physician to be chief army surgeon of the province where they were stationed. Dr. Schlimmer, a Dutchman, was appointed to go to Gilan, Dr. Fagergrin, a Swede, to Shiraz, and Dr. Astaniyu(?), of unknown nationality, to Tabriz. The first two received a salary of 150 tomans, the latter 250 tomans per year. Mirza Sadeq, who had studied medicine in Edinburgh as of 1846, was sent to Tabriz. Those Persians willing to become army doctors had to be licensed by Dr. Kazulani (?), the chief army surgeon. The latter died on February 2, 1852, and was replaced by Dr. Polak.¹⁰⁴

In addition to an improvement in the quality of medical staff, Amir Kabir also ordered the construction of an army hospital. According to Polak, this happened at his suggestion.¹⁰⁵

---

⁹⁷ Serena, *Hommes*, pp. 137-38.
⁹⁸ Rice, *Mary Bird*, p. 89.
⁹⁹ Serena, *Hommes*, p. 142; Collins, *In the Kingdom*, p. 276 (a small dispensary at Golhak).
¹⁰⁰ Wright, *The English*, p. 126; Rubin, *The Formation*, pp. 295-99.
¹⁰¹ Price, William. *Journal of the British Embassy to Persia*. 2 vols. in one (London: Thomas Thorpe, 1832), vol. 1 p. 33.
¹⁰² Drouville, *Voyage*, vol. 2, pp. 164-66.
¹⁰³ For details see Polak, *Persien*, vol. 2, pp. 211-12.
¹⁰⁴ Adamiyyat, *Amir Kabir*, pp. 327-28; Government of Iran, *Vaqaye'-ye Ettefaqiyeh*, vol. 1, p. 303 (nr. 56, 5 Jomadi I, 1268/26 February, 1852).
¹⁰⁵ Polak, "Medicinische Briefe," p. 140. Ebrahimnejad, "Theory and Practice," p. 171, mentions an anomymous Persian manuscript (*Resaleh dar khosus-e ta'sis-e mariz-khaneh*), written in the early 1850s, that proposed, amongst other other thing, the establishment of a military hospital. It seems likely that this text was written at the suggestion of the Amir Kabir, in which case it must

During the first half of the Qajar regime there did not exist any hospital in Persia, with the exception of the one at the shrine of Imam Reza at Mashad. In the pre-Qajar period there had been one or more hospitals (*mariz-khaneh*; *dar al-shafa'*, *bimarestan*) in several towns such as Isfahan and Tabriz, but they seem to have ceased operations during the eighteenth century.[106] However, in 1889, `Eyn al-Saltaneh mentioned the existence of the *Madraseh-ye Dar al-Shafa* or the Hospital School in Tehran, which had been constructed by Mohammad Shah (r. 1834-48). Its existence indeed is mentioned in 1851. There were a number of sick there as well as a photo shop. It would seem that this institution was not a proper hospital, but rather a kind of (philanthropic?) facility attached to a religious school and mosque.[107]

Whatever the truth of the matter, construction of the first State military hospital (*marizkhaneh-ye dowlati*) was started in 1850, and it was opened in January 1852. It also had a pharmacy and could house 400 patients. The first director was Mirza Mohammad Vali Hakim-bashi, and Dr. Kazulani, chief-doctor of the army, was responsible for medical treatment. The doctors with three students were busy everyday till noon, and the patients were satisfied with the service offered and left the hospital in good health, according to the government newspaper. From January 1852 till January 1853, 2,238 patients were treated in the hospital, mostly suffering from difficult (*sa`b*) diseases.[108]

E`temad al-Saltaneh reported that Naser al-Din Shah ordered the establishment of a hospital in 1857 in Tehran.[109] It was built outside Tehran at the instigation of Dr. Polak who had seen that sick soldiers were kept in dark cellar-like barracks, where they died like flies. Whether Polak referred to the first hospital that Amir Kabir had built in 1852, or whatever happened to that hospital is not known. Polak does not even refer to this hospital, although he had worked in it. Polak's original design was a roomy and light building, that formed a square with a spacious courtyard, in the middle of which was the inevitable pond. Around the building he had bushes and trees planted, while a wall

---

have been written in 1849, because construction work had started already in 1850.

[106] Floor, Willem and Faghfoory. *Dastur al-Moluk* (awaiting publication) Commentary q.v. `attarkhana; E`temad al-Saltaneh, *Mer'at al-Boldan*, vol. 1, p. 552; Asaf al-Dowleh, Mirza `Abdol-Vahhab Khan. *Asnad* 2 vols. ed. `Abdol-Hoseyn Nava'i and Nilufar Kasri (Tehran: Mo'asseseh-ye Motale`at-e Tarikh-e Mo`aser-e Iran, 1377/1998), vol. 1, pp. 20 (*marizkhaneh*), 39 (*dar al-shafa*); in general see Sajjadi, Sadeq. "Bimarestan," *Encyclopedia Iranica*, p. 257-59.

[107] `Eyn al-Saltameh, *Ruznameh*, vol. 1, p. 306; Sepehr, Mohammad Taqi Lesan al-Molk. *Nasokh al-Tavarikh* ed. Jamshid Kayanfar 3 vols. (Tehran: Asatir, 1377/1998), vol. 3, p. 1183. It was located opposite the Masjed-e Shah, part of it was situated in the Khiyaban-e Bodhorjmehr. Shahri, *Tarikh*, vol. 5, p. 700, n. 3

[108] Government of Iran, *Vaqaye`-ye Ettefaqiyeh*, vol. 1, p. 611 (nr. 102, 8 Rabi` II 1269/19 January, 1853) states that 1,238 patients were treated, but vol. 1, pp. 618-19 (nr.103, 10 Rabi` II, 1369/21 January, 1853) gives the higher number. On Dr. Kazulani, about whom I have not been able to find other particulars, see Ibid., vol. 1, pp. 34, 64, 260, 303 (his death) and Adamiyat, *Amir Kabir*, p. 327 who stated that he was the brother of Kazulani the chief painter (*naqqash-bashi*), who is not listed in Mohammad `Ali Karemzadeh-Tabrizi, *Naqqashan-e Qadim-e Iran* 3 vols (London, 1991).

[109] E`temad al-Saltaneh, *Montazam-e Naseri*, vol. 3, pp. 218, 255; Polak, "Medicinische Briefe," p. 140.

surrounded the site. The rooms were three and a half feet higher than the ground. The design was completely changed by the chief general during his absence, but Polak was able to get most of his way. Once the hospital had been built in 1857, the next battle began, how to get funds for its operation. The army doctors had an allocation for a large establishment, but spent most of it on themselves. Even the most necessary drug, quinine, they did not buy. The doctors shared the hospital's operational budget with the army's officers and were not interested in changing this arrangement. Polak's students, whom he had entrusted the management of food, clothing, instruments, and drugs, diverted the money for that for their own use. Instead of showing how a proper hospital might function, Polak got a demonstration of how Persia functioned. Nevertheless, it was not a wasted effort, because the students still learnt the concepts of hospital management, saw many patients, and learnt how much you could for the soldiers with small means. Hundreds of patients were treated at the hospital, and despite initial mistrust of the hospital, the sick gradually begged for admission. Because Polak was appointed the shah's personal physician he could no longer stay and the management was transferred to a Persian doctor. When he came back later he was shocked under what conditions patients were kept. It was like a scene from medical hell. "Patients with typhus and dysentery literally danced in their own feces and vomit." Also, all trees and bushes that he had financed with his own money had disappeared.[110] By 1860, it did not deserve the name of a hospital anymore, according to Häntzsche.[111]

Polak also had insisted to appoint a number of physicians as sanitary inspectors of army barracks. It was their task to ensure that preventive measures were taken to maintain proper hygienic conditions in the barracks, and to acquaint new recruits with preventive medical rules. To provide them with guidelines he had written instructions in Persian.[112]

The system became ineffective after Amir Kabir's fall from power, for in 1860, Häntzsche remarked that it was rare to find doctors attached to the troops, even in wartime. If there, these military physicians were badly paid, were insufficient in numbers and without any medicines.[113] According to official data, there were a number of army doctors and surgeons, however. In 1880 there were 106 of them. The chief army doctor (*ra'is al-atebba hakim-bashi-ye koll-e nezam*) was at the head of these army doctors, assisted by the chief doctor of the artillery corps (*hakim-bashi-ye tupkhaneh*), the chief surgeon (the *jarrah-bashi*), and the chief bookkeeper (*sar-reshtehdar-e atebba*). There were 10 doctors at the artillery corps, under a superintendent, the chief doctor of the artillery corps (*hakim-bashi-ye tupkhaneh*). There also was a new army hospital or *Dar al-Shafa'-ye Jadid-e Naseri-ye Tupkhaneh* with a staff of 15, consisting of two physicians, one surgeon, one chemist, one supervisor (*nazer*), four nurses (*parestar*); two cooks/washermen, and four guards.[114]

---

[110] Polak, *Persien*, vol. 1, 307-11. According to Elgood, *Medical History*, p. 512, the hospital was first put under the management of Dr. Polak and Dr. Schlimmer.
[111] Häntzsche, "Specialstatistik," p. 442.
[112] Polak, "Medicinische Briefe," p. 140.
[113] Häntzsche, "Specialstatistik," p. 442.
[114] E`temad al-Saltaneh, *al-Ma'ather*, pp. 349, 361. Sepehr, `Abdol-Hoseyn. *Mer'at al-Vaqaye`-ye Mozaffari va Yaddashtha-ye Mslek al-Mo'arrekhin* ed. `Abdol-Hoseyn Nava'i (Tehran: Zarrin,

In 1868, a new hospital was built for the army. The old one was now dedicated for civilian use and was placed under the management of Dr. Albo, who taught at the *Dar al-Fonun*. The old hospital became known as the *marizkhaneh-ye dowlati*.[115] A director and sub-director managed it. The staff consisted of three doctors, a manager (*mobasher*), a chemist (*davasaz*), two supervisors (*nazer*), one cook (*tabbakh*), one receiver, six nurses (*parestar*), one bathhouse attendant, one barber, and five washermen.[116]

The new military hospital was a small building with only a few rooms with about 20 beds. It was nicknamed 'the cemetery of the living.' There were no sick, for nobody came there. There was no physician, no nurse, no staff, and no drugs, because there was no money allocated for its operation, at least it was not made available to the hospital. The idea behind its creation was that the medical students at the *Dar al-Fonun* would receive part of their practical training at the hospital. However, after the death of the European professor, who only gave one course there, the project was abandoned. According to Mme. Serena, the shah had charged his relative `Ali Qoli Mirza E`tezad al-Saltaneh to manage the hospital, which is contradicted by Nafisi (see preceding paragraph). E`tezad al-Saltaneh, the shah's uncle, was, amongst other things, Minister of Science, Mines, and Telegraph with whom `Ali Akbar Khan had very close ties. For the operation of the hospital the shah had made an annual lump sum available for the treatment of 20 soldiers. `Ali Qoli Mirza used the funds for his own private use and let the hospital slowly deteriorate. There was only a small guard of soldiers. When Naser al-Din Shah wanted to make an inspection of the hospital after he had heard about its total failure and negligence, `Ali Qoli Mirza, having been forewarned ordered a number of soldiers to feign to be ill. This happened a few minutes before the shah's arrival and the soldiers were still fully dressed. The shah, however, was not taken in by this deception. He immediately ordered the so-called patients to be given the bastinado and to cancel the annual allocation, which was due a few days later. `Ali Qoli Mirza, however, provided the shah with a logical and credible explanation of the misunderstanding and continued to receive the annual allocation.[117]

There also was a military dispensary in Tehran, "exactly opposite the entrance to the [Golestan] Palace," where soldiers went to be treated for minor injuries.[118] The government Yearbooks (*Salnameh*) continue to list under the heading '*Tabib va Jarrah*' (under Ministry of War) a number of doctors that were attached to the army.[119] Asaf al-

---

1368/1889), pp. 97-98 (chief army surgeon Mohammad Nezam al-Hokama Tabib).

[115] Elgood, *Medical History*, p. 512. Wright, *The English*, p. 126 reports that the hospital was established with German help in 1869, but he does not provide any reference for that statement and it is nowhere mentioned in publications dealing with German-Persian relations.

[116] E`temad al-Saltaneh, *al-Ma'ather*, p. 405.

[117] Serena, *Hommes*, pp. 143-44; Nafisi, "Doktor `Ali Akbar Khan," p. 57. Curzon, *Persia*, vol. 1, p. 606, also relates this story without citing Serena.

[118] Collins, *From Pigeon Post*, p. 221.

[119] See, for example, E`temad al-Saltaneh, Mohammad Hasan Khan, *Dorrar al-Teyjan* (Tehran, 1308/1890), vol. 1, p. 8 (*atebba va jarrahan-e nezam*); Ibid., *Tarikh-e Salatin* (Tehran, 1898), vol. 2, p. 10; Ibid. *Nameh-ye Daneshvaran* (Tehran, 1321/1903), vol. 5, p. 10.

Dowleh mentioned the positive role of Mirza Molla Hoseyn Hakim-Bashi-ye Nezam-e Khorasan who took good care of the troops and who had a clean and well-provisioned dispensary in 1885 in Mashad.[120] Afzal al-Molk made similar remarks about Mirza Mohammad Nazem al-Atebba, the chief army surgeon, who also was credited with having established effective army dispensaries (*dava-khanehha*) for which he had been awarded a diamond ring.[121]

STATE CIVILIAN HOSPITALS

Despite the existence of one hospital for civilians in Tehran, as well as one in Mashad for the use of pilgrims only, around 1880, a Nestorian of Salmas maintained that there was neither a hospital nor a charitable dispensary at all in Persia, which clearly was wrong.[122] It is rather surprising to note that he did not mention either the American missionary hospital/dispensary at Urumiyeh. It is true that in the 1860s the Tehran hospital was a sorry excuse for such an institution, but that situation had changed in the 1870s.[123]

In addition to the new army hospital built in 1868, another civilian one had been built in 1874 or thereabouts. The new hospital was built after Naser al-Din Shah returned from his first tour to Europe. Hajj Mirza Hasan Khan Moshir al-Dowleh, the grand vizier, wanted to build a hospital in Tehran like the ones he had seen in Europe. He put `Ali Akbar Khan, a new graduate from the *Dar al-Fonun*, in charge of the construction of the *Marizkhaneh-ye Dowlati* (later Sina), and he remained in charge of the hospital till 1880. He then moved to Mashad, where Moshir al-Dowleh was the chief-administrator of the shrine complex and, at the latter's request established the Razavi Hospital there, which was financed from the shrine's foundation funds.[124]

In May 1889, `Eyn al-Saltaneh visited the new hospital that Eqbal al-Saltaneh had built in Tehran. He commented that it was very clean and proper.[125] But it would seem that this hospital did not remain operational. The 1317/1899 census of Tehran recorded the existence of only two unnamed hospitals, both in the Dowlat quarter.[126] The census probably referred to the old army hospital built in 1857, which then had become a civilian hospital, and the new army hospital built in 1874.

---

[120] Asaf al-Dowleh, *Asnad*, vol. 1, p. 176.
[121] Afzal al-Molk, *Afzal al-Tavarikh*, p. 139.
[122] Duval, Rubens. *Les Dialectes Néo-Araméens de Salamas* (Paris: F. Vieweg, 1883), pp. 52-53.
[123] Another Nestorian corrected this erroneous view in a book published 20 years later. Greenfield, *Verfassung*, p. 269.
[124] Elgood, *Medical History*, pp. 511-12; Nafisi, "Doktor `Ali Akbar Khan," pp. 56-57. The new hospital director became Mirza Mohammad Doktor Mo`tamed al-Atebba, who also taught Western medicine at the *Dar al-Fonun*, see Qasemi, *Danesh*, p. 7. The hospital fell under the jurisdiction of the Minister of Science, Hospital and Polytechnic (*Vazir-e `Olum va Dar al-Shafa va al-Fonun*), see Afzal al-Molk, *Afzal al-Tavarikh*, p. 5.
[125] `Eyn al-Saltameh, *Ruznameh*, vol. 1, p. 208.
[126] Sa`dvandiyan, Sirus and Ettehadiyeh (Nezam-Mafi), Mansureh. *Amar-e Dar al-Khelafeh* (Tehran: Nashr-e Tarikh, 1368/1989), pp. 353, 359, 451. For the location of the Dowlati hospital, west of the Meydan-e Tupkhaneh, see the map in Réza Moghtader, "Teheran dans ses murailles (1553-1930)," in Adle-Hourcade, *Téhéran Capitale bicentinaire*, p. 47, figure 2.

In 1904, at the suggestion of Hajj Sayyah a small hospital was established in Tehran to respond to the need for medical assistance created by the 1904 cholera epidemic. In collaboration with Mr. Naus, the Treasurer-General, and Mokhtar al-Saltaneh, the *mohtaseb* of Tehran, a building was rented and Feylosuf al-Saltaneh Mirza `Abdol-Karim was hired as its medical director, at a salary of 250 tomans per month. They also organized a system whereby sick people were transported to the hospital by droshke, all free of charge. Those that died were taken by the same service to the washers of the dead. The hackneys were paid one toman per patient. Dr. Morel, a French physician, assisted in the operation, in particular in managing the women's hospital that had been set up. Some wealthy individuals such as Moshir al-Dowleh provided further financial assistance.[127]

Shahri does not even list this hospital, which apparently must have been a temporary solution to an immediate problem (an epidemic), using a rented building. In fact, Shahri states that around 1912, there were only two Persian hospitals in Tehran, the Ahmadi (later Dowlati and ultimately Sina) and the Najmiyeh, in addition to the American and Russian hospital.[128]

By 1924, there were three government hospitals in Persia, all in Tehran. The largest and oldest was the Imperial Hospital (*marizkhaneh-ye dowlati*) with a nominal capacity of 50 beds, although this could be increased if funds were available. Most patients treated were those with acute malaria. During the summer many patients were treated in the garden under the trees. The staff consisted of a medical director, a surgeon, an assistant surgeon, a physician, an assistant physician, a surgeon aide and a physician aide, who dealt with patients who came for consultation. The nursing staff consisted of one trained nurse, two assistant nurses and 6 orderlies. The hospital had treated 499 hospitalized patients (450 men; 32 women; 17 children) during March 1923-March 1924. During the same period 6,450 outpatients were treated. Apart from in- and outgoing patients no database was kept.[129]

The Vaziri Hospital had been established in 1914, or thereabouts, with the funds of a philanthropist. It had never yet functioned properly, reason why the state took over its management in 1918. The hospital had 30 beds, for both medical and surgical cases. The director of the hospital was the chief medical officer at the same time. He also taught at the Medical School, as did the hospital's surgeon. Three students in their last year functioned as their assistants. There were eight nurses, two of which were female. During 1923-1924 the hospital admitted 344 patients and treated 1,104 outpatients.[130]

Progressive groups had agitated for the construction for a specialized women and children's hospital for a number of years. In particular, the women's journal *Shekufeh* had strongly argued for such a hospital.[131] Finally, the Women's Hospital, a small one with 20

---

[127] Sayyah, Hajj. *Khaterat-e Hajj Sayyah ya Dowreh-ye Khowf va Vahshat* ed. Hamid Sayyah (Tehran: Ebn Sina, 1347/1968), pp. 536-40.
[128] Shahri, *Tarikh*, vol. 2, p. 294.
[129] Gilmour, *Rapport*, p. 26.
[130] Gilmour, *Rapport*, pp. 26-27.
[131] *Shekufeh*, p. 199 (year 2, nr. 12, 23 Rajab, 1333/July, 23, 1915).

beds, had been established in 1918. It also served as training center for the Medical School for Women. Women were also admitted to give birth. During 1923-24, some 107 patients were admitted, 20 of which suffered from malaria. Some 1,342 outpatients were treated, of which 192 suffered from malaria. In 1921, the Medical School for Women had 13 students, who all belonged to the elite families; instruction was in French. They received a training of three years that was focused on women's diseases and obstetrics. On graduating the student received a diploma. They were not physicians, but more broadly trained than midwives.[132]

Table 5: Number of government hospitals outside Tehran and their capacity (1920)

Town	# Beds	Remarks	Nature
Enzeli	10 male + 5 female	Clinic + pharmacy	Municipality
Tabriz	30		Municipality
Hamadan	12	Only out-patients	Municipality
Mashad	(i) 70; (ii) 20; (iii) 6 male and 6 female	3 hospitals	Two Foundations (i) + (ii); British consulate (iii)
Mohammarah	20	-	Sheikh Khaz'al
Malayer	10	-	-

Source: Gilmour, *Rapport*, pp. 29-30.

There were also a number of hospitals that were established by private initiative. Gilmour does not mention them in his 1926 report, so they may have ceased operation some time before his fact-finding mission. In February 1886, Asaf al-Dowleh wrote that he intended to build a hospital in Tehran. The land had already been bought and land preparation had started. Unfortunately, there is no further mention of this hospital in Asaf al-Dowleh's published documents. He further had proposed to establish dispensaries in Sarakhs and Seistan and argued that such facilities should be established all over Persia.[133] In September 1897, the governor of Kerman, Bahjat al-Molk, had opened a hospital for the poor inside the citadel of Kerman, which had 20 beds as well as a nursing staff. The medical director was Hajji Mahmud Khan Kermani.[134] In 1904, `Abdol-Hoseyn Mirza Farmanfarma, when governor of Kermanshah, opened a newly built hospital in the town. However, when Farmanfarma was dismissed one year later the hospital was neglected and became dilapidated. When Farid al-Molk visited it in 1905 there were no patients in it, although its doctor was present. He told the new governor that Farmanfarma had given 70 tomans per month, which was insufficient. For the operating expenses of the hospital, excluding the salary of the doctor and the cost of charcoal were 100 tomans per month.[135]

---

[132] Gilmour, *Rapport*, p. 27.
[133] Asaf al-Dowleh, *Asnad*, vol. 1, p. 220.
[134] Sepehr, *Mer'at al-Vaqaye`*, pp. 169-70.
[135] Soltani, *Joghrafiya*, vol. 1, p. 533-34; Farid al-Molk Hamadani, Mirza Mohammad `Ali Khan. *Khaterat-e Farid* ed. Mas`ud Farid Qaragozlu (Tehran: Zavvar, 1345/1967), pp. 64-65, 228, 238, 223.

The Hamadan hospital was financed by a tax on transportation, and although a bare-bones operation it provided the patients better treatment than they would receive at home. There was no surgical service, even of the most elementary kind. The Mashad hospitals were totally neglected and had ceased to operate. In 1919, the president of the Sanitary Council made a pilgrimage to Mashad and at the time took steps to re-open the two old hospitals as well as to organize a public health service for the province of Khorasan. They still were operational when Gilmour made his fact-finding mission.[136] At that time, at the initiative of Dr. Ghani, a small hospital also was constructed in Sabzavar financed by the local community.[137] This hospital escaped Gilmour's attention, as did another one in Qazvin. In 1916, at the initiative of Hajj Mohammad 'Ali Amini the Amini Hospital had been built in Qazvin. It had 25-30 beds and a dispensary. For the operational cost Mr. Amini had endowed some villages to the hospital. It continued to function till 1927 when the endowment funds were not sufficient to keep it operational and reconstruction had to take place by the State.[138]

NON-GOVERNMENTAL HOSPITALS AND DISPENSARIES
The physicians attached to the British Legation in Tehran provided medical care to the poor and rich alike from the beginning of the nineteenth century. Missionary physicians soon followed this example. The American missionaries working among the Nestorian Christians in the Urumiyeh-Salmas area in 1835 established the first regular form of medical assistance. Much later other mission groups followed suit.

As of 1865, the Indo-European Telegraph Department (IETD) operated in Persia. Its many telegraph stations were managed mostly by British staff, some of whom kept an apothecary. It was in the first place for their own use. Despite the fact that the IETD employed a number of doctors to treat its personnel, at least one telegraph station manager also assisted needy villagers, who came from far and wide seeking medical help. For example, Sergeant Glover, who ran the telegraph station in Abadeh, also ran a dispensary, which had an apothecary with more than 300 different drugs. Sergeant Glover also had an excellent reputation as a puller of teeth. Although it was part of the IETD's policy to promote goodwill among the local rural population so as to ensure that damage to the telegraph line and poles was kept to a minimum, that goodwill went only so far. When, for example, Sergeant Glover's drugs were buried beneath the ruins of the telegraph station, which had been destroyed by a flood following heavy rain, the IETD refused to pay him compensation.[139] The IETD doctors also opened dispensaries in the towns where they were stationed, such as in the bazaar of Isfahan.[140] The quarantine station operated by the British Government in the Persian Gulf also provided medical

---

[136] Gilmour, *Rapport*, pp. 29-30. According to Hasanbeygi, *Tehran-e Qadim*, p. 210, the State Hospital was renamed after Ibn Sina (Avicenna) as the Sina Hospital in 1319Q/1901. He also has (p. 209) a picture of the hospital.
[137] Ghani, *Yaddashtha*, vol. 1, pp. 190-91.
[138] Varjavand, *Sima-ye Tarikh*, vol. 3, p. 1820.
[139] Collins, *In the Kingdom*, p. 109; see also pp. 162, 276; Rubin, *The Formation*, p. 299. Not all IETD employees had such dispensaries, and whether they had them or not, still suffered from various disorders, see, e.g., Waters, *Travel Reminiscences*, p. 39.
[140] Wright, *The English*, p. 126.

assistance to the local population, in particular the poor.[141] The goodwill that was created by this kind of medical assistance was so impressive that a commercial commission sent by the Government of India to Persia in 1904 remarked: "In my journey through Persia I have noticed the very great influence that a medical man possesses, and the good that he does; the appointment of a medical officer, with Hospital Assistants, at all head-quarters is desirable, and I would further suggest that the Consular Agents at Sirjan, Rafsinjan and Bampore be selected from the subordinate medical staff, and have dispensaries at these stations."[142]

By 1883, a dispensary with waiting rooms for either sex was operating in Isfahan, and managed by the British Church Missionary Society (CMS). "Another room had been set apart as a hospital where the more serious cases are treated surgically."[143] Mary Bird of the CMS opened a dispensary for Moslem women in the Isfahan bazaar in 1891, which, despite the opposition by the olama who forcibly shut it no fewer than five times between 1894-97, remained open due to popular support from her patients.[144] In 1896, the CMS opened a hospital with dispensary in Jolfa (Isfahan) and, between 1879-1900, it further established hospitals in Yazd (1901), Kerman (1901) and Shiraz (1923), in the latter case with financial assistance from Hajj Mohammad Hoseyn Namazi. In 1902, a clinic was opened in Isfahan itself, and later a hospital was built helped by a land gift from a local rich merchant. In 1924, the hospital in Shiraz was converted into a large hospital with financial assistance of the IETD.[145] Many of the Mission hospitals and schools had been made possible by the largesse of Persian merchants and other wealthy individuals, both Moslem and non-Moslem.[146]

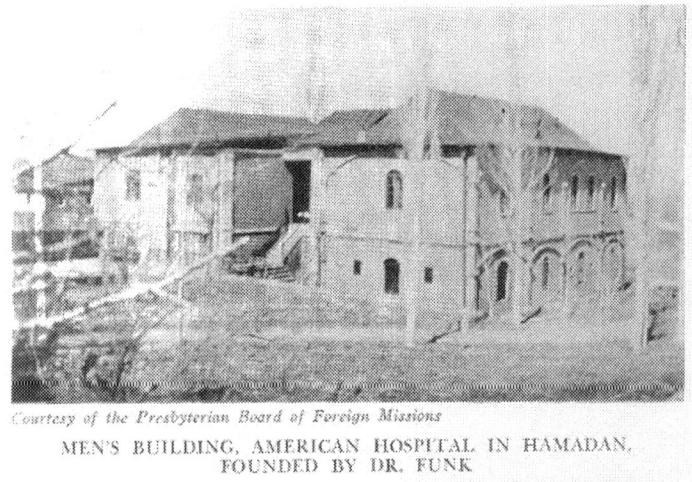

Figure 14: Men's building, American hospital in Hamadan.

---

[141] Sadid al-Saltaneh, *Bandar `Abbas*, p. 169.
[142] Gleadowe-Newcomen, A.H. *Report of a commercial mission to Persia* (Calcutta, 1904), p. 19.
[143] Wills, *In the land*, p. 164; Elgood, *Medical History*, p. 534.
[144] For the story of the clerical oppostion see Rice, *Mary Bird*, pp. 70-77
[145] Elgood, *Medical History*, pp. 534-35; N.N. "Current Topics," *Moslem World* 14 (1924), p. 182.
[146] Linton, *Persian Sketches*, p. 73; Rice, *Mary Bird*, pp. 133-34; Stuart, *Doctors in Persia*, p. 19.

Following the medical assistance provided by Dr. Grant after 1835, the American missionaries established a regular hospital in Urumiyeh in 1882 that was managed by Dr. Cochran. According to Aubin, as of about 1875, the American missionaries established a 15-bed hospital with dispensary in Tabriz, which initially mainly served the Armenian population. However, another source states that Drs. Holmes and Mary Bradford began their medical work in Tabriz only as of 1881, while it was only in 1913 that Dr. Lamme established a hospital in that town.[147] Another American protestant denomination opened a clinic in Tabriz in the early 1920s, which remained open till 1928.[148] As of 1882, the American missionaries had a doctor operating in Hamadan (Dr. E.W. Alexander later joined by Dr. G. Holmes), while Dr. Funk established a hospital in Hamadan in 1903. American missionaries opened their medical dispensary in 1881 in Tehran (Dr. N. Torrence, later joined by Dr. Mary Smith, the first female physician in Persia) and established a hospital therein 1893. A women's hospital was also built in 1897 in Tehran. Dr. Frame began his medical work in 1905 in Resht and built a hospital there in 1923; Dr. Blanche Wilson began her work in Kermanshah in 1905 and in 1922 a small hospital was established there. Dr. Cook started his medical work in Mashad in 1913 (later joined by Dr. Rolla Hoffman). The American missionaries had a total of about 188 beds by 1920 and treated more than 30,000 patients per year. They only charged money for drugs, if the patient was rich; the poor received both treatment and drugs free-of-charge.[149] Wilson reported that the Mission Hospitals and dispensaries treated tens of thousands of patients every year. They also provided education in hygiene and trained native physicians, especially at Urumiyeh.[150] The number of non-governmental hospitals was reduced after World War I. Due to the Russian Revolution the Russian hospitals were closed, while the French missionary service also stopped its operations. The German medical staff did not return, while the number of private (Russian and Armenian) physicians in the North increased. The situation of private hospitals in 1909 is represented in Table 6.

Table 6: Foreign Private Hospitals and Private Modern Physicians in Persia (1909)

Nationality	Type of organization	Location	Type of service	Staff
American	Presbyterian Mission	Urumiyeh, Tabriz, Resht, Tehran, Hamadan; Qazvin*, Kermanshah*	Hospital (plus apothecary) *polyclinic	11 physicians of which 2 female
British	British Government and Church	Tehran, Mashad, Torbat-e Heydari, Naserabad,	Small government hospital in	At least 10

---

[147] Aubin, *La Perse*, p. 45; Government of Iran, *Iran-Shahr* 2 vols. (Tehran: Unesco, 1964), vol. 2, pp. 1449-50.
[148] Sajjadi, "Bimarestan," p. 261.
[149] ʿEyn al-Saltameh, *Ruznameh*, vol. 1, pp. 377, 865; Government of Iran, *Iran-Shahr*, vol. 2, pp. 1449-51; Elgood, *Medical History*, pp. 511-12, 534.
[150] Wilson, *Persian Life*, p. 310.

	Missionary Society	Kermanshah, Bushire Isfahan, Kerman, Yazd, Shiraz	Torbat and Mashad. CMS had hospitals in Kerman and Yazd one for women, and one for men;	
Russian	Red Cross; Government; Road Company	Tehran; Mashad, Torbat-e Heydari; Tabriz; Urumiyeh	Small hospital (Tabriz) (Torbat) (Urumiyeh)	At least 4
German	Government	Tehran, Tabriz, Barforush, Resht, Hamadan, Senneh, Kermanshah	Legation physician and one that directs the government hospital. In all towns German apothecaries	2
French	Private; Lazarists#	Tehran, Tabriz, Bushire, Khosrova#	As teachers at the *Dar al-Fonun*, government service. Small hospital at Khosrova#	At least 4 + a Nestorian trained in France at Khosrova
Persian Moslem and Armenian	Private	Tehran, Tabriz, Bushire, etc.	In private practice or attached to foreign hospitals	At least 10

Source: Grothe, *Zur Natur*, pp. 131-32; Aubin, *La Perse*, p. 71 (The Lazarists had a small hospital of eight beds; the American hospital had 40 beds; the dispensary was open twice per week).

In 1900, the Yazd CMS hospital treated 35,600 patients, some of who even came from Baluchistan and Afghanistan to seek treatment, while in 1907 the American hospitals treated 30,000 patients.[151] Dr. Malcolm wrote that, "there was some truth in what one doctor said, that more than half the cases that came into the [CMS Yazd] hospital had come there in consequence of the Persian doctors' treatment. The remedy is generally worse than the disease."[152] The CMS operation in Kerman started in 1902 with a small hospital, with a male and a female section. In 1913 a bigger hospital was completed, mostly with funds and land gifts from the local Kermani community. In the 1920s the hospital was further enlarged and modernized.[153]

---

[151] Stileman, *The Subjects*, p. 75. Grothe, *Zur Natur*, p. 131.

[152] Malcolm, *Children*, p. 89; Stuart, *Doctors in Persia*, p. 7.

[153] A Friend of Iran, *"Dawdson," The Doctor*, p. 27, 34, 54-56, 58-59, 63; Rice, *Mary Bird*, p. 133-34. For a description of the modern equipment the Isfahan hospital had acquired by around 1920 see Stuart, *Doctors in Persia*, pp. 17-19.

The British CMS continued its operations in four locations where it had one hospital each:[154]

Isfahan	180 beds (120 for men and 60 for women)
Kerman	80 beds (60 for men and 20 for women)
Yazd	80 beds (60 for men and 20 for women)
Shiraz	50 beds (new hospital under construction)

The American Presbyterian Missionary Society operated seven hospitals by 1920:

Mashad	50 beds
Tehran	45 beds
Resht	25 beds
Hamadan	25 beds
Kermanshah	25 beds
Tabriz	100 beds
Urumiyeh	the hospitals had been destroyed during the war and medical services were carried out in two provisional buildings.

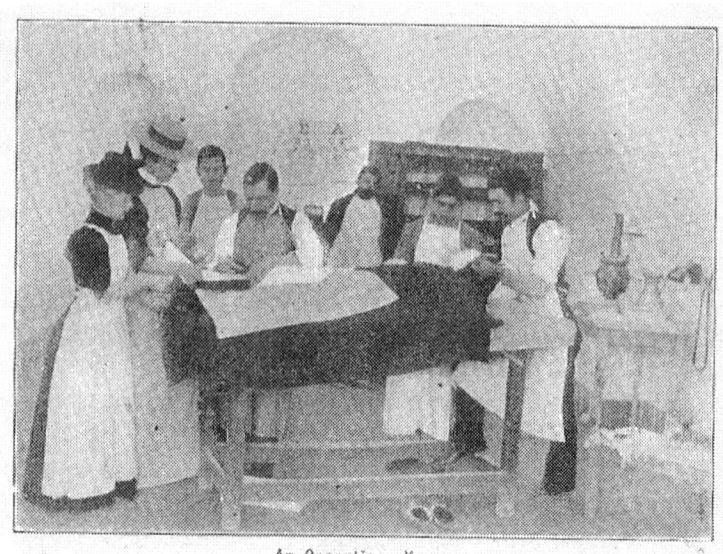

An Operation, Yazd.

Figure 15: An operation in the CMS hospital at Yazd.

Despite the long presence of the American mission in Urumiyeh in the town itself the Jewish and Moslem communities in 1892 were still "very conservative and wish no European help." Nevertheless, in 1904 the medical staff treated 12,754 patients of all

---

[154] See also Rice, *Persian Women*, pp. 261-62 as to the equipment of the CMS hospitals. The CMS also operated a dispensary in Shahr-e Kord from 1920-1923; see Amir Hoseini, Karim Nikzad. *Shenakht-e Sarzamin-e Char Mahall* (Isfahan, 1357/1979), p. 47.

creeds and ethnic groups, according to Speer.[155] The same kind of reaction was present in towns such as Yazd and Kerman.[156] However, initial stand-offishness if not hostility soon turned into acceptance and appreciation. There were still problems such as in 1908, when rumors were spread that operations were carried out in the hospital in Kerman that should not be done. A high-placed British individual even lent credence to these rumors and sent "a vindictive report" to London and, as a result, the CMS considered closing down the Kerman hospital. When the town's people learnt about the pending closure in the autumn of 1907 "a letter was written and signed by all the *mujtaheds* or leading mullahs, with 700 seals of merchants and townsfolk affixed." The CMS then decided to continue its Kerman operation.[157] Dr. Emmeline Stuart, who elaborated about the initial difficulties to overcome Moslem prejudice with regards to the Christian doctors, wrote around 1923, "No longer have we the same prejudices to contend with. No longer is the *istikhareh*, or omen, indispensable before patients submit to the treatment. It is now as a rule, only consulted by the more bigoted Moslems, or by those who do not really want to come into hospital, or who are afraid to undergo an operation."[158] When Dr. Dodson died of typhoid fever while caring for his patients in Kerman in 1937, "The Governor of the town, all the officials, and fifteen thousand people lined the narrow streets and went to the bare graveyard in the desert outside the town to do honour to the man who had served them for thirty-four years."[159]

The various British consulates also provided medical assistance to the poor. In most cases, Indian medical orderlies did the actual medical work. The dispensary in Mashad, which had one British doctor, treated about 6,000 patients per year. In Bushire, the British dispensary and small Residency hospital treated 13,000 outpatients in 1907. The British consulate's dispensary at Ahvaz treated almost one hundred patients per day.[160]

---

[155] Speer, *Hakim Sahib*, pp. 166, 270, 328-29 (in 1905 some 13,868 patients were treated).
[156] Malcolm, *Five Years*, pp. 55-59; A Friend of Iran, *"Dawdson," The Doctor*, pp. 20-21; Hume-Griffith, *Behind the Veil*, pp. 157-51
[157] A Friend of Iran, *"Dawdson," The Doctor*, pp. 55-52.
[158] Stuart, *Doctors in Persia*, p. 23.
[159] A Friend of Iran, *"Dawdson," The Doctor*, p. 73.
[160] Wright, *The English*, p. 126.

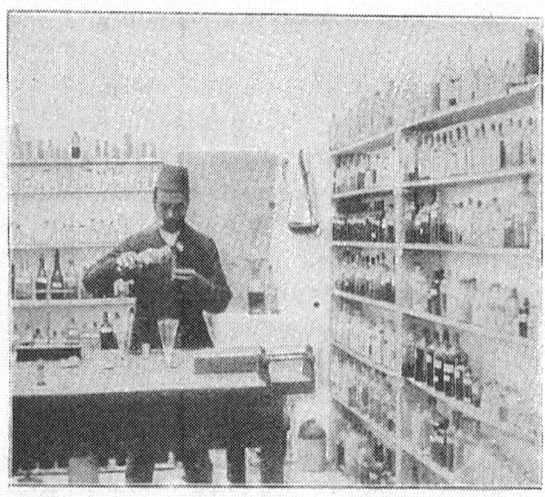

Figure 16: The CMS dispensary at Yazd.

The British APOC maintained its own medical service for its staff, although it also extended its gratis services (including dental treatment) to the local population who did not have any relationship with the Company. It operated two hospitals (one in the [oil] Fields, one in Abadan), of which the former was the most modern in Persia, as well as 12 separate dispensaries (nine in the Fields; one at Mohammarah, one at Bawardah, and one at the refinery). The Fields hospital had a capacity of 88 beds, a dispensary, two operating rooms (one for septic, the other for aseptic cases), a laboratory, and a radiology unit. The Abadan hospital had a capacity of about 100 beds, a dispensary, a dental surgery, an operation room, a pathological laboratory, a disinfection station and X-ray equipment. The number of patients treated in the Fields numbered more than 90,000 in 1926, while at Abadan the number was more than 140,000 in the same year. In the Fields the APOC employed a senior medical officer, two resident medical officers, a visiting medical officer, a consulting surgeon, a pathologist, and an ophthalmologist. These were assisted by 26 local nurses under a European matron and assisted by eight European nurses. A similar number of staff was employed at Abadan.[161]

Until November 1915, two German physicians (Dr. Ilberg and Dr. Becker) managed the Imperial Hospital. After their departure, Persian physicians ran the hospital. In 1917, the Russian used the hospital, its staff and equipment rather roughly, so that by 1918 the hospital could only receive 30 patients. The British government offered to assist with the management of the hospital and improve it, to which the Persian government agreed. As a result, between 1919-23, the British government helped to reorganize the government hospital at Tehran with 90 beds, which also supplied staff (Dr. Neligan, Dr. Scott), as well as medical stores and equipment, as did the APOC. However, because the Persian government did not provide any real support for the operation of the hospital, the unpaid and neglected Persian staff blamed the British for their problems. The British doctors,

---

[161] Williamson, *In A Persian Oil Field*, pp. 123-32.

however, were but advisers and had no decision authority. British involvement therefore became an embarrassment, reason why Great Britain withdrew its assistance in 1923.[162]

Apart from the medical facilities listed in Table 6, there also was a small hospital of 14 beds established by the Russian government on the island of Ashuradeh in 1848 to treat its naval staff as well as Russian consular staff in the Caspian littoral. Furthermore, Russia transformed the Sepahdar mansion in Qazvin into a hospital at the beginning of the World War I. The Sisters of Compassion managed it till 1918 when the Russians left, who handed it over to the British. The Russian Road Company also maintained a small hospital for its staff. It was transferred to the Persian government in 1925.[163] French nuns (*filles de charité*) also had a small hospital-dispensary in Tehran.[164]

The dispensaries and hospitals were almost empty during Ramadan, because the taking of medicine, or the use of drops into the eye, was tantamount to breaking fast. European doctors therefore had to be aware to tell the few patients that showed up to take their medicine twice a night instead of twice a day. Also, after Ramadan the dispensaries were full of patients who had overeaten at night after having eaten nothing during the day.[165] Although the patients were treated free of charge at the mission hospitals and dispensaries, they nevertheless felt that the physicians also gained something, viz., an enhanced spiritual position because of having done a good deed or *thavab*.[166] Rich Persian patients paid, of course, for their medical service and medicine. "In fact, what might be called the private practice of the doctors largely pays for the upkeep of the hospitals, with their thousands of patients."[167]

---

[162] Elgood, *Medical History*, pp. 546-49 (with details on the state of the building and staff, and how it developed later). Litten, *Persische Flitterwochen*, pp. 6, 242; Wright, *The English*, p. 127.
[163] Teymuri, Ebrahim. `Asr-e Bikhabari (Tehran, 1363/1984), pp. 269-71 (Russia also obtained a concession for the establishment of a hospital in Astarabad); Elgood, *Medical History*, p. 512; Varjavand, Parviz. *Sima-ye Tarikh va Farhang-e Qazvin*. 3 vols. (Tehran: Ney, 1377/1998), vol. 3, pp. 1818, 1822. There also was a temporary hospital in Urmiyeh, which was started in 1915 to combat the cholera epidemic. It was discontinued when the Russian troops left in 1918.
[164] Hassendorfer, "Les médecins français," p. 61.
[165] Malcolm, *Children*, p. 49.
[166] Malcolm, *Children*, p. 55.
[167] Rice, *Mary Bird*, p. 134 ("About two-thirds of the working expenses of the hospitals, apart from drugs, are paid locally.")

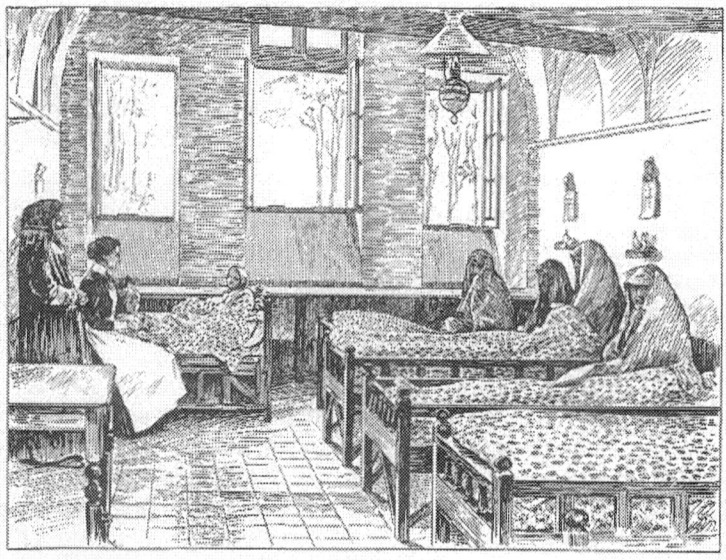

Figure 17: A women's ward of the CMS hospital at Jolfa.

QUARANTINE

A third delivery mechanism for modern Western medical science was that of increased public health awareness and sensitization. Although the growing capacity of the modern Western medical infrastructure was able to treat ever more patients after 1890, it was more important to try and prevent that infectious diseases occurred. Despite the outbreaks of localized as well as national epidemics the Persian government had not developed a system to contain the spread of disease. In 1809, Tancoigne observed that there was no system of quarantine in Persia.[168] Some form of quarantine was applied by individual governors, such as happened in 1821 at Shiraz during the cholera epidemic at Bushire[169] as well as during the plague of 1831. At that time, nobody from Tabriz, where the plague raged, was allowed to enter the town of Khoy, for example.[170] When, in 1852, cholera broke out, Amir Kabir imposed quarantine at the border with Iraq.[171] In November 1856, the government tried to stop pilgrims going from Kermanshah, where cholera had broken out, to Iraq, where the Turkish authorities had already imposed quarantine rules since 1854. The pilgrims were kept at the border for 10 days and then the Persian authorities wanted to keep them there for another 10 to 20 days. Food was running out, however, and

---

[168] Tancoigne, *A Narrative*, p. 244. Nevertheless, servants of the British mission coming from Tiflis had to "perform a quarantine," before they were allowed into Erevan. Morier, *A Second*, p. 335.
[169] Rich, *Narrative*, vol. 2, p. 224.
[170] Stocqueler, J.H. *Fifteen Months' Pilgrimage trough untrodden tracts of Khuzistan and Persia* (London: Saunders and Otley, 1832), vol. 1, p. 186.
[171] Adamiyyat, *Amir Kabir*, p. 326; for the ongoing international discussion on the need for quarantines as reported in the Persian press see Government of Iran, *Vaqaye`-ye Ettefaqiyeh*, vol. 1, pp. 500, 579; vol. 2, pp. 913, 2778 (*kerakhtin, qeranteyn, qerantineh*).

given the lack of order and organization the estimated 15,000 pilgrims forced their way into Iraq and several people, including soldiers, were killed.[172] In 1861, a non-commissioned officer who had been charged with containing a cholera outbreak stopped the Prussian embassy at Zarghan. He gave the embassy instructions which villages to avoid.[173] Since 1864, if not earlier, the British Political Resident had been practically vested with sanitary control of Bushire by the government of Persia. This also meant that all vessels calling on Bushire were quarantined at sea.[174] But such public health measures were the exception rather than the rule.

In 1868, the *Majles-e Hefz al-Sehhah* or Sanitary Board was formed under the presidency of Dr. Tholozan. The board was mainly composed of Persian physicians. Tholozan wrote a pamphlet on "how to diagnose cholera and what to do?" Polak had already drawn up such a document in 1858 for army officers to acquaint them with the symptoms of malaria, dysentery, typhoid fever and colds, and what to do about it. These were the main diseases of which soldiers died. Polak had been very pleased when the officers told him later that with use of his pamphlet they had managed to reduce mortality among their troops to an unheard of minimum.[175] Due to a total lack of support the Board's work was discontinued after six months. According to Abbas Khan, it was but a national debating club that had neither charter nor rules, and only met in case of need, such as when there was an outbreak in or near Tehran.[176] Tholozan did not accept this defeat and made a proposal to Naser al-Din Shah to improve public hygiene in a realistic manner. Tholozan was aware of the fact that most of the population lacked the means to bring about a change in both personal and public hygiene. However, certain changes were possible, changes that the government could enforce, or so he believed. His proposal consisted the establishment of a Public Health Council, of a ban on pilgrimage when there was an epidemic, a total ban on the transport of corpses to the holy sites, construction of public latrines and sewers, canalization of water towards the towns, construction of public washing places, construction of decent housing for the poor, renovation of caravanserais and public baths, and the appointment of public health doctors in the main towns of Persia. These items remained on the agenda for the improvement of public health and some of them were implemented towards the end of the Qajar reign, although most of them only were realized in the mid 1950s and thereafter.[177]

Although the Persian government did not adopt any of the measures that Tholozan had proposed, it would change its position somewhat a few years later. After the Great Famine of 1871-73 that had been accompanied by a cholera epidemic and the plague, Naser al-Din Shah at the urging of the European medical community led by Dr.

---

[172] De Gobineau, A. *Les Dépêches Diplomatiques.* ed. Adrienne Doris Hytier (Geneva-Paris: Droz-Minard, 1959), p. 34.
[173] Brugsch, *Reise*, vol. 2, pp. 164, 200.
[174] Lorimer, *Gazetteer*, p. 2533; Elgood, *Medical History*, pp. 515-16.
[175] Polak, *Persien*, vol. 1, p. 310.
[176] Ebrahim-Nejad, "La médecine européenne," p. 84; Kotobi, L'émergence," p. 267 both citing Dr. Tholozan, *Rapport à Sa Majesté le Chah sur l'état actuel de l'hygiène en Perse. Progrès à réaliser et moyens de les effectuer* (Tehran, August 1869) litho; Abbas Khan, *Taoun*, p. 129.
[177] Ebrahim-Nejad, "La médecine européenne," pp. 85-86.

Tholozan, decided to create a new institution that would be responsible for the country's public health. The board was first known as Board of Health (*Majles-e Sehhat*) and later as Sanitary Council (*Majles-e Hefz al-Sehhat*). Tholozan, who was the driving force behind the Council, was, in the words of Elgood, "indefatigable. He instituted a rudimentary quarantine system, revived the public vaccination service, which Dr. Cloquet had initiated. He dispatched into the provinces physicians, trained by him in the Dar-ul-Funun, armed with the necessary outfit to deal with epidemics in the villages."[178] However, these laudatory activities are not confirmed by other sources.

The International Sanitary Commission meetings of Istanbul (1866) and Vienna (1874) had obliged Persia to create a Board of Health in Tehran and to organize an effective public health service in the provinces. Despite Persian promises nothing much had been done. Ottoman Turkey had a great interest, as did Europe, in what happened in Persia, because of the spread of cholera. The Ottoman medical representative, Dr. Castaldi, who had been sent to Tehran to monitor Persian compliance did not leave off pressing the Persian government.[179]

It was only in 1876 that the Persian government finally gave in, because of an outbreak an epidemic of diphtheria in Tehran, cholera in Seistan, and of the plague in Khuzistan in March, where about 2,500 people, of which 1,800 in Shushtar, died. The governor of Bushire imposed quarantine, and also asked the British authorities to do the same at sea. In April 1876, a quarantine station had been opened on Abadan Island to control all traffic from the Shatt al-Arab, although the application of the quarantine was sloppy. In June 1876, Naser al-Din Shah instructed the creation of a public health or sanitary council (*Majles- hefz-e sehhah*) with a view to safeguard public health. To that end physicians were to convene once per week under the auspices of the Ministry of Science. They had to bring to the authorities' attention from all parts of Persia how to safeguard public health, to prevent the outbreak of diseases. From among this council, experienced physicians with the title of *hafez al-sehheh* had to be appointed to each city and province to promote public health and to treat people and to send reports on the state of health of the population and diseases to the central council.[180] These also had to begin with a compulsory campaign of smallpox vaccination and they had to report monthly about its results.[181]

The Council consisted of Persian and European physicians in equal numbers, under the chairmanship of `Ali Qoli Mirza. He held two meetings. The first one decided to establish two quarantine stations on Persian soil, viz. at Qasr-e Shirin and Bushire. A number of soldiers were stationed there, whose commander served as medical inspector at the same time. All arrivals from Ottoman territory were kept in a kind of sheep corral, where they had to pay 6 francs/tomans per day, if they were Persians, and twice as much if they were

---

[178] Elgood, *Medical history*, p. 518; Browne, E.G. *Arabian Medicine* (Cambdridge, 1924), p. 518.
[179] G.D. "Sanitätsreformen," p. 299; Lorimer, *Gazetteer*, pp. 2520-22.
[180] E`temad al-Saltaneh, Mohammad Hasan Khan. *Ketab al-Athar va'l-Ma'ather* (Tehran, 1306/1884), p. 56 [new] 115 [old]; Nafisi, "Doktor `Ali Akbar Khan," p. 57; Lorimer, *Gazetteer*, p. 2533; Elgood, *Medical History*, p. 519.
[181] E`temad al-Saltaneh, *Montazer*, vol. 1, p. 242; vol. 2, p. 343.

Ottoman subjects. Food and water had to be paid for extra and at excessively high prices. The length of stay depended on what kind of agreement could be reached with the commanding officer, and could last for months after the end of an epidemic. Munis Effendi, the Ottoman ambassador in Tehran, was able to put a stop to these proceedings in the fall of 1876. The second meeting decided to send a physician to Luristan where in March 1876 a severe pest epidemic had broken out. One year later the Persian doctor still had not reached Luristan, but it did not prevent him from sending fictitious reports based on hearsay. Because he was not paid the Persian doctor had attached himself to the suite of the Persian governor of Arabistan and traveled with him and thus was ensured of his daily needs.

After the two sessions the Board of Health ceased its activities, because the threats made by Munis Effendi had thwarted the popularity of medical reform. It was only in the spring of 1877 with the outbreak of the plague in Iraq and of cholera in Khorasan that at Dr. Castaldi's urgings the Sanitary Council was convened again. As of February 1877, each Sunday the Council met regularly presided over by `Ali Qoli Mirza. Drs. Tholozan and Castaldi as well as Persian physicians were members. Tea was drunk and water pipes were smoked, but not much business was done or discussed. The most concrete result was a too high tariff for quarantine operations, which was 10 times higher than the already too high Ottoman tariff. In addition, statistics were collected about mortality in the major cities by requiring the washers of the dead, who alone were permitted to perform the ritual washing, to provide that information on a weekly basis. Because of the existence of the telegraph the Tehran council was able to form an opinion about the state of public health of the entire country. From these early statistics it became immediately clear that the recently introduced disease of diphtheria had become a major problem. Similarly, smallpox also raged, and of 760 persons affected in Isfahan only 30 survived. The Sanitary Council continued to debate these phenomena without taking any action, however.[182]

Later Dr. Tholozan, the *hakim-bashi-ye hozur*, headed the sanitary council of Tehran. Other members were Dr. Kampusan Pir (Turkey) and Dr. Albo of the *Dar al-Fonun*. The members of the central council numbered 15 persons, and included leading traditional physicians who were hostile to Western medicine such as Mirza Mohammad Taqi Shirazi, Fakhr al-Atebba Kani and Mirza Ahmad Kashi. The council of Azerbaijan and West-Persia had members in Tabriz, Khoy, Maragheh, Urumiyeh, Sanandaj, Kurdistan, Zenjan, Qazvin, Resht, Hamadan, and Kermanshah. In Khorasan and Mazandaran there were members at Mashad, Sabzavar, Shahrud, Semnan, Astarabad, and Mazandaran. In Fars it had members in Shiraz, Isfahan, Kashan, Qom, Lorestan and `Arabestan, Yazd, Kerman, and Bushire.[183] That these physicians were indeed in place is confirmed by Basir ol-Molk, who, when in Mashad, wrote that, "this morning Mirza Mostafa, the doctor of the sanitary council (*hafez al-sehhah*), gave me four *methqal*s of iodide-potassium (*yodurudupatas*), one *methqal* of a hot medicine, 13 *nakhod* of epicacuanha (*epika*). I gave

---

[182] G.D. "Sanitätsreformen," pp. 299-300; Elgood, *Medical History*, p. 519-22; Kashani-Sabet, Firoozeh. "'City of the Dead': the Frontier Polemics of Quarantines in the Ottoman Empire and Iran," *Comparative Studies of South Asia, Africa, and the Middle East* 18/2 (1998), pp. 51-54.
[183] E`temad al-Saltaneh, *al-Ma'ather*, Appendix pp. 42-43.

8,000 [dinars] the price of the iodide (*yodur*) as written."[184] In Mashad, in 1882, an attempt was made, with the support of the governor, to initiate a public health program that included better hygienic conditions in public places and facilities.[185]

The council tried to meet regularly, but this was not always possible due to the fact that many of its members were court physicians, who had to accompany the shah on his many outings. Also, during summertime many moved to cooler parts and were not available for meetings in Tehran. When the council met, a report was prepared of its meeting, a summary of one of which was published in the newspaper *Danesh*. The paper reported that Mirza Hesam al-Din Tabib Hafez al-Sehhah-ye Shiraz had sent a report on cholera to the Council. He ascribed the occurrence of this disease to rice cultivation around Shiraz and the filthy state of its streets.[186] The same newspaper also discussed public health issues drawing upon the French publication *Journal d'Hygiene* as well as developments in medical science.[187] Apart from the appointment of these public health doctors nothing happened. Unfortunately, the health officers placed in the provinces were poorly trained, prepared or equipped. They had no training in public health, no laboratory, no drugs, and some officers left, because they had not been paid. Sometimes the public health officers tried to misuse their authority for their own benefit as in the case of a Persian quarantine doctor who "threatened to fumigate the people [British Indian caravaneers], unless they gave him money."[188]

Browne, who attended one of the meetings of the Board in the end of 1887, was favorably impressed with the quality of the discussion that was attended by 16 of the chief Persian physicians of Tehran, most of whom only knew Islamic-Galenic medicine. The death rate of Tehran and the chief provincial towns were read and discussed. Also, different treatments of ophthalmia and a case of lithotomy were discussed. However, he did not have much faith in the reliability in the reports on the causes of mortality, because these reports relied on information provided by the washers of the dead.[189]

The Sanitary Council failed to reach an agreement with the countries bordering Persia as to the establishment of quarantine posts. The discussions had led to nowhere due to lack of funds and differences of opinion.[190] The proper functioning of the quarantine system was also inhibited by the fact that provincial officials did not provide a reliable

---

[184] E'tesam al-Molk, *Safarnameh*, p. 170; also in Kermanshah (Soltani, *Joghrafiya*, vol. 1, p. 538), Semnan (Rafi`, *Tarikh-e Semnan*, p. 546), Kerman (Vaziri, *Joghrafiya*, p. 52), Qom (Afzal al-Molk, *Tarikh*, p. 146, Qasemi, *Danesh*, p. 20); Najm ol-Molk, *Safarnameh*, pp. 9, 54, 178 (Khuzestan), Shiraz (Qasemi, *Danesh*, p. 33), and Bushire (Ya Hoseyni, Sayyed Qasem, *Sad Sal-e Matbu`at-e Bushehr* [Bushire: Ershad-e Melli-ye Bushehr, 1374/1995], p. 232); Hamadan (Badi`i, *Yaddashtha*, p. 278; Afzal al-Molk, *Afzal al-Tavarikh*, p. 198); Pirzadeh, *Safarnameh*, vol. 1, p. 17 (Shiraz).
[185] Nezam al-Saltaneh Mafi, *Khaterat va Asnad*, vol. 1, pp. 27-29 and appendix 3 to this book.
[186] Qasemi, *Danesh*, p. 33 (nr. 9, 1 Dhu'l-Hejjah 1299/15 October, 1882)
[187] Qasemi, *Danesh*, pp. 41 (nr. 11, 1 Moharram 1299/13 November, 1882), 49 (nr. 13, 1 Safar 1300/12 September, 1882) regarding rabies, 55 (diphtheria)
[188] Benn, *Overland*, p. 117.
[189] Browne, *A Year*, pp. 107-08; Ibid., *Arabian Medicine* (Cambridge, CUP, 1921), p. 93.
[190] Lorimer, *Gazetteer*, pp.2533-45; Elgood, *Medical History*, pp. 522-23.

assessment of the local medical situation, even when the shah explicitly asked for it.[191] Some of the diseases continued to be imported, even after a system of quarantine was established at the border posts in 1876, because it was not applied effectively. Inside Persia itself there was no effective control,[192] because it was haphazard in nature and often imposed too late.[193] The effectiveness of the quarantine system was also undermined, because Dr. Tholozan was not very much in favor of such a system, and, in fact, he later even opposed it.[194] He nevertheless drew up regulations for the quarantine service and took steps for the establishment of a quarantine station at Khaneqin. This station was on the Ottoman-Persian border and the entry point for the caravans of pilgrims and of corpses coming from Persia with destination Karbala. This measure was also in response to international agreements that Persia had reached in 1870 and 1878 with the Ottoman Empire, *viz.*, that corpses could only be transported to Ottoman territory (Karbala) three years after the date of death, and that a sanitation control post would be established at the border.[195]

Persia joined the articles of the International Sanitation Commission (3 April 1893, and 30 October 1897) with regards to the Mecca pilgrims and the Persian Gulf regulations.[196] The Persian government imposed quarantine in case cholera occurred in Khuzistan, as occurred in September 1889 in Shushtar.[197] This was not always possible due to the lack of facilities and other means to have an impact. This was the case in July 1892, when the British consul urged to impose quarantine in Bandar `Abbas and Lengeh.[198] In 1897, when there was a rumor of possible outbreak of plague in the Gulf, Russia immediately sent a sanitary commission to Bandar-e Gaz to contain the disease if it showed itself.[199]

In 1904 the Persian Sanitary Council was re-established. It replaced the earlier council, which had grown into medical discussion society rather than a body of public health service. The function of the new Council was to reduce the spread of infectious diseases,

---

[191] Nateq, "Ta'thir," pp. 48-49.
[192] Gilbar, "Demographic Developments," p. 140; Kashani-Sabet, "'City of the Dead'," p. 53.
[193] Speer, *Hakim Sahib*, p. 165.
[194] Ebrahim-Nejad, "La médecine européenne," pp. 86-88, for his arguments. Tholozan also admitted to his compatriot Binder, Henry. *Au Kurdistan* (Paris: Quantin, 1887), p. 390-93 that he considered quarantine of limited value. Tholozan most likely just adhered to the conclusion reached by the 1874 Cholera Conference at Vienna, which recommended the abandonment of land quarantine for Europe, but insisted on the maintenance of sea quarantine, see Lorimer, *Gazetteer*, p. 2522 and Kashani-Sabet, "'City of the Dead'," pp. 54-55.
[195] Elgood, *Medical History*, p. 520; Wright, *The English*, p. 127. There were doctors who worked for the Sanitation Council, see Sepehr, *Mer'at al-Vaqaye`*, pp. 217 (Hamadan), 225 (author of a book on Public Health). For the functioning of quarantine system as seen from the Turkish side of the Persian border see Saad, Lamec. *Sechzehn Jahre als Quarantänearzt in der Türkei* (Berlin: Reimer, 1913).
[196] Greenfield, *Verfassung*, p. 273; Elgood, *Medical History*, p. 523.
[197] Nezam al-Saltaneh Mafi, *Khaterat va Asnad*, vol. 2, p. 45.
[198] Nezam al-Saltaneh Mafi, *Khaterat va Asnad*, vol. 2, pp. 119, 140 (Bushire and hinterland).
[199] Kalmykov, *Memoirs*, p. 96. The Russians also wanted to send the commission to the Gulf, which neither the British nor Persians wanted and led to the British taking control over the sanitary arrangements in the ports, see Lorimer, *Gazetteer*, p. 2547.

in particular of cholera and the plague, through Persia. It collected data, organized public health preventive measures, arranged for vaccinations and supervised the import and distribution of narcotic drugs. It further advised the Persian government on all matters concerning public health. Under the auspices of the Ministry of the Interior, the Council became the chief public health authority in Persia. Its members were composed of 12 Persian doctors, medical representatives of the ministries of Foreign Affairs and the Interior, the Customs Administration and the Police, two foreign professors from the Medical School, and doctors of the foreign Legations. There also were some honorary members who did not have a vote.[200]

In 1904, the quarantine system on the border with Iraq was severely tested and found wanting when one of the well-known olama of Najaf traveled with a large number of his disciples (*tollab*) on pilgrimage to Mashad. The quarantine staff at Kermanshah refused the group entry into the city and insisted that it took up lodgings in the quarantine station to determine that they had not been infected with cholera that was raging at that time in Najaf. The disciples told the health officials that, "the footsteps of His Eminence (*hezrat-e aqa*) are sacred and merciful, and wherever he sets foot the calamity will be lifted. There is no need for quarantine." When the health officials pointed out that His Eminence had been present in Najaf and Karbala and that it had not prevented the epidemic to strike there the disciples replied by giving them a severe trouncing with their sticks. After all, one does not question the word of a leading religious personality in Persia. Then they moved quickly into Kermanshah. The next day a few of them fell ill, and that same day 23 of them died. The remainder spread out and traveled to Borujerd, Isfahan, Hamadan and other places and nobody dared to stop them and thus the cholera spread. Finally, via Qom, they arrived at Tehran and spread the disease there. The rich and mighty took to the hills, the weak and the poor remained behind and many of them fell victim to the disease, "as is usually the case," Hajj Sayyah the source for this event wrote.[201]

Following an agreement with the Persian government in 1897, the quarantine service in the Persian Gulf was ensured by the Government of India, which had placed medical officers at the head of five Persian quarantine stations, which also had disinfecting equipment, viz., at Bushire, Mohammarah, Bandar `Abbas, Lingeh and Jask. Members from the Indian Medical Service staffed the stations; they were supervised by the Bushire Residency physician, but paid by the Persian government. They had no responsibility for the public health of the town where they were located, although there were British

---

[200] Government of Great Britain, *Geographical Handbook*, p. 409; Lorimer, *Gazetteer*, p. 2251 (because the Council was presided by a French doctor, who tended to disregard the official reports by the British Residency Surgeon and to give more weight to "the irresponsible reports" by a French doctor stationed in the Gulf, the British were not entirely pleased with the effectiveness of the council. This changed, when a Persian physician took over the council's presidency and Dr. Neligan, the British Legation physician, became its vice-president). The French were therefore also very much upset when, due to a disagreement between the French ambassador in Tehran and Dr. Schneider, the British Dr. George replaced the latter as president of the Coucil in 1906. Nategh, "Les Persans," p. 192; Elgood, *Medical History*, p. 526-29.

[201] Sayyah, *Khaterat*, pp. 535-36. In the first decade of the twentieth century, Ayatollah `Abdol-Hoseyn Lari declared that the system of quarantine and payment of the passport (*tadhkereh*) were an innovation (*bed`at*) and thus forbidden. Lari, "Shesh Resaleh," p. 225.

dispensaries in Bushire and Bandar `Abbas (as of 1906). Also, they had no means to stop Arabs fleeing epidemics on the other side of the Gulf to the Persian littoral. The chief medical officer was based in Bushire, in addition to the two regular physicians already there. He reported to the Sanitary Council. The fact that Persian Moslems had to get sanitary certificates from British doctors caused some resentment, even leading to anti-British demonstrations in 1899 in Bushire. It came therefore as no surprise that in 1928 that fiercely nationalistic Reza Shah took over the control of the quarantine system in the Persian Gulf from the British.[202]

The best descriptions of how the quarantine system functioned refer to the situation in Bushire, a location that most European travelers visited and thus had to experience its administrations. Because the British-Indian government had been delegated the responsibility to maintain and manage the quarantine system in the Gulf, the British residency surgeon in Bushire was port health officer, but enforcement of the quarantine rules was the responsibility of the Bushire customs authorities. The quarantine station was on the `Abbasak island in the bay of Bushire.[203]

Quarantine inspection took place on board. Ships with the plague had to carry a yellow flag; it took one hour from anchorage to Bushire.[204] Initially 10 days of quarantine were required for a ship coming from Karachi, but in early 1907 this was cut in half. The fast mail steamer did the trip in four days, thus leaving still one to one-and-half days to be spent on the quarantine island, before being allowed to land in Bushire. Bradley-Birt qualified his stay there as, "Purgatory." The quarantine station "is a rough, hastily finished building, yet containing all that is actually required for the short, but compulsory stay." Its staff consisted of two Persians. For the Asian traveler there were huts; there are no other buildings but an incinerator to destroy the clothes of the plague-stricken. "For the white man the doctor's examination is a mere formality; for the Asiatic it is little less perfunctory."[205] The difference in treatment between English and non-English had already raised hackles with de Vilmorin in 1895, when he noted that when the Persian governor had closed the port to all ships, including Persian ones, the British consul allowed English ships to enter, but not others.[206] Also, riots broke out in Bushire when in 1899 quarantine was imposed because plague had broken out, a disease unknown until then and therefore not yet feared. People therefore resented the sanitary regulations that they considered an imposition rather than in their interest.[207]

---

[202] Wright, *The English*, p. 127; Elgood, *Medical History*, pp. 526-27, 550. For details on the implementation of the agreement, including attempts by the Customs Service to take control over the sanitary arrangements in the Persian Gulf as well as related Russian shenanigans, see Lorimer, *Gazetteer*, pp. 2547-51.
[203] Lorimer, *Gazetteer*, pp. 349, 341.
[204] Norden, Hermann. *Under Persian Skies* (Philadelphia: McCrea Smith, n.d.), pp. 44-45.
[205] Bradley-Birt, F.B. *Persia, through Persia from the Gulf to the Caspian* (Boston: J.B. Millet, 1910), pp. 28-29 (for a description of the island), 32-34.
[206] De Vilmorin, Auguste Lacoin. *De Paris à Bombay par la Perse* (Paris: Firmin-Didot Co, 1895), p. 350.
[207] Elgood, *Medical History*, p. 524.

On the Caspian littoral quarantine stations were built in 1912 at Enzeli and Astara. The latter was destroyed in the aftermath of World War I, and was not operational anymore. There also was a station at Jolfa, while funds for a new one at Mashad-e Sar had been allocated. The station at Jolfa had one public health worker, but otherwise no details are known about the staffing or equipment, despite the fact that it was the most important station on the common border with Russia. There were no stations on the border with Afghanistan and British-Baluchistan (now Pakistan). There was no quarantine station on the Iraqi and Turkish border. The dangerous transport of corpses was controlled from Kermanshah where a medical officer gave a permit if the corpse was totally desiccated or if it had a certificate proving it had been interned for at least three years. Only when an epidemic broke out a sanitary post was established at Qasr-e Shirin.[208] In Enzeli, in 1907, a French doctor was stationed as quarantine officer. As in the case of Bushire depending on one's financial position treatment was different. "By his orders the steerage passengers were detained in quarantine on the ship. The cabin passengers were permitted to land and to remain under observation at the hotel under guard of sentries. ... Meanwhile the pilgrim, resenting their differential treatment, and imagining that we had been let off all quarantine, beat their guards, effected their escape to shore, and proceeded on their way inland."[209]

Table 7: Quarantine stations and their staff (1924)

Name station	Physician	Staff	Disinfection unit	Remarks
Mohammarah	1	12	Velox	Passengers 1st-2nd-3rd class
Bushire	2	14	Bowman	All classes of passengers
Bandar `Abbas	1	17	Velox	Needs repairs
Lengah	1	9	Velox –in bad state	Only 3rd class passengers
Jask	1	10	Velox	Lacks equipment
Enzeli	1	7	Dehaitre	Ineffective control
Astara	1	4	Dehaitre	Does not function
Jolfa	n.a.	1	n.a.	n.a.
Kermanshah	n.a.	n.a.	n.a.	n.a.
Qasr-e Shirin	-	-	-	No quarantine building or control

Source: Gilmour, *Rapport*, pp. 20-24.

---

[208] Government of Great Britain, *Geographical Handbook*, pp. 412-13; Watelin, *La Perse*, p. 68 (at Astara, the quarantine station was housed in a collapsible dwelling). There had been a sanitary post in Nasratabad (Seistan) in 1906 as well as a sanitary barrier in Khorasan formed by Russia in Khorasan, for details see Elgood, *Medical History*, p. 528.

[209] Ross, *A Lady Doctor*, p. 13.

Although the European members of the Sanitary Council were not above using that body for political rather than pursuing public health objectives, new Persian members, doctors trained in Western medicine, wanted to make the council more effective. One requirement was that the Council had its own adequate budget. The Persian members were able to convince their government to levy a tax on the transport of corpses to Iraq as well as to allocate 10% of the tax on horses and carriages in 1911, which the Council intended to use for gratis smallpox vaccination campaigns.[210] After 1921, the council was transferred from the Ministry of the Interior to that of Education. The council met once a month, or more during times of epidemics. A program for a national health service had been developed, but it was only executed in Tehran.[211] Sanitary commissions had been formed in five provincial towns and 48 medical officers (in 1925) had been appointed in a number of towns.[212]

LICENSING OF PHYSICIANS

Apart from the license requirement introduced by Amir Kabir in 1851, which fell into disuse after his execution, until 1882, all Persian doctors (whether Moslem, Jewish, or Christian) as well as European doctors, practiced in Persia without having to pass an examination, or even to get permission to practice.[213] At that time, the government of Persia recognized the fact that there were too many quacks and charlatans, who were offering medical services, without having sufficient knowledge of medicines and diseases.

> In Tehran and other cities of Iran, the people who had no religion or conscience would begin treating people when they had learned something about medical herbs and the names of a few diseases, and as such, would kill people in this way. Therefore, His Imperial Majesty ordered that a major Board (*majles-e bozorg*) should be established and, in this body, the scientists and those who have good experience in this field should examine all those who want to practice medicine. In this way, separate those who are killing people and those who are not. If anybody begins a medical practice and starts treating people without having the license (*neshan*) and permission (*ejazeh*) of this Board, the person will be strongly punished.[214]

Whether it was the result of this royal order or not I do not know, but the 'licensing' of physicians also seems to have been practiced in the provinces. At least that is the conclusion that one may draw from Asaf al-Dowlch's remarks in a document dated April 20, 1870. He wrote that doctors who had neither knowledge, nor experience or training

---

[210] Elgood, *Medical History*, pp. 531-32.
[211] Government of Great Britain, *Geographical Handbook*, pp. 409; Gilmour, *Rapport*, pp. 57-61.
[212] Gilmour, *Rapport*, pp. 20.
[213] Greenfield, *Verfassung*, p. 270. Gilmour, *Rapport*, p. 33 mentioned that the doctor gave his apprentice a kind of diploma at the end of the training period, while Rasooli, *The Life Story*, p. 19, wrote that the local authorities would give a Persian doctor permission to practise.
[214] E'temad al-Saltaneh, Mohammad Hasan Khan. *Ketab al-Athar va'l-Ma'ather* (Tehran, 1306/1884), p. 115; Qasemi, *Danesh*, p. 7 (nr. 2, 7 Sha'ban, 1299/24 June, 1882) for further details; Government of Great Britain, *Geographical Handbook*, pp. 408-09.

were treating patients. He therefore had given orders to ban all those considered to be unfit to be a doctor from practicing. Application of this order was conferred upon Aqa Sayyed Ja`far Hakim-Bashi. After the latter's approval Asaf al-Dowleh also would personally test a doctor's expertise after which a license would be granted.[215]

It is unknown how many doctors there were in Persia, who had received and passed an education in Western medical studies by the end of the nineteenth century. In 1894, of the 27 medical students (amongst which one woman) at the American Missionary Hospital at Urumiyeh 14 were already practicing medicine.[216] In addition, there must have been at least fifteen Persian doctors who had received their training in Europe and some 50 that had received medical instruction at the *Dar al-Fonun*.[217] This number of doctors clearly was not enough to provide modern health care. This also struck Naser al-Din Shah when he made a trip to Mazandaran in 1882. He had been struck by the lack of medical care in the region visited, where the local population suffered from several diseases. Therefore, on his return to Tehran, he issued a writ charging Mirza Ahmad Tabib, grandson of Mirza Ahmad Hakim-bashi-ye Tonakeboni, to provide the effected population with the necessary medical treatment.[218]

Some private European physicians also had established themselves in Persia or came there for short visits. In particular the visits by two ophthalmologists at the request of Zell al-Soltan drew the attention of the elite. Mokhber al-Dowleh also invited a physician from Europe, who was a student of Kalazosky (?) and an ophthalmologist. He made 3,000 tomans/year, worked five hours per day and had two days off per week (Friday and Saturday).[219] To their number should be added the doctors working in mission hospitals, foreign legations, and foreign agencies.

Apart from several court physicians, Naser al-Din Shah also employed a royal dentist,[220] who also supplied his services to some other members of the elite, such as Naser al-Din's brother, who had 11 teeth drawn at one session, and later two more.[221] There seems also to

---

[215] Asaf al-Dowleh, *Asnad*, vol. 2, p. 45.
[216] Speer, *Hakim Sahib*, p. 185. In 1906, there were two Western trained doctors in Ardabil, see Aubin, *La Perse*, p. 108 (Dr. Sissak Moujikian trained at Istanbul and a Chaldean protestant doctor trained at Chicago); see also Safari, *Ardabil*, vol. 3, p. 477.
[217] Ekhtiar, *Dar al-Funun*, pp.177-99. According to the newspaper *Danesh* (nr. 2, 7 Sha`ban, 1299/24 June, 1882) there had been a total of 42 medical graduates from the *Dar al-Fonun* in 1882, while there were 4 medical students at that time, see Qasemi, *Danesh*, pp. 7-8.
[218] Qasemi, *Danesh*, p. 22 (nr. 6, 16 Shavval, 1299/31 August, 1882)
[219] `Eyn al-Saltaneh, *Ruznameh*, vol. 1, p. 737 (student of the famous Kalehzuski); E`temad al-Saltaneh, *Ruznameh*, pp. 1101-03 (regarding the visit of the famous eye doctor Galachuski), and by the ophthalmologist Collins, who wrote a book about his visit. Collins, Edward Treacher. *In the Kingdom of the Shah* (London: T.F.Unwin, 1896).
[220] `Eyn al-Saltaneh, *Ruznameh*, vol. 1, p. 904; vol. 2, p. 1323; E`temad al-Saltaneh, *Ruznameh*, pp. 109, 200, 237, 548, 600, 614, 618, 757, 998; Wishard, *Twenty Years*, p. 266 ("For many years, M. Hybonnet, dentist to the Court, was the only one in Tehran"); E`temad al-Saltaneh, *al-Ma'ather*, p. 390; Ibid., *Ruznameh*, p. 26 (*chahar-shanbeh* 28); Hassendorfer, "Les médecins français," p. 61.
[221] `Eyn al-Saltaneh, *Ruznameh*, vol. 1, p. 336; vol. 2, p. 1073; E`temad al-Saltaneh, *al-Ma'ather*, p. 390 (he was one of the European court physicians or *atebba-ye khasseh-ye ferangi*).

have been a female dentist in Tehran in the late 1880s. Basir al-Molk noted in his Diary that went to the house of the dentist, who was a woman named Mme Valet (?), the sister of Mr. Vakstal.[222] However, most members of the elite initially did not make use of the European dentist, according to Mostowfi.[223] One of them did, however, and provided interesting information about the cost of dental help in 1896 in Tehran. "It was agreed upon that I would pay a fee of 20 tomans for the treatment. One tooth, number one, one toman. He would charge for one set of teeth with spring (*fanar*) 30 tomans and without spring 25 tomans. The fee to fill two numbers of teeth] is 8,000 and 9,000; the cleaning of two numbers [of teeth] is 5,000 and 3,000 [dinars]. The drawing of two teeth number two is 2,000 and 1,000."[224] The CMS, and probably also the other missionary dispensaries, also offered the service of dental extractions. This was not without its cultural misunderstandings. Mary Bird wrote that, "A report is abroad that I want to collect teeth for sets, so I carefully give every one I extract to its owner! It is taken away, washed with water and camphor, and placed in a hole in a wall where the sun will fall on it, so that the patients will not be toothless in the next world!"[225]

Although by the end of the Qajar period there was no dental school in Persia, there were nevertheless some locally trained dentists in Tehran, who only had to pass a simple examination.[226] In 1906, there was M. Alexander, who had been trained in the office of Dr. Matin a-Saltaneh. At that time the newspaper *Tarbiyat* published a number of articles on the importance of dentistry and dental hygiene.[227] In Ardabil, the first modern dentist only started to practice around 1920.[228] In 1922, Dr. Stump, the long-time sole European dentist in Persia and first lecturer in dentistry in the Medical School wrote an article in which he lamented the sorry state of dental health and of the dentist profession in Persia.[229]

Until 1911, Persian doctors and dentists received their certificate from doctors and/or hospitals whom they had trained with. These constituted the bulk of 'modern' trained doctors. In addition, there were some Persians who had received training in Europe, whose small number grew after 1900. Apprentices of Persian doctors and assistants trained in the various foreign hospitals obtained permits to practice. In 1911, the *Majles* passed a law obliging aspiring doctors and dentists to pass an examination at the government Medical School.[230] These licensed doctors formed the bulk of the medical

---

[222] Basir al-Molk, *Ruznameh*, pp. 479-98 (or Valtop [?]). She received 2.5 *qran*s for the visit. I have not been able to find any information on these persons.
[223] Mostowfi, *Sharh*, vol. 1, p. 529; E'temad al-Saltaneh, *Ruznameh*, pp. 84, 663.
[224] Sadid al-Saltaneh, Mohammad `Ali Khan. *Safarnameh-ye Sadid al-Saltaneh*. ed. Ahmad Eqtedari (Tehran:Behnashr, 1362/1983), p. 138.
[225] Rice, *Mary Bird*, p. 118.
[226] Neligan, "Public Health," part III, p. 742; Wishard, *Twenty Years*, p. 266.
[227] "Mohsenat-e dandan az asli va `ariyeh," in the newspaper *Tarbiyat*, vol. 3, pp. 2058-59 (year 6, nr. 693, 15 Dhu'l-Qa`deh, 1323/11 January, 1906), see also "Ahammiyat-e kar-e dandan va dandansazi," Ibid., vol. 3, pp. 2145-46 (year 6, nr. 404, 12 Jomadi I, 1324/5 July, 1906).
[228] Safari, *Ardabil*, vol. 3, p. 486.
[229] Stamp, Dr. "What do teeth do?" *`Alam-e Nesvan* 2 (November 1922), pp. 6-10; Elgood, *Medical History*, p. 537.
[230] Government of Iran, *Majmu`eh-ye Qavanin ... dar chahar dowreh-ye taqniniyeh*, pp. 393-96 (Persian text of the *Qanun-e Tebabat* dated 3 Jomadi II 1329/11 June, 1911). For the French text

professional class. Most of those who had studied medicine abroad had gone to France, less to Beirut, Great Britain, United States, or Germany. All foreign doctors had to register their diplomas at the Ministry of Public Instruction and then were also licensed, irrespective whether they worked for foreign legation, missionary hospitals, foreign companies, or as private practitioners. The latter category of doctors hardly existed prior to the Russian Revolution, but thereafter a considerable number of Russians and Armenians with European diplomas settled and practiced in northern Persia. The new law also abolished the post of lecturer in Islamic-Galenic medicine in the Medical School, thus formally breaking with its medical tradition.[231]

The reason for opting for a gradual modernizing approach was that Persia just did not have enough Western trained doctors. The reality was that most doctors were those trained in the Islamic-Galenic system and it was not realistic to forbid them to practice. The law, therefore, provided a grandfather clause. If you had practiced outside Tehran for more than 10 years and thus had shown that your treatments had not been harmful you were allowed to continue to practice. Traditional doctors who had practiced in Tehran for more than five but less than 10 years were required to pass a government examination within a period of three years. Some *Majles* deputies had argued that the law should apply to the country as a whole, because otherwise quacks that were not allowed to operate in Tehran would "go to the provinces and there engage in murder." But the view that there should be an immediate clear cut with the past throughout the country did not win out. It was also argued that in Tehran more specialists would practice who needed modern drugs, which, if used improperly, might be harmful.[232]

Those arguing for the gradualist approach were borne out by reality because the law was not even applied in the provinces, where its implementation proved to be impossible at that time. In Bushire, there were "few medical practitioners, of whom only three employ European methods and drugs, the remainder remaining faithful to Avicenna and Galen. Female superstition still requires the presence of the medicine-man, expert in casting out malicious Jinns."[233] In Gilan, for example, the doctors and chemists were not even aware of the new 1911 laws regulating their profession. When in 1919, 'Isa Sadeq, the Superintendent of Education, tried to execute the law he was accused of acting as if he still were in the period of absolutism of the past and doctors started a media campaign (in the papers, rumor mongering, calls to politicians) to make Sadeq stop his unwanted interference.[234] According to Mostowfi, "The well-known physicians of the period were generally old-fashioned doctors. Only a few had a wide reputation and were in demand due to their surgical skills. Generally speaking, people preferred the old-fashioned doctors.[235] In a small provincial town such as Damghan there were only two licensed

---

see Gilmour, *Rapport*, pp. 34-36. The American hospitals are explicitly mentioned and assigned a role in this law, because unlike the other foreign hospitals, they trained Persian doctors and nurses.
[231] Neligan, "Public Health," part III, p. 742; Good, "The Transformation," p. 72.
[232] Government of Iran, *Modhakerat-e Majles, Dowreh-ye Dovvom-e Taqniniyeh*, pp. 1576-80.
[233] Government of Great Britain, *Trade Report 1913-14*, p. 1.
[234] Sadeq, *Yadegar*, vol. 1, p. 202.
[235] Mostowfi, *Sharh*, vol. 1, p. 528. For a picture of a famous Jewish physician, see Friedrich. *Persien in Wort und Bild* (Berlin: Schneider, 1926), p. 132. This also explains why the shahs

(*mojaz*) physicians, who mostly practiced traditional medicine and prescribed mostly herbal drugs.[236]

Nevertheless, progressive women's publications such as *Shekufeh* (Blossom) and *Danesh* (Knowledge) made an effort to point the advantages of modern Western medicine over traditional Persian medicine. These papers not only argued in favor of modern diagnostic and therapeutic methods, but also ridiculed the use of omens (*falbin*) through the printing of caricatures and articles.[237]

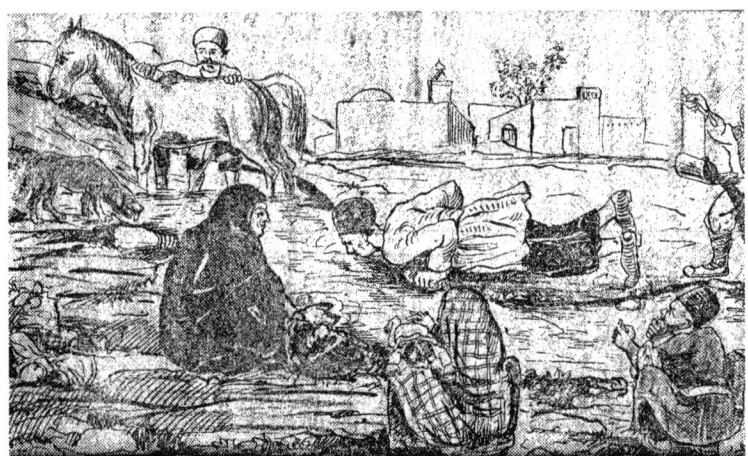

Figure 18: Caricature showing unhygienic conditions (Bohlul newspaper).

In 1924, a total of 905 doctors were licensed to practice in Persia. Of these, 253 had a diploma (this number includes European and American doctors residing in Persia); the remaining 652 had been authorized to practice as a result of the 1911 law. Of these, very few had any notion of modern Western medicine, although some enjoyed a good reputation. This number of official doctors translated into one doctor per 11,000 inhabitants. However, of the 905 doctors, a total of 323 practiced in Tehran, so that, excluding Tehran, there was one doctor per 16,800 inhabitants in 1924. The corresponding figure for Tehran was one per 680 inhabitants. Given the inadequate health situation in Persia it is clear that these doctors did not serve the population at large. Also, at the same time there was a much larger number of unregulated practitioners of folk medicine operating in Persia, who served the bulk of the population. Few of the Western trained Persian physicians took surgery as a specialty.[238] By 1920, only one or two

---

continued to use Persian doctors, because they felt more confortable with them. E'temad al-Saltaneh, *Ruznameh*, p. 916 wrote about the newly arrived Dr. Schneider, "Let's wait and see how many of us will be on his list of victims."

[236] Keshavarz-Damghan, *Sad Darvazeh*, p. 244 (Neyz al-Hokama and Sharif al-Atebba).

[237] See *Danesh*, pp. 40, 36 (*Shekufeh*, pp. 33-34 (year 1, nr. 9, 3 Jomadi II, 1331/May 10, 1913).

[238] Gilmour, *Rapport*, pp. 33-36 (including the text of the law); Linton, *Persian Sketches*, p. 80. In Kermanshah there were 20 doctors, five of whom had diplomas, the remaining 15 did not. Soltani, *Joghrafiya*, vol. 1, p. 535; Varjavand, *Sima-ye Tarikh*, vo. 3, p. 1818 (about 3-4 authorized doctors, most of whom non-Moslem). In fact, in Maragheh none of the traditional doctors were licensed to

women had taken up Western medicine as a profession. Quite a few, however, had become good nurses after training in mission hospitals.[239]

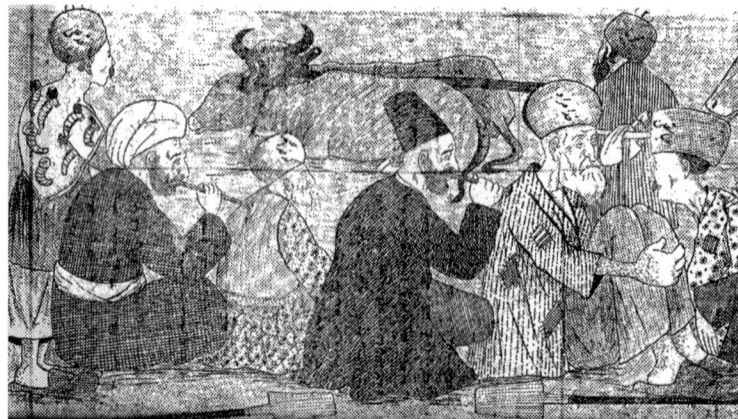

Figure 19: Caricature showing cupping and leeching (Bohlul newspaper).

LICENSING OF CHEMISTS

By the end of the Qajar period drugstores (`attari) still were numerous, but their nature had not changed much. What had changed was that more modern chemist shops had also been established. This was but the result of the progress made by modern Western medicine that used chemical products, often in powder form, rather than herbal products. The *Dar al-Fonun* also trained its students in the science of pharmacology, the first five of whom were outstanding. One of them, Mirza Kazem Mahallati Shimi, became teacher in chemistry and natural sciences at the school. The purpose of training in pharmacology was, amongst other things, to promote the establishment of modern pharmacies in Persia.[240] I do not know whether any of the *Dar al-Fonun* graduates opened a pharmacy, but in 1897, the grand vizier, Amin al-Dowleh, opened a pharmacy in the Chaleh Meydan quarter. The shop was staffed with a doctor and a salesperson, and provided gratis medical treatment and drugs to the poor.[241]

The doctors opposing Western drugs struck a cord with the populace. This was not just an economic question, for towards the end of the nineteenth century there also was a growing anti-Western spirit in Persia. As a result, when Dr. Schwerin, who was the head of the pharmacology department of the *Dar al-Fonun*, opened a retail pharmacy in Tehran this was met with a violent demonstration, probably of the 'spontaneous' kind.[242] Nevertheless, this demonstration did not stop Dr. Schwerin from continuing his business. Other chemists soon followed his example and also established *dava-khaneh*s or *apoteyk* in Tehran. Another professor of the *Dar al-Fonun*, Dr. Maulion, also opened a chemist

---

practice. Some them, therefore, opted for training to be able to pass the state exam, see Good, "The Transformation," pp. 68, 71-72.
[239] Rice, *Persian Women*, pp. 252-53.
[240] Ekhtiyar, *Dar al-Funun*, p. 234.
[241] Sepehr, *Mer'at al-Vaqaye`*, p. 194.
[242] Shahri, *Tarikh*, vol. 4, p. 327-28.

shop, and later a number of Armenian doctors (Petrosiyan, Papaziyan, and Garnik), who had been trained in Beirut and Switzerland, followed suit.[243] In Tabriz, there was since 1889 a pharmacy operated by Loqman al-Mamalek (Mo'in al-Atebba), physician of Mozaffar al-Din Mirza, the crown prince. He received an annual subsidy of 2,000 francs from the French government to operate his school, the *Loqmaniyeh*, and his pharmacy. In 1907, there was a French pharmacy in Tabriz operated by Mr. Renard, but it is not clear whether it was the same or an additional one.[244] Around that time Mirza Musa Khan Hakim-Bashi, a graduate of the *Dar al-Fonun*, established the first chemist shop in Qazvin, next to his doctor's practice. Later, the first Armenian doctor in Qazvin, Dr. Vartan Hakopiyan did the same.[245] The Persian government had hired two French pharmacologists by 1903, who had set up a laboratory in the *Takiyeh-e ye Dowlat* where they taught their courses. In addition, Dr. Schneider had convinced Mozaffar al-Din Shah also to attach a French pharmacist to his court, as part of his medical team. In 1926, Neligan, concerning the situation in Tehran, wrote, "Chemists' shops are numerous."[246] Whereas this category of trade did not yet occur in the census of 1886, in 1929 there were no less than 148 of such shops in Tehran.

Table 8: Number of chemist shops in Tehran and their distribution over the city quarters (1929)

Name quarter	# Shops	# Masters	# Workers	# Helpers
Ark	24	22	42	6
Dowlat	37	33	49	4
Hasanabad	10	11	8	2
Sangalaj	26	16	18	8
Qanatabad	6	5	7	-
Mohammadiyeh	9	8	7	2
Sharq	3	3	5	-
Bazaar	25	19	43	11
'Owdlajan	12	12	14	1
Shahr-e Now	-	-	-	-
Total	148	137	111	34

Source: Baladiyeh, *Salnameh-ye Dovvom*, pp. 78-79.

It is of further interest to note that there were no chemist shops in Shahr-e Now, the poorest quarter of Tehran, while their largest number was in the more affluent quarters such as Ark, Dowlat, Sangalaj and Bazaar.

Because of new government regulations some of the better chemists did not sell poisons or narcotics to the public without a doctor's prescription, while they also kept records of

---

[243] Hasanbeygi, *Tehran-e Qadim*, p. 205; *Tarbiyat*, index q.v. *Muliyun, Davakhaneh*, and *Davasazi*.

[244] Aubin, Eugène. *La Perse d'aujourd'hui* (Paris: Armand Colin, 1908), p. 46; Nategh, "Les Persans," pp. 192, n. 13, 194.

[245] Varjavand, *Sima-ye Tarikh*, vol. 3, p. 1818.

[246] Neligan, "Public Health," part III, p. 742; Nategh, "Les Persans," p. 192 (the French captain Gustave Lecomte was hired at 15,000 francs per year; he also was obliged to establish a chemical laboratory and teach students pharmacology); Hassendorfer, "Les médecins français," pp. 61; Government of France, *Rapports Commerciaux des agents diplomatiques et consulaires de France* – Année 1914 no. 1079 Perse (Paris, 1914), p. 40.

sales. They also sold modern medical instruments and other medical necessaries. Forbes-Leith mentioned, for example, the existence of a number of Armenian drugstores in Hamadan, where he was able to buy "a limited number of instruments, such as scalpels, sinus and artery forceps, surgical scissors, and a supply of lint and bandages," as well as some drugs and powdered brimstone for a campaign against scabies around 1920.[247]

In October 1919, the government issued a rule regulating the business of the sale drugs (`attari`). Only those who had been licensed by the Ministry of Public Instruction were allowed to be engaged in this business. You had to (i) have a diploma in pharmacology issued by a university in Europe, or (ii) have worked for at least five years in a recognized chemist shop, or (iii) pass an examination of practical pharmacology. Only those who held European university diplomas were allowed to be chemists in Tehran. Outside the capital the examinations were still applied.[248] As in the case of doctors, the law regulating the chemist's profession was not applied in the provinces either. The chemists like the doctors also severely criticized Sadeq's actions and brought political pressure to bear and, as a result, he got nowhere either in applying the new regulations to chemists.[249] In Damghan, at that time, there were only two druggists, who did not have Western drugs and only sold herbs and their experience.[250]

In 1922, a poorly equipped school of pharmacology was opened as part of the Medical School. Students needed to have a state certificate showing they had an elementary school education as well as two years of having worked in a pharmacy. During their study, which included botany, herbal pharmacology, chemistry and physics, they also needed to be employed in a state certified pharmacy.[251] This "westernization' of a branch of the medical infrastructure that customarily also dispensed medical advice and medicine meant that slowly, but certainly this aspect of their work was brought to an end. The increased use of chemical instead of herbal medicine also reduced the role of the drugstores (`attar`), while promoting that of the modern chemist shops.[252]

The past so-called hostility of some Persian physicians to Western drugs did not constitute a hindrance for the growing import of these products. In 1909, the most desired imported chemical drugs were:

1. Double carbon acid natron. It was mostly imported from Russia and cost 2.40 to 2.80 Mk per *mann-e Tabriz*, while its price in Russia was 1.20 Mk.

---

[247] Forbes-Leith, *Checkmate*, pp. 89-90; see also the ad published in various issues of the women's periodical *Danesh*. Neligan, "Public Health," part III, p. 742. In 1926, there were 19 chemist shops in Kermanshah. Soltani, *Joghrafiya*, vol. 1, pp. 535-36.
[248] Gilmour, *Rapport*, pp. 36-38 has the French text of this law. The *Majmu`eh-ye Qavanin* does not include the Persian text of this law, at least in my copy. These good intentions to regulate pharmacies had already been announced in 1906, see *Tarbiyat*, vol. 3, p. 2266.
[249] Sadeq, *Yadegar*, vol. 1, pp. 202-03.
[250] Keshavarz-Damghan, *Sad Darvazeh*, p. 244. A similar situation existed in Ardabil, where the first apothecary was started in th 1930s. Safari, *Ardabil*, vol. 3, pp. 486-87.
[251] Gilmour, *Rapport*, pp. 16.
[252] Good, "The Transformation," p. 73.

2. Scottish pills[253] from Glasgow, where they cost 40-50 Pf. The local price was 3-3.30 Mk, while the transportation cost alone were 4.80-5 Mk, and therefore it was not sold much.
3. Magnesia sulfirica; mostly imported from Russia. Its price was 2.80 Mk, while in Germany it cost 15 Pf. Per kg. The British also exported it in blue bottles of 250g and 500 g. Because of the small units and transportation cost, the unit costs were higher and therefore it sold little.
4. Sulphuric acid, natrium acid, saltpeter, chlorine alkali, etc. were only imported from Russia, because the European transporters raised many difficulties.
5. Santonon, quinine, tartaric acids, etc. were sold in large quantities. As mass products they had to be cheap and therefore the profit rate was only 3-5%. Recently, Prototi & Co. (Milan) had marketed a quinine powder that contained 40% quinine and 60% cinchonin with much success. One *methqal* (4.6 g) of this product was sold in a sachet and a glass at 36 Pf.
6. Cuvin capsules, pink pills, and an array of other medical drugs, of which France was the major exporter, also sold well.
7. Empty medical gelatin capsules,[254] which can only be sold at very low prices just like quinine. The wholesale price for 1,000 packages containing each 100 capsules; cost 500 Mk, although discounts had to be given.[255]

Because the Persian market offered good prospects for sale many European firms tried to offer their products for sale. In the 1911 German "Commercial Guide for Persia" (*Handelsratgeber für Persien*) there was a separate section on medical chemical drugs, with subsections for drugs (*davajat-e tebbi*; six firms), pharmaceutical products (*alat baraye-e davasazi*; six firms), disinfection products (*adviyeh zedd-e 'afuni*; four firms), herbal drugs (*davajat-e nabati*; six firms), insecticides (*asbab baraye talaf kardan-e khatarateh*; four firms), conservatives (*mavad ma'muleh baraye hefz-e felzat az rang*; two firms), bandages (*parcheh va navar baraye maramar*; six firms), and hospital products (*parchehha-ye nazuk jehat-e marizkhaneh*; two firms). There also were 10 firms that advertised medical and dentistry instruments, including disinfection apparatus.[256] Germany, which trailed Russia and Great Britain in the export of medical chemical drugs

---

[253] According to Hermann Schelenz, *Geschichte der Pharmazie* (Berlin: Springer, 1904), p. 579, so-called Scottish pills were already in use in the eighteenth century and according to one report they "strengthen the brain and senses, get rid of dizziness and head aches, open up constipation, induce sputum, and evacuate all superfluous fluids. It is the best drug for traveling. They do not require rule or diet. You can eat and drink with them whatever you want." Thanks to Doris Mir-Ghaffari (Halle University) for unearthing this reference. As to constipation pills (*habbeh-ye shahi*) see also Polak, *Persien*, vol. 2, p. 220.

[254] These were a medical product, consisting of a solid or elastic casing (most often made of gelantine) that was filled with an active ingredient. Most widely available were the so-called solid gelatine capsules. These were cylindrical capsules consting of two parts that were filled with the active ingredient and then were mechanically merged (*zusammengesteckt*). Hence the German term *Steckkapseln*. (*Wörterbuch für Arzneimittel*). Thanks to Doris Mir-Ghaffari (Halle University) for unearthing this reference.

[255] Küss, W. *Handelsratgeber für Persien* (Berlin, 1911), pp. 115-16.

[256] Küss, *Handelsratgeber*, part II, pp. 2-5, 48 (surgical instruments, artificial eyes, glasswork, etc).

to Persia, had become the second major exporter by 1914, after Great Britain. In particular, cheap German quinine and salts sold well. France mainly sold special products such as serums, vaccines, and medical herbs.[257] One British firm, "Burrough, Wellcome & Co. make a special feature of their Persian trade. They send European travellers al over the country and freely circulate Persian leaflets, giving an account of drugs and their properties."[258] In 1914, the Persian government, at the request of the governor of Isfahan, granted tax-exemption to the drugs and instruments purchased by the CMS hospital in that town, "by making an annual grant of £50."[259]

VACCINATION

Despite the various attempts to begin smallpox vaccination since 1809, it was only 102 years later that some concrete action was taken to realize this long desired objective. As of 1911, the *Majles* had allocated 10% of the vehicle tax for the execution of a vaccination campaign. This amount was never fully transferred, and I have been unable to find when, where, and how many of the first vaccinations in the twentieth century were realized.[260] The vaccination service received £2,000 per year in 1923-24. Vaccination was not compulsory. Initially, the cow-pock vaccine was transported from Paris, but due to the variation in temperature the vaccine was not always active on arrival in Persia. As of 1922, the Pasteur Institute in Tehran produced the vaccine. By then, there were a total of 202 official vaccinators, of which 22 in Tehran, and 180 in the provinces, of which 17 itinerant ones. The vaccinators were physicians who received a pay of £3 per month; the itinerant ones received £7.10*s*. Payment was only given after vaccinations had been executed. Vaccinations were done during spring and fall, during the other two seasons the weather was too inclement (too cold or too hot). According to the unverified numbers supplied by the vaccinators the following number of people had been vaccinated between 1919-1924. It was not known how many of the vaccinations had been successful.[261]

Table 9: Number of persons vaccinated against smallpox (1919-24)

Period	# Persons vaccinated
1919-20	44,619
1920-21	62,095
1921-22	41,024
1922-23	66,338
1923-24	75,662

Source: Gilmour, *Rapport*, p. 31.

---

[257] Government of France, *Rapports Commerciaux des agents diplomatiques et consulaires de France* – Année 1914 no. 1079 Perse (Paris, 1914), p. 40.
[258] Ross, *A Lady Doctor*, p. 94.
[259] Rice, *Mary Bird*, p. 134.
[260] Government of Iran, *Majmu`eh-ye Qavanin ... dar chahar dowreh-ye taqniniyeh*, p. 302 (text of the *Qanun-e hefz al-sehheh va abeleh-kubi* dated 5 Dhu'l-Qa`deh 1328/8 November, 1910). Nategh, "Les Persans," p. 192 mentions that in 1905, Dr. Scheider was one of the co-founders of a vaccinology institute, about which I have not been able to learn more.
[261] Gilmour, *Rapport*, p. 30-31. It was still didicult initially to convince villagers to accept vaccination, see, e.g., Homayuni, *Molk-e Anbir-amiz*, p. 93. In some towns, people remember that one of the new type of doctors was "an injection doctor." Good, "The Transformation," p. 72.

PASTEUR INSTITUTE

In 1921, with French assistance, the Pasteur Institute was opened. It made vaccines, served as a general medical laboratory for the medical profession, carried out independent research, and offered courses in bacteriology to the Medical School.[262]

Despite the changes in training and regulations, Persian medical practice still remained mainly medical, using mostly herbal drugs. Surgery was still something basically left to the traditional surgeons (*jarrah*). There were very few doctors (*hakim*) trained in modern surgery techniques and not many practiced it. Because the medical profession was in a transitional stage, the old hot-cold paradigm still guided much of medical diagnostics and therapy.[263] This was not only because many old doctors did not know any better, but also because the patients of modern doctors expected and insisted on it. Nevertheless, Persian doctors and patients had embraced the latest European and American medicines (antipyrin, phenacetin, aspirin, calomel, boric acid, zinc sulphate, sublimate, salines, and quinine) with a vengeance. "The country is flooded with samples and circulars. The names of certain reputable forms, however, are well known and their preparations highly esteemed."[264] The establishment of a public pathological laboratory also improved medical practice.[265]

The reformist press accompanied the government's hesitant steps to change people's minds and attitudes and develop the necessary modern medical infrastructure of Persia with a view to improve public health in the country with articles on the importance of hygiene, information about diseases and advances in medical science. The women's periodical *Shekufeh* (Blossom), for example, stated in its masthead that it was a newspaper devoted to subjects such as "manners, literature, child hygiene, housekeeping, and childcare."[266] It was a subject that in particular picked up around 1900, including in cartoons. Both the general and the feminist press made the occurrence of, for

---

[262] Neligan, "Public Health," part III, p. 742; Gilmour, *Rapport*, pp. 27-29.
[263] Wood, M.M. *Glimpses of Persia* (London: CMS, 1922), p. 59; Mostowfi, *Sharh*, vol. 1, pp. 527-28; Mosaddeq, Gholam Hoseyn. "Jarrahi-ye Novin-e Orupa'i dar Iran," *Ayandeh* 15 (1368/1989), p. 464. There was among the elite a growing understanding of what modern surgery could do, as is clear, for example, from the articles on appendicitis in the newspaper *Tarbiyat*, Index q.v. *Apandisit*.
[264] Neligan, "Public Health," part III, p. 742; Küss, *Handelsratgeber*, part II, pp. 2-5, 48 (for the major German firms); Good, "The Transformation," p. 73. According to `Eyn al-Saltaneh, *Ruznameh*, vol. 1, p. 262, writing in 1889, antipyrin tablets had recently arrived from the USA.
[265] Neligan, "Public Health," part III, p. 742.
[266] See, for example, the first private newspaper in published in Persia, *Tarbiyat* 3 vols. (Tehran: Ketabkhaneh-ye Melli, 1377/1998), which has a large range of medical subjects ranging from individual diseases and doctors to medical techniques and remedies, Index q.v. *Amraz, Bimari, Teb, Tebabat* and the individual names of the various diseases and physicians. See also a more politically oriented newspaper such as *Ruznameh-ye Anjoman-e Tabriz* 2 vols. (Tehran: Ketabkhaneh-ye Melli, 1376/1997), Index q.v. *Atebba, Amraz, Hefz al-sehhah, Ta`un, Qaranteyn,* and *Vaba* as well as the women's periodicals *Shekufeh* and *Danesh*, Table of Contents, pp. eleven to twenty-four and Index. Kashani-Sabet, Firoozeh. "'City of the Dead': the Frontier Polemics of Quarantines in the Ottoman Empire and Iran," *Comparative Studies of South Asia, Africa, and the Middle East* 18/2 (1998), p. 56.

example, venereal disease a main public health concern in its publications.[267] It also treated other factors that contributed to a less optimal public health situation such as child marriage,[268] prostitution,[269] prevention of the contamination of water supply,[270] child rearing,[271] and information on vaccination and major diseases such as malaria, tuberculosis, and typhoid.[272] Books also were published that focused on both personal and public hygiene,[273] while government publications also pressed home the importance of this issue.[274] However, measures to improve public and personal hygiene still left to be desired, as did the measures taken by the government, which were totally inadequate to the task.

According to Dr. Neligan, writing in 1926, after 19 year's of experience in Persia, including as a member of the Sanitary Council:

> The young diplomés prefer to remain in Tehran or in one of the larger towns. There is a great need of well-trained doctors, especially in the country districts, and there is no source of supply of men adequately equipped, in the modern sense of the word, for quarantine work, for special posts during epidemics, for the newly organized and enlarged army, or as municipal and provincial health offices. The difficulties of the public health authorities at Tehran in dealing with emergencies or in obtaining accurate information may well be imagined.[275]

---

[267] *Tarbiyat*, Index q.v. *Amraz-e jeldi, Suzanak, Sifilis*, and *Kuft*; *Shekufeh*, p. 147 (year 2, nr. 20, 7 Dhu'-l-Qa`deh 1332/September 21, 1914); `*Alam-e Nesvan* 1 (September 1923); Ibid., 1 (September 1922), pp. 36-42.

[268] *Tarbiyat*, Index q.v. `*Aqd va nekah*; `*Alam-e Nesvan* 6 (July 1923), p. 6. Child marriage, child care, health, hygiene and a host of other issues were already debated since about 1900 in the press and were also brought to the attention of the Parliament (*Majles*) by women's organizations as soon as it had been created, see Afary, Janet. *The Iranian Constitutional Revolution, 1906-1911* (New York, Columbia UP, 1996), pp. 177-208; *Shekufeh*, q.v. *Ezdevaj* and *Zanashu'i*. Child marriage was also a major theme of contemporary fiction; see Kamshad, H. *Modern Persian Prose Literature* (Cambridge: CUP, 1966), pp. 60-72.

[269] `*Alam-e Nesvan* 1 (September 1922), pp. 29-34. Prostitution was a theme that resounded very much in contemporary fiction as well; see Kamshad, *Modern Persian Prose*, p. 60f. See on its prevalence Floor, Willem, "Some Notes on Mut`a," *ZDMG* 138 (1988), pp. 326-31.

[270] *Tarbiyat*, Index q.v. *Ab, Ab-e ashameydani, Ab-anbar* and *Hammam*; *Shekufeh*, q.v. *Behdasht*; `*Alam-e Nesvan* 1 (May 1932), pp. 5-17 (repeating the old proposal to cover the open waterduct system of Tehran to keep out contaminants); Ibid., 1 (January 1925), pp. 408.

[271] *Tarbiyat*, Index q.v. *Atfal*; *Shekufeh*, Index q.v. *Atfal*; `*Alam-e Nesvan* 3 (January 1922); Ibid., 4 (March 1922), pp. 36-42; Ibid., 1 (November 1923), pp. 13-14.

[272] *Tarbiyat*, Index q.v. *Abeleh, Abeleh-kubi, Tebb-e nowbeh, Sel, Homay-e motbeqeh, Hesbeh, Tifu'id* and *Vaba*; *Shekufeh*, Index q.v. *Abeleh, Eshal, Tifus, Sorkhjeh, Ta`un, Vaba*; `*Alam-e Nesvan* 6 (July 1922), pp. 3-7 (typhoid); Ibid., 3 (January 1922), pp. 5-9 (malaria); Ibid. 3 (May 1931), pp. 111-16 (malaria); Ibid., 5 (September 1931), pp. 193-200 (tuberculosis); Ibid., 3 (May 1932), pp. 104-08 (tuberculosis and cancer).

[273] See Ali N_-Rouze, "Essai de bibliographie persane," *Revue du Monde Musulmane* 60 (1925), pp. 29-34.

[274] See, for example, Jahed, Amir. *Salnameh-ye Pars* (Tehran, 1926-41).

[275] Government of Great Britain, *Geographical Handbook*, pp. 408-09.

Although a new generation of physicians had been trained and were in training, both abroad and in Persia, they were not able to transform the conditions of public health in Persia during the next thirty years.[276] After all, the major problem was lack of public and personal hygiene, and more doctors, even when better trained, with better drugs and with more hospitals, were neither the answer to that problem nor a substitute for it.[277]

PUBLIC HEALTH MEASURES BY THE MUNICIPALITY OF TEHRAN
The measures taken by the central government to modernize the public health sector remained mainly restricted to Tehran, and were, if not haphazard, certainly ineffective. The first steps dated from the days of Amir Kabir. In 1851, he had pamphlets drawn up to inform the population about what caused contagious diseases like cholera and what to do to prevent them. He also informed them not to throw their rubbish and offal into the streets, and not to pollute the drinking water, all of which caused disease. The mayor (*kalantar*) of Tehran appointed staff (*rika*) to keep the streets clean.[278] Because icehouses were not properly cleaned, and did not use clean water to make ice, Amir Kabir had a wall built around them.[279] To make streets cleaner he further initiated a program to pave them, and started with those around the Ark, the royal palace complex. The same program also was initiated in Tabriz.[280] However, after Amir Kabir's fall and execution, his successor put a stop to all these improvements and things became as before, filthy. Probably inspired by this example, or may be at the command of Amir Kabir, the mayor or *kalantar* of Tehran asked Persian doctors to write pamphlets how to prevent and how to deal with cholera. About ten years later, E'tezad al-Saltaneh, the Minister of Education, asked a leading court physician, Mohammad Taqi Shirazi, to write a treatise on cholera. This was probably done within the context of the discussions of the Sanitary Council, which, as has been discussed, was mainly an ineffectual debating society.[281] However interesting these initiatives may have been, they left no trace, for there was neither implementation nor other follow-up, as is clear from the lack of preventive measures against cholera.

---

[276] See, for example, Najmabadi, Mahmud. "Nakhostin pezeshki amukhtegan-e Irani dar Sewis," in Iraj Afshar ed., *Namvareh-ye Doktor Mahmud Afshar* 12 vols. (Tehran: Mowqufeh-ye Doktor Mahmud Afshar, 1367/1988), vol. 4, pp. 2162-69; Mosaddeq, Gholam, "Jarrahi-ye Novin," pp. 464-66; Afshar, Iraj. 'Dar bareh-ye Doktor Yusef Mir," in Ibid., vol. 4, pp. 2169-82; Dashti, `Ali, "Dar bareh-ye Doktor Yusef Mir," in Ibid., vol. 4, pp. 2177-79; Mir, Mohammad `Ali and Mir, `Ali Mohammad. "Yadi az Doktor Yusef Mir Irevani," *Ayandeh* 17 (1370/1991), pp. 41-45; "Khaterat-e Vahid," *Vahid* 21-31 (1352-54/1973-75); Eqbal, Yaghma'i. "Doktor Mohammad Hasan Khan Hakim al-Dowleh," *Amuzesh va Parvaresh* 42 (1351/1972), pp. 358-64; Government of Iran, *Iran-Shahr*, vol. 2, pp. 1399-1452.

[277] For an analysis and appreciation of this public health issue in post-Qajar Persia see Good, "The Transformation," pp. 69-82.

[278] Government of Iran, *Vaqaye`-ye Ettefaqiyeh*, vol. 1, p. 68 (nr. 14, 7 Rajab 1267/8 May, 1851).

[279] Government of Iran, *Vaqaye`-ye Ettefaqiyeh*, vol. 1, p. 82 (nr. 17, 17 Rajab 1267/18 May, 1851).

[280] Adamiyyat, *Amir Kabir*, pp. 328-29.

[281] Ebrahimnejad, Hormuz. "Un traité d'épidémiologie de la médecine traditionelle persane," *Studia Iranica* 27 (1998), pp. 83-106.

The second time that steps were taken to clean up the city dated from the time of Naser al-Din Shah's return from his first visit to Europe in 1873. Among the modern institutes that had been created was the new police force (*nazmiyeh*), under the Italian-Austrian official, de Monteforte. At the latter's recommendation the department of control of public thoroughfares (*edareh-ye ehtesab*) was absorbed by the police department. The *ehtesab* department had as one of its tasks to keep the roads clean (*tanzif*) in the administrative part of Tehran, *i.e.*, around the royal palace. To that end the department employed a sanitation staff with 100 donkeys to transport the refuse from their zone of operation. It was further the *tanzif*'s task to clear toxic and other dangerous items from the moat around Tehran to avoid that the stagnant water became a health hazard. The population also was instructed to respect cleanliness of the public roads and to desist from throwing all kinds of refuse into the streets. House owners were responsible to keep the area in front of their house clean. Naser al-Din Shah regularly criticized the *ehtesab* for not doing a good job and to clean up their act and the streets. Despite these spasmodic bouts of royal interest the streets of Tehran were of a doubtful cleanliness. In fact, a new source of revenue had been created, while from a point of view of public hygiene there was not much improvement in the situation.[282] Similar steps to clean the streets as well as to relocate the tannery were initiated in Mashad in 1882, but do not seem to have had a lasting impact. In effect, it is not even known whether, and to what extent, the decision taken to keep the town clean was actually carried out.[283]

`Eyn al-Saltaneh reported that in 1890 an effort was made to clean the streets of Tehran by charging homeowners one toman per square meter of street frontage. But he already expressed doubts about the viability of the plan, before it even had been executed, and it came to naught, because he later described the filthy condition of the Tehran streets.[284] The notion that public and personal hygiene and the incidence of disease were related had by that time also become accepted by members of the elite such as `Eyn al-Saltaneh. Basir al-Saltaneh reported that on March 27, 1888 Naser al-Din Shah had given instruction to clean up the city, and that Amin al-Soltan, the grand vizier, commented, "now we have become doctors (*hakim-bashiha*)."[285] In 1897, a new attempt was made to clean up the city. Karim Agha, Monazzam al-Saltaneh, *vazir-e nazmiyeh va ehtesabiyeh*, made a major effort to clean and pave the streets to which end he printed affiches and also asked for financial support from the homeowners. He paved the Khiyaban-e Marizkhaneh and the Khiyaban-e Darvazeh-ye Shemiran. After a short while the city became quite clean, but soon it reverted to its old filthy state.[286]

Further steps had to wait till the establishment of a constitutional government in Persia in 1906, and even then it took some years before new measures were taken. Despite the fact

---

[282] Floor, Willem. "Securité, Circulation et Hygiene dans les rues de Teheran a l'époque Qajar, in: in Adle, Charyar et Hourcade, Bernard eds. *Téhéran Capitale bicentenaire*, Institut Francais de Recherche en Iran, 1992 (Bibliotheque iranienne, vol. 37), pp. 194-97; `Eyn al-Saltameh, *Ruznameh*, vol. 1, pp. 491, 903 (despite the *ehtesabiyeh* the streets are still filthy).
[283] Nezam al-Saltaneh Mafi, *Khaterat va Asnad*, vol. 1, pp. 27-29 and appendix 3 to this book.
[284] `Eyn al-Saltaneh, *Ruznameh*, vol. 1, pp. 256, 561, 651-52, 846, 903; vol. 2, p. 1055.
[285] `Eyn al-Saltaneh, *Ruznameh*, vol. 2, p. 1055; Basir al-Molk, *Ruznameh*, p. 457.
[286] Sepehr, *Mer'at al-Vaqaye*`, pp. 188, 212; `Eyn al-Saltaneh, *Ruznameh*, vol. 2, p. 1254.

that in 1907 the *Majles* had adopted the Municipality Law requiring amongst other things provincial governors "to pay strict attention to ... public health and sanitation ... and act with utmost speed in the case of epidemics. Physician, nurses, drugs, and equipment must be sent to the epidemic areas by the governor."[287] The problem was that apart from political problems, Persia did not have the money to implement this law. In fact, it was only in 1910 that the *Majles* adopted the imposition of a new transportation tax (*navaqel*) part of which would be used for to pave the roads of Tehran. Due to difficulties in the implementation of this tax not much money was available to achieve its intended results. In 1911, the *Majles* adopted a new law (*Nezamnameh-ye Tahdid-e Taryak*) that only became effective in 1913. In that same year, Persia signed the Hague Convention of 1913. As a result the production, trade and manufacturing of opiates was restricted. This new rules would result in regulation and supervision of cultivation to the export of opium in all its stages with the intent to reduce opium consumption in Iran itself.[288]

Apart from some efforts to 'clean up' some streets of Tehran towards the end of the nineteenth century, the first concentrated and comprehensive national effort to improve living conditions in the city was the Municipal Act of 1913.[289] The Tehran municipality had somewhat more success with its decision to charge a new tax on abattoirs (1913), while stipulating that only in abattoirs animals could be slaughtered. The purpose of this measure was to reduce the quantity of entrails that were thrown into the streets by household 'butchers.' A few months later (1914) new sanitary regulations were published that had to be respected by the abattoirs and butcher shops, although no staff was appointed to enforce the new rules. It was also decided to move Tehran's abattoir outside the city to Farahabad, just south of Tehran. The site was not an adequate one, however. It was next to a cemetery, water was in short supply, and the building itself was inconvenient. Therefore, in 1925, the municipality decided to move the abattoir to Niyazabad, a site and building that allowed respecting sanitation requirements.[290]

Another hygienic problem were the stables inside the Tehran city walls in which cows were kept for their milk and meat. The considerable amount of dung and other refuse produced by these cows was such that the Municipality of Tehran decided in 1914 to order the relocation of these stables to a location outside the city.[291] The Municipality also constructed washrooms in the poorest quarter to enable women to wash their clothes. Outside the building there was a large reservoir for the first wash, and afterwards the women went inside to do the second and last wash. The idea was to reduce the pollution

---

[287] Government of Iran, *Majmu`eh-ye Qavanin ... dar chahar dowreh-ye taqniniyeh*, pp. 87-108; see also Kashani-Sabet, "'City of the Dead'," p. 56 regarding the existence and objectives of the Municipal Society (*Anjoman-e Baladiyeh*) in 1907.

[288] On the implementation of this law and its effect see Floor, Willem. *A Fiscal History of Iran in the Safavid and Qajar Period* (New York: Bibliotheca Persica, 1999), pp. 400-04, and Ibid., *Agriculture in Qajar Iran* (Washington, DC: Mage, 2003), pp. 459-60.

[289] Ayatollah `Abdol-Hoseyn Lari declared that the municipality (*baladiyeh*) was acceptable as long as it focused on public health issues, but not if it allowed the establishment of coffeehouses and gambling dens and the like. Lari, "Shesh Resaleh," p. 225

[290] Floor, "Securité," p. 197; Gilmour, *Rapport*, p. 56.

[291] Floor, "Securité," pp. 197-98.

of the drinking water, because prior to that time women washed the clothes anywhere, including in the uncovered water mains (*jub*s).[292] Furthermore, regulations were drawn up for the making and storage of ice, and a municipal medical officer needed to inspect the ice before it could be taken from storage. The Tehran Municipality also regulated barbers. Public health officials had to inspect all barbershops, and barbers had to sterilize their tools after each client. The Municipality also made printed instructions available to barbers how to properly do venesection. Finally, the Municipality published regulations for the 162 public bathhouses (150 for Moslems, 12 for Armenians). In 1914, public baths had been exempted from the payment of property tax to induce them to respect hygienic rules. However, there were no rules for the change of water, which was only done at the explicit instruction of the medical officer. Normally, the scum that collected on the surface was skimmed off three times per day, while the deposit at the bottom of the reservoir was cleaned out every morning. There also were rules concerning the bathhouse staff and their clothing and these had to pass a medical examination.[293]

To see to the implementation of the various regulations as well as to maintain public health the Tehran Municipality had divided the city into 10 zones, with one public health official per two zones. It was their task to inspect all food supplies for sale, in particular, milk, bread, meat, and fish. They also had to inspect the shops themselves and verify whether the sales staff did not have infectious and/or skin diseases as well as the general cleanliness of the shops. They also had to inspect all public building such as mosques (ablution facilities, latrines), schools, public baths, caravanserais, hotels, government offices, and prisons as well as the public water supply and its conduits. Furthermore, they had to inspect the sites where the dead were washed and ensure that hygienic measures were in place, that conditions in cemeteries and the transport of corpses did not damage public health as well as that the conditions in the streets in general were satisfied. Finally, they had to see to it that nobody practiced medicine without authorization, to inspect barbershops and verify the application of the rules.

The Tehran health service was headed by a medical officer, who was assisted by one officer for each of the five officially recognized quarters. In 1922, with the reorganization of the municipality a medical service was established. Several treatment service centers for the poor were opened: "six for general diseases, one for women's diseases, one for venereal diseases, and a dental clinic. A municipal hospital with 100 beds was also opened. Tehran also had a lunatic asylum (*dar al-majanin*), a poor-house, an orphanage, and a crèche for foundlings, all administered by the municipality."[294]

Gilmour was not much impressed with the actual result of the hygiene measures or with the effectiveness of the public health officials. It would take long to list the many deficiencies listed by Gilmour, but suffice it to say that there were not enough funds and

---

[292] Gilmour, *Rapport*, p. 56; for a picture see David Fraser, *Persia and Turkey in Revolt* (Edinburgh-London: Blackwood, 1910), p. 274.
[293] Gilmour, *Rapport*, pp. 62-64 (steps were also taken to construct public latrines, for use when those in mosques and the like were closed). The women's periodical *Shekufeh*, pp. 147-48 (year 2, nr. 20, 7 Dhu'l-Qa`deh 1332/September 21, 1914) also had been clamoring for such rules.
[294] Government of Great Britain, *Geographical Handbook*, pp. 409; Gilmour, *Rapport*, pp. 57-61.

means for the public health officials to be really effective, even if they had wanted to. Also, many of the implementation arrangements for the public health measures did not exist, while there was not even a program for the education of the public at large. As a result, the steps taken by the Municipality were but the very beginning of a long process that is still going on. Meanwhile, Tehran had some new institutions and buildings, but it was still a very dirty and unhygienic city where the population at large as well as their service providers had not the slightest idea about the importance of hygiene, and what they could do to improve things.[295]

Bushire was one of the few towns where soon after the adoption of the Municipal Act a self-supporting municipal organization had been established by 1913. It undertook various public works such as the rebuilding of the seawalls. Furthermore, "new roads were laid down and steps were taken for the lighting of the town and the main road leading to the suburbs in 1913. Donkeys, in insufficient numbers, are used to remove the accumulated rubbish. The municipality owns a prison and pays some 40 policemen recently provided with uniforms, blue for winter and khaki with red facings for summer. The central administration has accepted the principle that municipal taxes should be spend in the location that raises them."[296] Because of the First World War and its aftermath the works started by the Municipality had been discontinued. In 1920, "a capable and energetic Persian" headed the municipality and he worked hard to improve living conditions in the town. However, despite his efforts, the British consul concluded that, "Bushire was as a whole and especially its center a filthy place.[297]

As far as medical service was concerned there were a few traditional Persian doctors and healers. "Apart from the dispensary maintained by the Indian Government, there is no government medical aid of any kind, no statistics that would be of value are available to show the extent of the ravages of the diseases."[298] To improve medical service, the British had made a beginning with the construction of a hospital and a free dispensary in Bushire in 1913. The funds for the hospital had come from voluntary contributions from local merchants. Not only the Municipality's work program had experienced a delay, so had British hospital plans. "By the end of 1920 work had started by the residency mason and under the supervision of the British Executive Engineer for the Gulf Ports," and the first storey was almost complete by September 1921.[299] It was only in April 1923, that the Bushire Charitable Hospital was occupied. "It was quite an improvement on the present building where the residency surgeon carried on his work under adverse conditions. The latter and his staff do practically the whole of the medical work of the town."[300] However,

---

[295] Gilmour, *Rapport*, pp. 59-62. The Tehran municipal example was slowly followed elsewhere with mixed results in Kermanshah, Soltani, *Joghrafiya*, vol. 1, p. 549, 553-61.
[296] Government of Great Britain, *Trade Report 1913-14*, pp. 1, 6 (Because of public health concern there was continued removal of garbage).
[297] Government of Great Britain, *Trade Report 1920-21*, p. 1.
[298] Government of Great Britain, *Trade Report 1921-22*, p. 2.
[299] Government of Great Britain, *Trade* Report 1920-21, p. 1; Ibid., *Trade* Report 1920-21, p. ii. ; Wright, *The English*, p. 127.
[300] Government of Great Britain, *Trade* Report 1921-22, p. 1; also Ibid., Trade Report 1922-23, p. 3 which notes no change, and no cholera or other infectious diseases during that year.

> many essentials were lacking, e.g., electric light, water supply, cookhouses, quarters for staff and a sanitary drainage system. Electric light has since been installed, two engines purchased and thanks to the AIOC a free supply of kerosene oil and petrol for power has been obtained. A drain into the sea and a large Ab-anbar (rainwater storage tank) has also been constructed. But until the quarters of the staff have been built the hospital can only be considered to be an 'outdoor' dispensary.... No marked improvement can be recorded in the state of the Town.... However, that the whole of the European population and the more wealthy Persian families all reside either at Naidi 2 _ miles or at Bushire 6 miles south of the Town itself. These residential areas are comparatively clean and healthy and most of the houses contain a second storey to catch cool breezes from the sea in the summer.[301]

Although in other towns less progress was made with public health measures there were nevertheless signs of change. In Astarabad, for example, in March 1917 the local government asked the Russian consul for help to clean the streets. Fifty Russian soldiers forced shopkeepers in the bazaar to clean the passageways, which led to a closure of the bazaar. When the governor protested the Russians sent 50 soldiers who swept the streets in the town and the bazaar and put up public lighting.[302] In Kerman, Dr. Dodson noticed in 1918 that in the wake of the famine influenza and cholera raged. But he was cheered that he found during his house calls, "that his steady teaching had begun to sink in, and many even of the poor people were burning infected clothing and taking other precautions." He also was instrumental in convincing the governor of Kerman, a patient of his, to introduce hygienic and health-inducing ergonomic rules for carpet production.[303] This and other similar public health measures were in consonance with the programs of some of the political parties active in Persia at that time.[304]

It would take another generation before the improvement in public hygiene started to make a difference in the disappearance of endemic diseases.[305] Although the government wanted to improve health conditions in the country it had neither the funds nor the infrastructure to

---

[301] Government of Great Britain, *Trade Report 1923-24*, p. 1.
[302] Anonymous, *Mokhaberat-e Astarabad* 2 vols. eds. Iraj Afshar and Mohammad Rasul Daryagasht (Tehran: Tarikh-e Iran, 1363/1984), vol. 2, p. 534 (nr. 8).
[303] A Friend of Iran, *"Dawdson," The Doctor*, pp. 60-62. For details see Verinder, A. *The Cry of the Children* (London: CMS, 1922); Floor, Willem. *Labour Unions, -Law and -Conditions in Iran (1900-1941)*, Occasional Paper no. 26, (Durham University, 1985).
[304] Ettehadiyeh (Nezam-Mafi), Mansureh. *Maramnamehha va Nezamnamehha-ye Ahzab-e Siyasi-ye Iran dar Dovvomin Dowreh-ye Majles-e Showra-ye Melli* (Tehran: Tarikh-e Iran, 1361/1982), pp. 52, 127, 163. Even in a small town like Ardabil some public health measures were taken. Moshir al-Hokama was the public health officer and inspected the public baths, the slaughterhouse and the ditches. Safari, *Ardabil*, vol. 3, p. 479.
[305] Floor, Willem. "The market police in Qajar Persia, the office of darugheh-yi bazar and muhtasib," *Die Welt des Islams* 13 (1971), pp. 212-29; Ibid., "Securité, Circulation et Hygiene dans les rues de Teheran a l'époque Qajar," in: Adle, Charyar et Hourcade, Bernard eds. *Teheran*, (Institut Francais de Recherche en Iran, 1992 - Bibliotheque iranienne, vol. 37), pp. 173-198.

make that happen. The allocated budget for the entire health sector for the year 1923-24 was only £27,000 of a total state budget of £5.7 million, or less than half a percent.[306] Also, the model it had chosen (a few expensive hospitals and a limited number of highly trained and expensive doctors) was not able to reach the majority of the population and thus address the root cause of the problem. The latter was not only in need of medical assistance, but above all in need of education. For having the wrong ideas about what caused disease and thus how to prevent them was more of an obstacle than the outbreak of disease itself. As Merritt-Hawkes pointed out in the early 1930s, "Education comes slowly, and there is too general a belief that the magic sun cures all evil. That is a tenacious national belief quite regardless of the facts."[307] Under the Pahlavi dynasty a beginning was made to improve public health, but it was only in the 1950s that nationwide and sustained medical campaigns were initiated to eradicate endemic diseases and to improve public and personal sanitation based on modern scientific knowledge.[308]

---

[306] Gilmour, *Rapport*, pp. 16-16.
[307] Merritt-Hawkes, *Persia*, p. 104.
[308] Government of Iran, *Iran-Shahr*, pp. 1399-1452; Schayegh, Cyrus. "Sport, Health, and the Iranian Modern Middle Class in the 1920s and 1930s," *Iranian Studies* 35 (2002), pp. 341-70.

CONCLUSION

Most of the data used in this book are from European sources, but there is a difference with other fields of life experience such as politics where parochial interests played a much greater role and hence information from European sources shows more bias. Most of the sources used were written by practicing doctors, many of whom knew the languages of Persia, its people and institutions. Many of them also had trained Persians to become physicians, and a number of them were even quite familiar with Islamic-Galenic medicine. Their observations therefore were often colored by a thorough and sympathetic understanding of the difficult process that Persians had to go through to adopt and adapt to a different paradigm, one that seemed to be at odds with what they had held dearly up till then. The litany of seemingly ridiculous, ignorant, and backward ideas, practices and beliefs has not been presented here to pass judgment on Persian medicine and its practitioners. Rather, in the words of Dr. Lichtward, "One mentions all these details of the present-day practice of ancient medicine, not to condemn, but merely to record."[1] The Persian sources that have been used (mainly by patients or friends and family members of patients) rather than contradicting the picture suggested by European sources confirm it.

All sources agree that health conditions in Qajar Persia were bad due to unsanitary conditions in either workplace or at home. Water sources generally were unclean and vectors for disease. There were neither public health services nor a notion of hygiene. Given these unsanitary conditions it was no surprise that endemic diseases as well as the occasional outbreak of the plague, cholera and other infectious diseases afflicted the Persian population. The most prevailing diseases included malaria, rheumatic affections, eye diseases, diseases of the digestive organs, and venereal diseases.

Not only did people not have any idea about the most basic ideas of hygiene, but neither did the prevailing systems of medical knowledge. One may distinguish three: Islamic-Galenic medicine, folk medicine and Prophetic medicine. These three systems co-existed in Qajar Persia, but unlike in medieval times there was an almost seamless transition from one to the other. The tension that had existed between Galenic medicine and Islam in the Middle Ages was something of the past. Galenic medicine, in fact, had become Islamic medicine. Medicine as practiced in Qajar Persia therefore was a blend of pre-Islamic Persian folk medicine, the Galenic concepts of the humors and temperaments that had entered into popular parlance in both urban and rural areas, and the overarching principle of divine or supernatural causation as represented by Prophetic medicine.

People applied the hot-cold dichotomy of Islamic-Galenic medicine universally; even those who had no idea that something like Islamic-Galenic or humoral medical theory existed. However, that was all it was; a convenient division of diseases that suggested that the doctor knew what he was talking about, which he did not. Moreover, it shows that folk medicine had adopted Islamic-Galenic medicine rather than the other way around. The professed practitioners of the latter discipline may have theorized humorally,

---

[1] Lichtwardt, "Ancient Medicine," p. 84.

and they did very little of that, but they acted by trial-and-error, very much as folk doctors did. The division between the three schools of medicine therefore may seem to be a bit artificial given their merging in practical terms, but it is necessary to show that the labels used (such as Islamic-Galenic) do not always reflect the nature or quality of the goods that they purport to offer. Moreover, even a superficial survey of articles and books, in particular those that profess to provide an overview of Persian medicine, show that they are all based on theoretical Islamic-Galenic medieval works and entirely ignore medical reality.

The reality was that folk medicine provided the majority of the population with medical care and it would continue to do so down to the mid-twentieth century. Galenic-Islamic medicine, which generally is still believed to have been the major medical system serving the population, was of little importance. The number of its practitioners was small, and their services were only available to those who could afford so, which was Persia's elite.

The introduction of modern western medicine into Qajar Persia in the early 1800s changed the way Persians thought about medical matters and how they practiced it, although it would take one-and-half century before western medicine really made its major and definite impact. There was some opposition against Western medicine among the medical professionals. This opposition came from some practitioners of the Islamic-Galenic system and only against the use of Western medical drugs. This was due to the fact that European doctors only challenged part of the medical establishment and tradition. They did not compete with the spiritual and popular healers, in fact, in certain and a growing number of cases, they rather enhanced their effectiveness, and in some cases even used them. Folk medicine mostly ignored Western medicine, although many of its practitioners absorbed the odd Western drug and practice into their arsenal, as they had done centuries earlier with Galenic medicine. Its practitioners continued to do their work and neither tried to denounce or embrace western medicine. This was partly due to the fact that they were mostly illiterate, and partly because they were not challenged by western medicine until the 1950s.

Not all Islamic-Galenic doctors opposed Western medicine, and even those that did, only opposed certain aspects thereof. For Western doctors were mainly concerned with *tebb-e yadi*, the hands-on medical practice. Persian Galenic doctors usually refrained from that type of therapy. The success of Western doctors was in surgery and even gynecology, areas that Galenic doctors left to practitioners of folk medicine.[2] The competition started with general practice and internal medicine, which was the domain of Galenic medicine. These opponents had no real scientific arguments against western medicine and could only refer to the lore of the ancients as their defense or to the foreignness of western medicine. Western doctors here also were able to offer better treatment and drugs, but they used chemical products, allegedly dangerous, nay even poisonous products, reason why Galenic doctors attacked that aspect of Western medicine, counting on people's ignorance to win their battle. Although they themselves had accepted the use of certain Western medicines they insisted that these had to be made inside Persia rather than in the

---

[2] This did not mean that they did not write about it; in fact, they did so rather profusely, see, for example, Cyril Elgood, *Safavid Medical Practice* (London: Luzac, 1970), pp. 208-33.

infidel West. Willy-nilly, Galenic practitioners started to use western medicines and methods, because even if they disagreed with western medicine and its drugs the latter's effectiveness could not be denied. The borrowing of western methods and medicines, however, often was without proper understanding of its methods and their proper use. Hajji Baba's chief-physician's request to steal the Frankish doctor's pill is illustrative in this respect. As a result, Galenic medicine that made the only oppositional noise was the one that was relegated to the dustbin of history unlike folk medicine that persists till today. New rules and institutions promoted western medicine, even if its results (Persian hospitals) sometimes looked like a caricature to western medical men.

The drive for change of the public health situation in Persia was driven by a small but over time growing number of reformers. The country's power elite wanted reforms (educational, military, industrial, political) to make Persia a stronger and more independent nation, and that movement also favored promoting modern medical knowledge. Initially these reforms had a mainly military objective, i.e. to enable Persia's army to be better trained, armed, and physically capable to deal with outside threats. However, in the second half of the nineteenth century this became part of a broader drive for modernization and overall and comprehensive change of Persian society. Clearly, not everybody agreed with the reformers and that was true for sectors other than the medical one as well.

As a result of the efforts by both Persians (doctors and political reformers) and Westerners towards the end of the nineteenth century Western medical concepts were gaining ground in all major towns, for a small, although growing, number of physicians had been educated in Europe and others who were medical graduates of the *Dar al-Fonun* or of the missionary hospitals. Also new laws and regulations were adopted to limit the practice of traditional medicine and to promote modern Western medicine. How limited the impact of these new ideas was may be clear from the fact that as late as 1924, there were only 253 physicians with diplomas from accredited schools, many of who were Europeans attached to their embassies or agencies, commercial or missionary. The government had only established a small number of hospitals, which mainly served the army. More effective and larger in number were the hospitals established and managed by missionary groups. Apart from some efforts to 'clean up' some streets of Tehran towards the end of the nineteenth century, the first concentrated and comprehensive national effort to improve living conditions in the city was the Municipal Act of 1913. Nevertheless, the resulting activities still fell far short of what was required to create better public hygienic conditions in the urban areas.

The penetration of medical knowledge and systems through missionaries may even have been more important than anything else, including government regulations. The missionary medical facilities provided state-of-the art medical service, trained a large number of medical practitioners (doctors, nurses) and ingrained ideas of hygiene among those whom they served. The government hospitals were fewer in number, less well equipped and staffed, and their service was of lower quality and less comprehensive in scope.

Meanwhile, most of the political and scientific-reformist attention stayed focused on a very expensive medical delivery system. That is, a system that was based on the use of highly trained, but costly doctors working in highly expensive hospitals. This meant that their services remained limited to a small segment of society. In this connection it is interesting to quote part of a satirical article from a newspaper from the small town of Qazvin in 1927. Under the heading "The difficulty of drugs and healthcare in Qazvin" the paper defined the term pharmacy and doctor as follows:

> Pharmacy: in Qazvin this means two to three shops of which the price of the European (*ferangi*) drugs are [so high that they are] with the recording angels (*ba keram al-katebeyn*) and all the sick people, whether rich or poor, cannot afford to buy.
> Doctor: thus people are called in Qazvin who write prescriptions in French and who do not take into account the purchasing power of the poor and miserable; a large number of the poor have died because they could not afford the high price of medicine have stopped using it.³

The majority of the population continued to be mainly served by folk medical practitioners. In the second half of the twentieth century folk medicine healers (ranging from herbalists and faith healers to bonesetters.) continued their practice in particular in the rural and tribal areas, but modern Western medicine has definitely become the major system of medicine that is being applied in Persia.⁴

Even the application of vaccination campaigns remained limited in size, as did other preventive measures, such as public hygiene. It was only starting in the 1950s that campaigns to eradicate endemic diseases were initiated and that battle was only won in the 1970s.⁵

---

³ Varjavand, *Sima-ye Tarikh*, vol. 3, p. 1823.
⁴ See, for example, Soltani, *Joghrafiya*, vol. 1, p. 537; Amir Hoseini, Karim Nikzad. *Shenakht-e Sarzamin-e Char Mahall* (Isfahan, 1357/1979), pp. 44-47; Jozani, *La beauté*; Safinezhad, Javad. *Talebabad* (Tehran: Daneshgah, 1345/1966), pp. 430 (*fal-gu'i*), 410-14 (medical superstitions), 491-94 (jinns, *pari*s, *div*s); Alberts, Robert Charles. *Social Structure and Cultural Change in an Iranian Village* 2 vols. (thesis University of Wisconsin, 1963), vol. 2, pp. 906-44.
⁵ Faghih, Mohammad Ali. "Behdari," *Encyclopedia Iranica* vol. 4, pp. 101-02. For an overview about the changes brought about in a small provincial town see, for example, Badri Zahireddini, *Medizinische Topographie der iranischen Stadt Malayer* (thesis Erlangen-Nürnberg, 1966).

Appendix 1

Mansur Sheybani's Eyes – a case-study of sorts

In his Diary, Basir al-Molk, an important government official in the time of Naser al-Din Shah, made entries with regards to the treatment of his son's, Mansur, eye-disease. Basir al-Molk did not elaborate on the type of eye disease, and did not even refer to it by name. Although we have to guess what kind of affliction it was, the short notations in his diary throw some interesting light on the nature of medical therapeutic methodology. For easy reference I have inserted the page numbers of Basir al-Molk's Diary between brackets in the translated paraphrased text.

On 6 Ramazan 1304 (May 29,1887) Basir al-Molk noted that it is now two days that Mansur's eye hurt. The next day (May 30), he did not leave the house because of the intense pain in Mansur's eye. He sent for Nur Mohammad who bled Mansur. Basir al-Molk also stayed home on May 31, because of Mansur's pain. Nur Mohammad came in the afternoon and opened Mansur's eye. Basir al-Molk was totally upset. On June 1, Mansur's condition was bad and his eye was troubled (*maghshush*). Nur Mohammad came every day to treat Mansur. Yusef went and brought Khanom Nahneh, the wife of Mirza Hoseyn Zenjani, the sister of Mirza Masih Zenjani of the Owlad-e Mirza Ketab-e Allah. She recommended applying a plaster (*moshama'*). Nur Mohammad concurred. They applied a plaster and Mansur's situation got a bit better. The next day (June 2) Nur Mohammad opened the eye and it was a bit better. From to-day *shadanj* (?) was put in the eye. [258] On June 14, Basir al-Molk did not leave his house. In the morning Nur Mohammad came and gave a prescription and left. On June 15, Basir al-Molk took Mansur to the house Mo'taman al-Atebba to have him treat Mansur's eye. [259] On 1 Shavval 1304 (June 23, 1887) Nur Mohammad came and applied a plaster to Mansur's temple, gave a prescription and left. Two days later (25 June, 1887), Nur Mohammad came and told Basir al-Molk that there was an Indian sayyed who treated eyes. Basir al-Molk told him to bring the sayyed. Mirza `Abdol-Hoseyn also was there. They discussed things for some time. The sayyed wrote [a prescription] for a [mercury] pill. The ingredients were fetched, brought and made. Mansur ate three of these pills. He also gave a prescription for the eye. Mirza `Abdol-Hoseyn also wrote [some ingredients for a medicine] on that prescription. They left to get the drugs. The next day (June 26) Basir al-Molk sent again for the Indian sayyed, who made an eye medicine and put it into Mansur's eye. He took one toman as a fee (*haqq al-qadam*) for two visits and left. In the afternoon Nur Mahmud came; he administered the medicine, gave a prescription and left. A sayyed, the brother-in-law of the late Mirza Sayyed Razi came, looked at the eye and left. On June 28, Basir al-Molk put the Indian sayyed's medicine in Mansur's eye. It did not seem to do much. The next day (June 29), Nur Mahmud came, and Basir al-Molk used his medicine. He then sent for a female eye-physician, simply referred to as the wife of Mirza (*zan-e Mirza*). She came and gave a red and white medicine to put in Mansur's eyes. [261]. Almost one month later (2 Dhu'l-Qa`deh 1304/23 July, 1887) Basir al-Molk sent again for Sayyed Kahhal, the eye-doctor, and Hajji Sayyed Ahmad, son of the late Hajji Sayyed Mohammad Rowzehkhvan. Apparently the earlier treatment had had no result. The sayyed gave Mansur snuff (*anfiyeh*) and also a prescription for more of it. The snuff was fetched, but because it was of bad quality he had it returned. [This was probably given to make Mansur vomit] [268] The next day (July 24) Sayyed Kahhal came. A new medicine, consisting of juice of aloes (*sabr-e zard*) mixed with girl's milk (*shir-e dokhtar*, i.e., milk from a lactating mother who teats a girl)[1] was put in Mansur's eyes. The sayyed also gave *kondos* snuff (glasswort or a sterntatory). [268]. Two days later (July 26), Basir al-Molk sent for Sayyed Kahhal but he did not come, because he had taken a purgative (*moshel*). He gave, however, a medicine to put into Mansur's eye in the evening. Basir al-Molk wrote him to come, but the Sayyed replied to stick to the medicine. In the evening Basir al-Molk put the medicine in Mansur's eyes, while Mansur also ate one *methqal* (4.6 grams) of black myrobalan (*halileh-ye siyah*). [269]. Three days later (August 1), Sayyed Kahhal came and changed the medicine. He said this is the first day that I have administered this to Mansur, and it should take the granulation (*daneh*) out of his eye in five days. He also mentioned two other [unnamed] medicines that Basir al-Molk had to get. The next day (August 2) the doctor (Sayyed Hakim) returned. Basir al-Molk gave him the medicine and the magnet (*maqnatis*) that Reza Khan had bought yesterday. He said he had to examine it and took it with him. Reza Khan also had bought copper-oxide (*lasorkh*) and gave it to the doctor. The next day (August 3) the Sayyed came and gave medicine in which he had mixed the two drugs bought yesterday. Basir al-Molk gave him three tomans. [270]. The same day, Saraj al-Atabba came, who had been sent by Amin-e Hezrat. It was agreed that he would wait to see how things went. The next day (August 4), Sayyed Hakim came back from Shah `Abdol-`Azim and immediately gave Mansur his medicine. Basir al-Molk told the Sayyed about Saraj al-Atebba's consultation, and told him that it had been agreed to give Mansur calomel. He said, that if it did not help he would himself take care of it. Two days later (August 6), Sayyed Hakim came and put the medicine in Mansur's eye; he then ate lunch and left. [271]. The next day (August 7), the Sayyed came and poured the medicine into Mansur's eyes. The following day (August 8) he did the same. The day thereafter (August 9), the day Sayyed Hakim came. He had changed the medicine. For the right eye he gave a white medicine and for the left eye a red one. [272]. On August 10, Mirza `Abdol-Hoseyn came; it was agreed that Basir al-Molk give calomel for Mansur to eat. He left and made a pill that Mansur ate. Each pill had less than one 0.047 g (*gandom*) of calomel. The next day (August 11), Mirza `Abdol-Hoseyn said Mansur' eyes need an aggressive [*hesabi*] treatment. [273]. Three days later (August 14) Saraj al-Atebba came to see Mansur's eyes. He said, "to-night we will apply *surmeh* on the eyes." He gave yellow and red medicine with essence of quince (*lo`ab*), to drop in Mansur's eyes at night. The next day (August 15), Mirza Sheikh `Ali Saraj al-Atebba gave a prescription. The next day (August 16), he returned. Mansur felt bad. We stopped the calomel pill; he had eaten one in the morning and felt bad. Saraj al-Atebba gave a gargling drug (*gharghareh*) and left. Basir al-Molk sent for Hajji Sayyed Ahmad; he gave a gum disease (*pay-e dandan*) medicine and Mansur

---

[1] "Milk of a mother of a boy baby is 'warm,' while that of a mother of a girl is 'cold.' The latter is used in making soothing poultices and it is put into the ear to cure earache, and when it is mixed with the powdered berries of the wild barberry, it is believed to reduce inflammation." Donaldson, *The Wild Rue*, p. 192. According to Polak, "Medicinische Briefe," p. 139, "mother milk is sold here like cow milk by the pint. Old people, those with a decrepit constitution, and convalescing patients drink mother milk here, sometimes 130 *methqal*s [598 grams], about 150 Drachms; I often saw the most ambigious results, in particular in the case of a person convalescing from breast pain. Mostly it worked as a light purging."

improved; he also put medicine into Mansur's eyes. Mansur was quiet that night. In the afternoon Sayyed came and spoke some words of no account and left. He looked at the eye and then said, "I had not seen the eye. Now, we probably may cure it." The next day (August 17), Sayyed Hakim came; Saraj al-Atebba also came. They had applied the Sayyed's treatment. Sayyed Hakim came to Basir al-Molk's office and left a note saying that Mansur's right eye should be cured in the next 40 days. [274]. The next day (August 18), Sayyed Hakim came and left. Meanwhile, Sayyed Hakim had written a note to Basir al-Molk that he wanted 20 tomans. The following day (August 19), Sayyed Hakim came and gave a purgative (*moshel*) pill; he stayed and had lunch, then left. From his home he wrote Basir al-Molk a note to give the money. On 1 Dhu'l-Hejjah 1304/August 21, 1887 Mansur was bad. The pill that the Sayyed had given yesterday had resulted in much bowel movement and Mansur felt bad. Basir al-Molk did not sent for the Sayyed, but for Hajji Mirza Habibollah Hakim-bashi. He treated the bowel movement (*mezaji*); then left and said, "now we have to treat temper (*mezaj*)." He did not say anything good regarding the eye. [275]. Two days later Mirza's wife came, she said her bit and it was agreed that she would cure him in the next fortnight. [276] On August 24, Mansur got a little better. The child's eye had become troubled (*magshush*). That day it was the seventh or eighth day that it had become troubled. He said that his eye was infected (*dan zadeh*). Yesterday he had been taken to the house of `Arus NahNeh `Abdollah. To-day he also had been taken there. After sunset Nahneh Ostad Hasan came; she lanced one eye of the child and put egg yolk on it. Two days later (August 26), Mansur and some others went to make a pilgrimage at Shah `Abdol-`Azim. His eye infection (*daneh*) was better now they all said. [277]. On September 3, 1887 Basir al-Molk got a prescription for a poultice (*zomad*) for the child's eye. [279]. On September 17, the shah asked how is your child doing? [283]. On 5 Moharram, 1304/ October 4, 1887, Mirza's wife (*zan-e mirza*) healed an inflammation [?] [literally: killed the sparrow (*gonjeshk*)] in Mansur's eye. [285]. One week later (October 12), Mirza's wife promised to heal Mansur's eye one week later, and if not, Basir al-Molk would change doctors. [288]. To-day (October 22) Mansur felt indisposed, and ran a fever (*tebb*) in the afternoon. I sent for Zeyn al-`Abdin Khan; he did not come. The next day (October 23) he had malaria (*nowbeh*). In the morning, Mirza Sayyed Mohammad Hakim came and gave a medicine and an enema. He got better. In the evening Mansur had again fever and malaria. On October 24 Aqa Sayyed Baqer, came with his brother Mirza Khalil. He gave violet snuff for Mansur. When Basir al-Molk came home, Mansur had a severe fever; during the night he started to transpire and it became clear that he had malaria [292] On October 28, Hajji Mirza Abu'l-Qasem Saruji came; he stated that in 10 days Mansur's eye would be better and dripped medicine [in his eye]. [293] On 5 Safar, 1304/November 3, 1887, the infection (*daneh*) in his eyes was opened with the point of the lancet, liquid came, and he immediately saw the *akhund*'s face. [295]. A surgeon came to see Mansur's eye on November 5; he poured oil in it. [296]. On November 13 Basir al-Molk tried to see Tholozan with Mansur, but he was not in. [298]. On 1 Rabi` I, 1304 (November 28, 1886) Mansur had a headache and a bit of fever. The next day Mansur had a strong fever; he transpired from night till morning. On November 30, in the afternoon Basir al-Molk sent for Sayyed Fathollah Mirza Habibollah to treat Mansur's eye. [302] On December 12 and 14, Mansur went with his mother to the Shah `Abdol-`Azim shrine. [304-05] On 22 Rabi` II, 1304 (January 18, 1887) Basir al-Molk went to see the chief British physician; he and a colleague examined Mansur's eye carefully, and told him that if he wanted them to heal it they would. [312]. To-day (January 31) Mirza Heydar `Ali Khan came to see Mansur [316] On February 6, Mirza Farajollah Khan came to see Mansur [317] [It is not known why this piece of good news from the British doctors was not pursued, but Basir al-Molk is silent about the matter. Shortly thereafter he moved for one year to Malayer.] In that town there was an American doctor whom he went to see on 1 Sha`ban 1305/April 13, 1888 to see whether he could heal Mansur's eyes, but he did not learn anything new. [342]. [During his stay in Zenjan he corresponded with Mansur (pp. 347, 355, 358, 360, 362, 365, 366, 367, 377, 379-85, 387-90, 394-97, 400-03), but Basir al-Molk did not make any note on his son's health situation] On his return to Tehran after one year, Basir al-Molk reported on 28 Shavval, 1306/June 26, 1889 that the eye-surgeon (*jarrah-e cheshm*) Hajji Mirza Abu'l-Qasem came to treat Mansur's eye. [421]. On July 8, 1889 Hakim `Ashur started to treat Mansur's eye. He also came three days later to see Mansur. He gave him his previous digestive (*monzej*) and left [425]. To-day (July 18) was Mansur's for a purging and he did not eat [426] Hashem Hakim came to-day (July 17, 1889); he advised to change Mansur's treatment and left [426] This is the last time that Basir al-Molk reported on his son's illness. His diary came to an end on 28 Rajab 1307/March 20, 1890 or about 8 months later.

What is of interest of the chronological description of Mansur's illness, at least in my view, is the fact that (i) there was no real examination of Mansur's eyes and thus no diagnosis and that the treatment started, of course, with bleeding; (ii) there was no method, but for an empiricist, *i.e.*, a trial-and-error one; (iii) some of the physicians clearly did not know what they were doing, given the fact that two of them prescribed a different medicine for the left and the right eye; (iv) there usually was more than one physician involved in Mansur's treatment and they were changed regularly; (v) there was a realization that the patient's temper (*mezaj*) had to be stabilized.

Appendix 2

Table: Published medical works written by European teachers at the *Dar al-Fonun* between 1852-1888

Teacher	Title	Date of publication
Polak	*Mo'alejat va Tedabir-e Amraz-e Nowbeh va Eshal* (On the treatment of malaria and diarrhea),	1269/1852
Polak	*Bist Bab dar Tashrih* (twenty chapters on anatomy).	1269/1852
Polak	*Vaba'iyeh* (On cholera).	1269/1852.
Polak	*Tashrih-e Badan-e Ensan* (Human anatomy).	1270/1853
Polak	*Zobdat al-Hekmah* (The essence of medical science).	1272/1855
Polak	*Alaj al-Aqasam* (Treatment of illnesses).	1273/1856
Polak	*Ketab-e Jarrahi* (On surgery).	1273/1856
Polak	*Patuluzhi* (Pathology)..	1277/1860
Polak	*Jala al-'Oyun* (Ophthalmology).	1300/1882
Polak	*Somusat va Taryaq* (Poisons and Antidotes).	1304/1886
Polak	*Ketabcheh-ye Tebb-e Nezami* (Military Medicine).	?
Polak	*Kahhali* (Ophthalmology).	?
Schlimmer	*Serr al-Hekmah* (the Secret of Medicine).	1279/1862
Schlimmer	*Zinat al-Abdan* (On skin diseases).	1279/1862
Schlimmer	*Shafa'iyeh* (On remedies).	1284/1867
Schlimmer	*Loghatnameh* (Persian French dictionary)	1291/1874
Schlimmer	*Qava'ed al-Amraz* (Pathology).	1292/1875
Schlimmer	*Ashab al-Taviyeh* (Pharmacology)	?
Schlimmer	*Meftah al-Khavas* (On the use of medications)	?
Schlimmer	*Jala' al-'Oyun* (Ophthalmology)	?
Tholozan	*Zobdat al-Hekmah* (The essence of medical science)	1280/1863
Tholozan	Ornithorus Tholozanus (Parasitology)	
Albo	*Jarrahi va Darsha-ye Klinik* (Surgery and clinical medicine)	1305/1888
Albo	*Terapetik* (Therapeutics),	1283/1888

Source: Ekhtiar, *Dar al-Funun*, pp. 312-13; Schlimmer, *Terminologie*, pp. 229; Qasemi, *Danesh*, p. 37 (Albo publication).

Table: Manuscripts of medical works written by European teachers at the *Dar al-Fonun* between 1852-1888

Teacher	Title	Date
Polak	*Bimariha-ye cheshm* (Eye diseases)	?
Polak	*Patuluzhi* (Pathology)	?
Polak	*Tashrih* (Anatomy)	?
Polak	*Tashrih-badan-e ensan* (Anatomy of the Human Body)	1053
Polak	*Jarrahi* (On Surgery)	1311
Polak	*Jarrahi va darsha-ye keliniki* (Surgery and clinical lessons)	1306
Polak	*Jala' al-'oyun* (Ophthalmology)	1287
Polak	Resaleh-ye mo'alejeh-ye marz-e vaba (On the treatment of cholera)	1269
Polak	*Zobdat al-Hekmah* (Essence of medical science)	1279
Polka	*Resaleh dar jarrahi* (Treatise on surgery)	1302
Schlimmer	*Adviyeh va noskheha* (Drugs and prescriptions)	?
Schlimmer	*Asbab al-Tadviyeh* (Drugs)	1292
Schlimmer	*Amraz al-Sebyan* (Children diseases)	?
Schlimmer	*Patuluzhi* (Pathology)	?
Schlimmer	*Tohfeh-ye Naseri* (Naseri's Gift)	?
Schlimmer	*Tashrih-e madeh-ye 'asabi* (Anatomy of the nervous system)	1294
Schlimmer	*Jala' al-'oyun* (Ophthalmology)	1277
Schlimmer	*Zeinat al-abdan* (ornament of physiology)	1313
Schlimmer	*Serr al-hekmah* (Secret of medical science)	?
Schlimmer	*Shafa'iyeh* (Curative medicine)	1274
Schlimmer	*Qarabadeyn* (Pharmacopoeia)	1292

Schlimmer	*Qava'ed al-Amraz* (Canons of disease)	?
Schlimmer	*Meftah al-Khavas* (Key to Properties)	1277
Schlimmer	*Montakhab al-shafa'iyeh* (Selected treatment)	1305
Tholozan	*Abeleh kubi* (Vaccination)	1279
Tholozan	*Badaye' al-Hekmah-ye Naseri* (Marvels of medical Science)	1279
Albo	*Bayan-e marz nashi az khurdan-e gusht-e khuk va jarrahi-ye nezami* (Symptoms due to eating of pork and military surgery)	1300
Albo	*Terapetik* (Therapeutics	?
Albo	*Jarrahi* (Surgery)	?
Albo	*Jarrahi va darsha-ye kelinik* (Surgery and clinical lessons)	1306
Albo	*Tebb-e Jadid or Darsha-ye kelinik* (Modern medicine and clinical medicine)	?

Source: Arjah et al., *Ketabshenasi*; Schlimmer, *Terminologie*, pp. 229.

Table: Published medical works written by Persian teachers or students at the *Dar al-Fonun* between 1882-1897

Persian teacher/instructor	Title	Date of publication
`Ali Akbar Nafisi	*Pezeshknameh* (Medical therapy)	1317/1897
`Ali Ra'is al-Atebba & Dr. Khalil Khan Saqafi	*Javaher al-Hekmat* (On pathology)	1305/1887
Idem	*Amraz-e A`sab* (Neurological disorders)	?
Idem	*Amraz-e Nesvan* (Gynecology)	?
Idem	*Amraz-e Atfal* (Pediatrics)	?
Idem	*Ziya al-`Oyun* (Ophthalmology)	1300/1882
Abu'l-Hasan Bahrami	*Patuluzhi* (Pathology)	1300/1882
Idem	*Terapiyutik* (Therapeutics)	1305/1887
Idem	*Hezf al-Sehheh* (On health)	1312/1894

Idem	*Tashrih* (Anatomy)	1312/1894
Idem	*Fiziyuluzhi* (Physiology)	1315/1897
Hoseyn Khan Nezam al-Hokumeh Hanjan	*Meftah al-Adviyeh-ye Naseri* (Guide to medications)	?
Dr. Khalil Khan Saqafi	*Ma`refat al-Ruh* (On psychology)	1306/1888
Idem	*Resaleh'i dar jarrahi* (a treatise on surgery)	
Dr. Kermanshahi	*Amraz-e Moqarebati* (On venereal disease)	?
Idem	*Bimarishenasi* (Pathology)	?

Source: Ekhtiar, *Dar al-Funun*, pp. 314-16; Nafisi, "Doktor `Ali Akbar Khan," p. 63 (also for other medical books by Nafisi);

Appendix 3

Decisions of the Sanitary Council of Khorasan

Pursuant to the Royal Order a council met consisting of government officials and physicians that discussed all aspects of the state of public health of the people of Khorasan. The issues that were discussed and agreed upon and that need to be banned and forbidden in the interest of the public health of the people of this province are as follows:

First, once per week or twice per month, all doctors in the city have to convene in council and discuss the state of public health in the province. Whenever a new disease manifests itself in the city and its environs it has to plan its treatment and inform Hasan Khan, public health officer (*Hafez al-Sehhah*) for Khorasan, who on behalf of that council will inform the Sanitary Council of Tehran and request suggestions and instructions.

Second, all lepers have to evicted from the city altogether and to be relocated in the fortress of Kalat or some other secure place. Special [drinking] water [places] and bathhouses have to be prepared for them so that they will have no contact with other people.

Third, it will be strictly forbidden that clothes and old things, and the like are washed in the running streams and water reservoirs of the city, because most diseases are transmitted by these activities.

Fourth, people should not drink water from water reservoirs without a tap, and all city water reservoirs have to be equipped with a tap.

Fifth, a number of staff and a few head of mules are needed to clean the streets; they will be paid wages. Their main task is to remove the filth from the streets; therefore, each day they have keep the streets clean from filth and transport it outside the city. [27]

Sixth, because most of the refuse and filth comes from covered passageways, all these passageways have to be done away with, so that all streets are open to the sun.

Seventh, all the ditches of the bathhouses have to disappear. Undertakings have to be obtained that their owners will remove the wastewater from the city by digging subterraneous canals (*qanat*), because these items are a major cause of filth.

Eighth, latrine pits that are situated in the streets have to be forbidden and done away with entirely; no pits must be allowed in the streets.

Ninth, all physicians have to hold a meeting concerning the matter of the druggists. In the entire city a few experienced druggists have to be selected. Persons without the necessary knowledge are not allowed to sell drugs and thus to lead people to perdition.

Tenth, wells that are dug for drinking water are mostly near, if not adjacent to a latrine. It goes without saying, that its filth will pollute the water well. This [practice] is totally forbidden; latrines and water wells have to be dug at wide distances from one another, so that the drinking water is pure and not contaminated.

[in the margin of the letter] Rokn al-Dowleh, this needs to be executed in this manner and with sufficient and faithful attention; the beglerbegi [mayor] of the city has to give strict orders that he will strive in the same manner concerning the cleaning of the city of Mashad and each day a daily report has to be submitted. Done in 1300 Quy'il (1882, Sheep Year). [28]

Source: Nezam al-Saltaneh, *Khaterat va Asnad*, vol. 2, pp. 27-28.

BIBLIOGRAPHY

Abbott, K.E. "Notes Taken on a Journey Eastwards from Shiraz to Fessa and Darab, Thence Westwards by Jehrum to Kazerun, in 1850." *JRGS* XXVII (1857), p. 149-184.

Abu'l-Hasan Khan, Mirza. *A Persian at the Court of King George 1809-10. The Journal of Mirza Abul Hassan Khan.* translated and edited by Margaret Morris Cloake (London: Barrie & Jenkins, 1988)

Adamec, L. ed. *Historical Gazetteer of Iran*, 4 vols. (Graz: Akademische Verlag, 1981).

Adamiyat, Fereydun. *Amir Kabir* (Tehran: Khvarezmi, 1348/1969).

Adams, Isaac. *Persia by a Persian* (n.p., 1900).

Adler, Elkan Nathan. *Jews in Many Lands* (Philadelphia: Jewish Publication Society of America, 1905).

A Friend of Iran, *"Dawdson," The Doctor. G.E. Dodson of Iran* (London: Highway Press, 1940).

Afshar, Iraj. 'Dar bareh-ye Doktor Yusef Mir," in Iraj Afshar ed., *Namvareh-ye Doktor Mahmud Afsha*r 12 vols. (Tehran: Mowqufeh-ye Doktor Mahmud Afshar, 1367/1988), vol. 4, pp. 2169-82.

Afzal al-Molk Kermani, Gholam Hoseyn. *Tarikh va Joghrafiya-ye Qom*. ed. Hoseyn Modarresi Tabataba'i (Qom, 1396Q/1976).

Aitchison, J.E.T. "Notes on the products of Western Afghanistan and of North-Eastern Persia," *Transactions of the Botanical Society* (Edinburgh) XVIII (1890).

Amir Hoseyni, Karim Nikzad. *Shenakht-e Sarzamin-e Char Mahall* (Isfahan, 1357/1979).

Anonymous [John Malcolm], *Sketches of Persia, from the journals of a traveller in the East* 2 vols. (London, 1828).

Anonymous, "Ärtze und Arzneiwissenschaft in Persien," *Mitteilungen der K.K. Geographischen Gesellschaft* XLVIII (Vienna, 1905), p. 97.

Ardakani, Hoseyn Mahbubi, *Tarikh-e Mo'assesat-e Tamaddon-e Jadid dar Iran* 3 vols. (Tehran: Daneshgah, 1368/1989).

Arjah, Akram- Hadiyan, Farideh- Soltanifar, Sadiqeh- and Chehrekhand, Zahrah eds. *Ketabshenasi-e Nosakh-e Khatti-ye Pezeshki-ye Iran* (Tehran: Ketabkhhaneh-ye Melli, 1371/1992).

Arnold, A. *Through Persia by Caravan* (New York: Harper & Brothers, 1877).

Asaf al-Dowleh, Mirza `Abdol-Vahhab Khan. *Asnad* 2 vols. ed. `Abdol-Hoseyn Nava'i and Nilufar Kasri (Tehran: Mo'asseseh-ye Motale`at-e Tarikh-e Mo`aser-e Iran, 1377/1998).

Aubin, Eugène. *La Perse d'aujourd'hui* (Paris: Armand Colin, 1908).

Babin, C and Houssay, F. "A Travers La Perse Méridionale," *Le Tour du Monde* 64 (1892).

Baker, James E. "A few remarks on the most prevalent Diseases and the Climate of the North of Persia," appendix to Herbert, Report on the present State of Persia and her Mineral Resources, House of Commons, Parliamentary Papers, *Accounts and Papers* 1886, 67, pp. 323-26.

Baladiyeh-ye Tehran (Servis-e Ma`aref va Ehsa'iyeh va Nashriyat). *Dovvomin Salnameh-ye Ehsa'iyeh-ye Shahr-e Tehran* (Tehran, 1310/1931).

Barton, James L. *Story of Near East Relief 1915-1930 An Interpretation* (New York: MacMillan, 1930).

Basir al-Molk Sheybani. *Ruznameh-ye Khaterat*. eds. Iraj Afshar and Mohammad Rasul Daryagasht (Tehran: Donya-ye Ketab, 1374/1995).

Bélanger, Charles. *Voyage aux Indes-Orientales*. 2 vols. (Paris: Arthus Bertrand, 1838).

Benjamin, S.G.W. "Farm Life and Irrigation in Persia," *The Cosmopolitan* 9/June (1890), pp. 131-44.

Binder, Henry. *Au Kurdistan* (Paris: Quantin, 1887).

Bird, Isabella (Mrs. Bishop). *Journeys in Persia and Kurdistan*, 2 vols. (London, 1891 [London: Virago Travellers, 1988]).

Bradley-Birt, F.B. *Persia, through Persia from the Gulf to the Caspian* (Boston: J.B. Millet, 1910).

Brittlebank, William. *Persia During the Famine* (London: Basil Montague Pickering, 1873).

Browne, E.G. *A Year Amongst the Persians* (London: A. & C. Black, 1970).

Brugsch, Heinrich. *Die Reise der K.K. Gesandtschaft nach Persien 1861-1862*, 2 vols. (Berlin: J.C. Hinrichs, 1863).

———. *Im Lande der Sonne. Wanderungen in Persien* (Berlin: Algemeine Verein f. Deutsche Literatur, 1886).

Buckingham, J.S. *Travels in Assyria, Media and Persia* (London, 1829 [Westmead: Gregg Int., 1971]).

Chirikov, E.I. *Putvoj zhurnal russkogo komissara-posrednika po turetsko-persidskomu razgranicheniyu* (St. Petersburg, 1875) translated by Abkar Masihi as *Siyahatnameh-ye Mosiyu Cherikof.* ed. `Ali Asghar `Omran (Tehran: Jibi, 1358/1979).

Chodzko, Alexandre. "Le Ghilan ou Les Marais Caspiens," *Nouvelles Annales des Voyages*, N.S. 2 (1850), pp. 285-93.

Churchill, S.T.A. "Sacrifices in Persia," *The Indian Antiquary* 20 (1891), p. 148.

Clarke, H.T. "Sketches on the State of Medical Knowledge in Persia," *London Medical and Surgical Journal* 2 (1837), pp. 707-10.

Cochran, James P. "Treatment of the Sick and Insane in Persia," *The American Journal of Insanity* 56 (1899), pp.105-07.

———. "Letter from Persia," *Medical Press of western New York* 2 (1887), pp. 83-85.

Collins, Edward Treacher. *In the Kingdom of the Shah* (London: T.F.Unwin, 1896).

Collins, Henry. W. *From Pigeon Post to Wireless* (London: Hodden and Stoughton, 1925).

Colvill, W.H. "Sanitary Report on Turkish Arabia," *Transactions of the Bombay Society* N.S. 11 (1872), pp. 32-73.

Danesh in: *Shekufeh beh enzemam-e Danesh. Nakhostin nashriyehha-ye zanan-e Iran* (Tehran: Ketabkhaneh-ye Melli, 1377/1998).

Dashti, `Ali, "Dar bareh-ye Doktor Yusef Mir," in Iraj Afshar ed., *Namvareh-ye Doktor Mahmud Afshar* 12 vols. (Tehran: Mowqufeh-ye Doktor Mahmud Afshar, 1367/1988), vol. 4, pp. 2177-79.

De Bode, C.A. *Travels in Luristan and Arabistan*. 2 vols. (London: J. Madden & Co, 1845).

De Fontenelle, Julia. "Das Apothekerwesen in Persien," *Das Ausland* 1838, pp. 119-20.

De Freygang, Madame. *Letters from the Caucasus and Georgia* (London: John Murray, 1823).

De Gobineau, A. *Trois Ans en Asie (de 1855 A 1858)* 2 vols. (Paris, Bernard Grasset, 1923).

———. *Les Réligions et les Philosophies dans l'Asie Centrale* 2 vols. (Paris: G. Crès et Cie., 1923).

———. *Les Dépêches Diplomatiques.* ed. Adrienne Doris Hytier (Geneva-Paris: Droz-Minard, 1959).

Dequevaullier, Dr. "Notice sur le docteur Ernest Cloquet," in *Notices sur le docteur Ernest Cloquet* (Paris, 1856), pp.8-23.

De Windt, Harry. *A Ride to India across Persia and Baluchistan* (London: Chapman & Hall, 1891).

Dieulafoy, Jane. *La Perse, la Chaldée et la Susiane* (Paris: Hachette, 1887).

Dols, Michael W. "Islam and Medicine," *History of Science* 26 (1988), pp. 417-25.

Donaldson, Bess Allen. *The Wild Rue. A Study of Muhammadan Magic and Folklore in Iran* (London: Luzac & Co, 1938).

Drouville, Gaspard. *Voyage en Perse pendant les années 1812 et 1813*. 2 vols. (Paris, 1819 [Tehran: Imp. Org. f. Social Services, 1976).

D'Vaume, Dr. "La lèpre dans le Kurdistan Persan," *Bulletin de la Société d'Anthropologie de Lyon* 5 (1886), pp. 158-62.

Eastwick, Edward B. *Journal of a Diplomate's Three Years' Residence in Persia*. 2 vols. (London, 1864 [Tehran: Imp. Org. f. Soc. Services, 1976]).

Ebrahimnejad, Hormoz. "Introduction de la médecine européenne en Iran au XIXe siècle," *Sciences Sociales et Santé* 16/4 (décembre 1998), pp. 69-96.

-. "La médecine d'observation en Iran du XIX siècle," *Generus* 55 (1998), pp. 33-57.

———. "Un traité d'épidémologie de la médecine traditionelle persane: *Mofarraq ol-Heyze va'l-Vaba* de Mirza Mohammad-Taqi Shirazi (ca. 1800-1873), *Studia Iranica* 27 (1988) pp. 83-107.

———. Theory and Practice in Nineteenth-Century Persian Medicine: Intellectual and Institutional Reforms," *History of Science* 38 (2000), pp. 171-78.

———. "Religion and Medicine in Iran: from Relationship to Dissocation," *History of Science* 40 (2002), pp. 91-112.

Edmonds, C.J. "Luristan: Pish-e Kuh and Bala Gariveh," *Geographical Journal* 59 (1922), pp. 335-56, 437-53.

Ehtesham al-Saltaneh. *Khaterat*. ed. Sayyed Mohammad Mehdi Musavi (Tehran: Zavvar, 1366/1987).

Eichwald, Eduard. *Reise auf dem Caspischen Meere und in den Caucasus Unternommen in den Jahren 1825-1826*. 2 vols. (Stuttgart und Tübingen: J.G. Cotta, 1834).

Eilers, Wilhelm. *Die Al, ein persisch Kindbettgespenst* (Munich, Bayerische Akademie der Wissenschaften, 1979).

Ekhtiar, Maryam Dorreh. *The Dar al-Funun: Educational Reform and Cultural Development in Qajar Iran* (unpublished thesis, New York University 1994).

Elgood, Cyril. *Medical History of Persia, and the eastern caliphate* (Cambridge: CUP, 1951).

Eqbal, `Abbas. "Abeleh-kubi," *Yadgar*, vol. 4/3 (1326/1947), pp. 68-72.

Eqbal, Yaghma'i. "Doktor Mohammad Hasan Khan Hakim al-Dowleh," *Amuzesh va Parvaresh* 42 (1351/1972), pp. 358-64.

E`temad al-Saltaneh, Mohammad Hasan Khan. *Ruznameh-ye Khaterat*. ed. Iraj Afshar (Tehran: Amir Kabir, 1345/1967).

———. *Mer'at al-Boldan* 4 vols in 3. ed. `Abd al-Hoseyn Nava'i and Mir Hashem Mohaddeth (Tehran: Daneshgah, 1368/1989).

———. *Montazam-e Naseri*. 3 vols. (Tehran, 1300/1883).

———. *Ketab al-Athar va'l-Ma'ather* (Tehran, 1306/1884).

E`tesam al-Molk, *Safarnameh-ye Mirza Khanlar Khan E`tesam al-Molk*. ed. Manuchehr Mahmudi (Tehran, 1351/1972).

Ettehadieh, Mansureh."Patterns in urban development; the growth of Tehran (1852-1903)," in Bosworth, Edmund and Hillenbrand, Carole eds. *Qajar Iran. Political, Social and Cultural Change 180-1925* (Edinburgh, Edinburgh UP, 1983), pp. 199-212.

`Eyn al-Saltaneh, Qahraman Mirza Salur. *Ruznameh-ye Khaterat*. 10 vols. eds. Mas`ud Salur and Iraj Afshar (Tehran: Asatir, 1376/1997).

Farmanfarma, Firuz Mirza. *Safarnameh-ye Kerman va Baluchistan*. ed. Mansureh Ettehadiyeh (Nazem-Mafi) (Tehran: Babak, 1360/1981).

Farmanfarma, `Abdol-Hoseyn Mirza. *Siyaq-e Ma`ishat dar `Ahd-e Qajar*. 2 vols. eds. Mansureh Ettehadiyeh and Sirus Sa`dvandiyan (Tehran: Tarikh-e Iran, 1362/1983).

Fasa'i, Hajj Mirza Hasan Hoseyni. *Farsnameh-ye Naseri*. 2 vols. ed. Mansur Rastgar Fasa'i (Tehran: Amir Kabir, 1378/1999).

Feilberg, C.G. *Les Papis* (Copenhagen: Nordisk, 1952).

Ferrier, J-P. "Lettre [sur le docteur Cloquet]," in *Notices sur le docteur Ernest Cloquet* (Paris, 1856), pp. 23-24.

Feuvrier, J.B.: *Trois ans à la Cour de Perse*. (Paris: F. Juven, 1900).

Floor, Willem. "Securité, Circulation et Hygiene dans les rues de Teheran a l'époque Qajar," in: Adle, Charyar et Hourcade, Bernard eds. *Téhéran Capitale bicentenaire*, Institut Français de Recherche en Iran, 1992 (Bibliotheque iranienne, vol. 37), pp. 173-198.

———. "Bloodletting," *Encyclopedia Iranica*.

Forbes-Leith, A.C. *Checkmate and Fighting* (London, 1927 [New York: Arno, 1973]).

Fraser, J.B. *Narrative of a Journey into Khorasan in the Years 1821 & 1822* (London, 1825 [Delhi: Oxford UP, 1984]).

———. *Travels and Adventures in the Persian Provinces and the Southern Banks of the Caspian Sea* (London: Longman, Rees, Orme, Browne and Greene, 1826).

Garrison, F.H. "Persian medicine and medicine in Persia." *Bulletin of the Institute of the History of Medicine* 46 (1933), pp. 129-53.

G.D. "Sanitätsreformen in Iran. *Globus. Illustierte Zeitschrift für Länder- und Völkerkunde* 31 (1877), pp. 299-300.

Ghaffari, Mohammad `Ali. *Khaterat va Asnad-e Mohammad `Ali Ghaffari, Na'eb-e Avval-e Pishkhedmat-bashi*. eds. Mansureh Ettehadiyeh and Sirus Sa`dvandiyan (Tehran: Tarikh, 1361/1982).

Ghani, Qasem. *Yaddashtha-ye Doktor Qasem Ghani* 9 vols. ed. Sirus Ghani (Tehran: Zavvar, 1367/89)

Gilbar, Gad G. "Demographic Development in late Qajar Persia, 1870-1906," *Asian and African Studies* 11 (1976), pp. 125-56.

Gilmour, John. *Rapport sur la situation sanitaire de la Perse* (Geneva, League of Nations, 1924).

Goldsmid, Sir Frederic J. *Eastern Persia, An Account of the Journeys of the Persian Boundary Commission 1870-71-72*, 2 vols. (London: MacMillan & Co, 1876).

Good, Byron J. "The Transformation of Health Care in Modern Iranian History," in Michael E. Bonine and Nikki Keddie eds. *Modern Iran. The Dialectics of Continuity and Change* (Albany: State University of New York Press, 1981), pp. 59-82.

Government of France, *Rapports Commerciaux des agents diplomatiques et consulaires de France* – Année 1914 no. 1079 Perse (Paris, 1914).

Government of Great Britain, "Report by consul-general Jones on the condition of the industrial classes in Tabrees," Tabriz October 15, 1870, House of Commons, Parliamentary Papers, *Accounts and Papers* [A & P], vol. 68 (1871), pp. 417-22.

———. "Report on the condition of the working classes in Bushire", by Major Smith, Lingah, November 11, 1870, House of Commons, Parliamentary Papers, *Accounts and Papers* [A & P], vol. 68 (1871), pp. 401-04

———. "Report by Mr. Jenner on the condition of the working classes in Persia," Tehran, 2 November 1870, House of Commons, Parliamentary Papers, *Accounts and Papers* [A & P], vol. 68 (1871), pp. 395-400.

———. "Report by Mr. Hakeem on the working classes [in the Bandar `Abbas area]," Bassadore, October 22, 1870. *Parlamentary Papers, Accounts and Papers* [A & P], pp. 404-08.

———. *Report on the trade of the consular district of Bushire 1913-14*, as well as of the years 1915-16, 1920-21, and 1921-22.

———. *Geographical Handbook Series - Persia* (September 1945).

Greenfield, J. *Die Verfassung des persischen Staates* (Berlin: Franz Vahlen, 1904).

Grothe, Hugo. *Wanderungen in Persien* (Berlin, Alg. Verein f. Deutsche Literatur, 1910).

Hakim ed-Dovleh (Mohammad Hassan Khan). *Grossesse, accouchement et puériculture en Perse* (Paris: thesis, 1908).

Hale, F. *From Persian Uplands* (New York: E.P. Dutton, n.d.).

Häntzsche, J.C. "Specialstatistik von Persien," *Zeitschrift der Gesellschaft für Erdkunde zu Berlin* 1869, pp. 429-49.

———. "Lepra in Persien," *Virchows Archiv* 27 (1863), pp. 180-83.

———. Physikalisch-medicinische Skizze von Rescht in Persien, *Virchows Archiv* 15 (1862), pp. 538-54.

Haqiqat, `Abdol-Rafi`. *Tarikh-e Semnan* (Tehran: Farmandari-ye Koll-e Semnan, 1352/1973).

Hasanbeygi, Mohammad Reza. *Tehran-e Qadim* (Tehran: Mansuri, 1377/1998).

Hassendorfer, Colonel. "Les médecins militaries français fondateurs et organisateurs de l'Enseignement Médical et de la Santé Publique en Iran," *Histoire de la médicine* 4/7 (1954), pp. 57-63.

Heinrich, Gerd. *Auf Panthersuche durch Persien* (Berlin: Reimer/Vohsen, 1933).

Holmes, W.R. *Sketches on the Shores of the Caspian, Descriptive and Pictorial.* (London: Richard Bentley, 1845).

Höltzer, Ernst. *Persien vor 113 Jahren* ed. Mohammad Assemi (Tehran: Vezarat-e Farhang va Honar, 2535/1976).

Homayuni, Sadeq. *Molk-e `Abir-amiz. Farhang va Mardom-e Fars, "Sarvestan"* (Shiraz: Beh Nashr, 1377/1998).

Hume-Griffith, M.E. *Behind the Veil in Persia and Turkish Arabia* (Philadelphia, J.B. Lippincott, 1909).

Janab, Sayyed `Ali. *Ketab al-Isfahan* (Isfahan 1303/1924) litho.

Jaubert, P. Am. *Voyage en Arménie et la Perse* (Paris: Pélicier et Nepveu, 1821).

Javadi, Shafi`. *Tabriz va Peyramun* (Tabriz: Bonyad-e Farhangi-ye Reza Pahlavi, 1350/1971).

Jozani, Niloufar. *La Beauté Menacée* (Paris-Tehran: IFRI, 1994).

Kalmykov, Andrew D. *Memoirs of a Russian Diplomat. Outposts of the Empire, 1893-1917* (New Haven, Yale UP, 1971).

Kashani-Sabet, Firoozeh. "'City of the Dead': the Frontier Polemics of Quarantines in the Ottoman Empire and Iran," *Comparative Studies of South Asia, Africa, and the Middle East* 18/2 (1998), pp. 51-58.

Kennion, R.L. *By Mountain Lake and Plain, Sport in Eastern Persia* (Edinburgh-London: Wm. Blackwood & Sons, 1911).

Keshavarz-Damghan, `Ali Asghar. *Sad Darvazeh. Mokhtasari as Tarikh va Joghrafiya-ye Damghan* (Tehran, 1352/1973).

Khan Ali, *Choléra en Perse. Prophylaxie et traitement* (Paris: thesis, 1908).

Khan, Mesrop Nevton. "Talismanic Superstitions of Persia," *Gunter's Magazine* VI/2 (September ,1907), pp. 179-93

Knanishu, J. *About Persia and its People* (Rock Island, Ill 1899).

Korf' F. *Pro'ezd' chrez' Zakavkaskii krai* (St. Petersburg, 1838) translated by Eskander Dhabihan as Kurf, Barun Fyudur. *Safarnameh* (Tehran: Fekr-e Ruz, 1372/1993).

Kotobi, Laurence-Donia. "L'émergence d'une politique de santé publique en Perse Qâdjâre (XIX-XXe siècles)," *Studia Iranica* 24 (1995), pp. 261-83.

Kotzebue, Moritz von. *Narrative of a Journey into Persia in the suite of the Imperial Russian Embassy in the year 1817* (Philadelphia: Carey & Sons, 1820).

Küss, W. *Handelsratgeber für Persien* (Berlin, 1911).

Landor, E. Henry. *Across Coveted Lands* 2 vols. (New York: Scribners, 1903).

Lari, Sayyed `Abdol-Hoseyn. "Shesh Resaleh-ye Siyasi va Ejtema`i," ed. Sayyed `Ali Mir Sharifi in Rasul Ja`fariyan, *Mirath-e Eslami-ye Iran* 10 vols. (Qom: Ketabkhaneh-ye mar`ashi-Najafi, 1377/1998), vol. 9, pp. 203-90.

Larrey, Baron H. "Notice sur le docteur Ernest Cloquet," in *Notices sur le docteur Ernest Cloquet* (Paris, 1856), pp. 3-6.

Lichtwardt, H.A. "Ancient Therapy in Persia and England," *Annals of Medical History* 6 (1934), pp. 280-84.

———. "Ancient medicine in modern Persia." *Ann. Med. Hist.* 7 (1935), pp. 81-84.

———. "Western Medicine in Iran," *Muslim World* 32/3 (1937), pp. 236-41.

Linton, J.H. *Persian Sketches* (London: CMS, 1923).

Loeb, Laurence D. *Outcaste. Jewish Life in Southern Iran* (New York: Gordon and Breach, 1977).

Loghman ed-Dowleh, Mohammed Hussein Khan Moïn ol-Atebba. "Salek" *Etude du bouton d'Orient*. (Paris: thesis, 1908).

Lorimer, J. G. *Gazetteer of the Persian Gulf* (Calcutta, 1915 [Gregg: Westmead, 1970]).

Lycklama à Nijeholt, T.M. *Voyage en Russie, au Caucase et en Perse*. 4 vols. (Paris-Amsterdam: Arthus Bertrand-C.L. van Langenhuysen, 1873).

Mahdavi, Mo`ezz al-Din. *Dastaha'i az panjah sal owza`-ye ejtema`i-ye nim-qarn-e akhir* (Tehran, 1348/1969).

Malcom, Napier. *Five Years in a Persian Town* (London: John Murray, 1905).

Malcolm, Mrs. Napier. *Children of Persia* (Edinburgh: Oliphant, Anderson & Ferrier, 1911).

Massé, Henri. *Croyances et Coutumes Persanes* 2 vols. (Paris: Maisonneuve, 1938).

Merritt-Hawkes, O. A. *Persia – Romance & Reality* (London: Nicholson & Watson, 1935).

Millingen, Frederick. *Wild Life Among The Koords* (London: Hurst and Blackett, 1870).

Mir, Mohammad `Ali and Mir, `Ali Mohammad. "Yadi az Doktor Yusef Mir Irevani," *Ayandeh* 17 (1370/1991), pp. 41-45.

Mohandes, Hajji Mohammad Mirza-ye. "Raport-e Mamlekat-e Khorasan ba ba`zi molheqat-e an. ed. Qodratollah Rowshani," *Mirath-e Eslam*, vol. 6, pp. 499-581.

Money, R. C. *Journal of a Tour in Persia during the years 1824 & 1825* (London, 1828).

Moore, Benjamin Burges. *From Moscow to the Persian Gulf* (New York: G.P. Putnam's Sons, 1915).

Morier, James. *A Journey through Persia, Armenia and Asia Minor in the Years 1808 and 1809* (London: Longman, Hurst, Rees, Orme, and Brown, 1812).

-. *A Second Journey through Persia, Armenia, and Asia Minor ... between the years 1810 and 1816* (London: Longman, Hurst, Rees, Orme, and Brown, 1818).

———. *Hajji Baba of Isfahan* (numerous editions).

Mosaddeq, Gholam Hoseyn. "Jarrahi-ye Novin-e Orupa'i dar Iran," *Ayandeh* 15 (1368/1989), pp. 464-66.

Moshtaq Kazemi, Morteza. *Ruzgar va Andisheha* 3 vols. (Tehran: Ebn Sina, 1350/1971).

Mostowfi, `Abdollah. *Sharh-e zendagani-ye man*, 3 vols. (Tehran: Zavvar, n.d.).

Mullen, T. F. "Cholera in Persia," Appendix C to Part I of Government of India, *Administration Report of the Persian Gulf Political Residency and Muscat Political Agency* for the Year 1889-90, pp.15-18.

Nafisi, Sa`id. "Doktor `Ali Akbar Nafisi Nazem al-Atebba," *Yadgar* 3/4 (1325/1946), pp. 52-65.

Najmabadi, Mahmud. "Hakim Shelimer Felamanki, *Rahnama-ye Ketab* 13 (1349/1970), pp. 574-80.

———. "Nakhostin pezeshki amukhtegan-e Irani dar Sewis," in Iraj Afshar ed., *Namvareh-ye Doktor Mahmud Afsha*r 12 vols. (Tehran: Mowqufeh-ye Doktor Mahmud Afshar, 1367/1988), vol. 4, pp. 2162-69.

Najm ol-Molk, `Abdol-Ghaffar. *Safarnameh-ye Khuzestan*. ed. Mohammad Dabir-Siyaqi (Tehran: Elmi, 1342/1963).

Nategh, Homa. "Les Persans à Lyon," in Balaÿ, C. Kappler, C. and Z. Vesel eds. *Pand-o Sokhan* (Paris-Tehran: IFRI, 1995), pp. 191-99.

Nateq, Homa. "Ta'thir-e ejtema`i va eqtesadi-ye bimari-ye vaba dar dowreh-ye Qajar," *Tarikh* 1/2 (2536/1977), pp. 30-62.

Nazare Aga (Ardachir Khan). *Contribution à l'étude des conférences sanitaires internationales dans leurs rapports avec la prophylaxie des maladies pestilentielles en Perse* (Paris, thesis 1903-04).

Neligan, A.R. "Public Health in Persia. 1914-24," *The Lancet* Part I; Part II-March 27, 1926, pp. 690-94; Part III-April 3, 1926, pp. 742-44.

Nezam al-Saltaneh Mafi, Hoseyn Qoli Khan, *Khaterat va Asnad*. 2 vols. eds. Ma`sumeh Nezam-Mafi, Mansureh Ettehadiyeh (Nezam-Mafi), Sirus Sa`vandiyan, and Hamid Ram Pisheh (Tehran: Tarikh-e Iran, 13612/1982).

N.N. "Esfand Mah va Abji Kuchek," *Ettela`at-e Mahaneh* 107 (Bahman 1335/1956), pp. 34-35.

Norden, Hermann. *Under Persian Skies* (Philadelphia: McCrea Smith, n.d.).

Nweeya, Samuel K. *Persia and the Moslems* (St. Louis, 1924).

Olivier, G.A. *Voyage dans l'Empire Othoman, l'Egypte et la Perse*. 6 vols. (Paris: Agasse, 1802-07).

Orsolle, E. *Le Caucase et La Perse* (Paris: Plon, Nourrit et Cie., 1885).

Perho, Irmeli. *The Prophet's Medicine. A Creation of the Muslim Traditionalist Scholars* (Helsinki, Finnish Oriental Society, 1995).

Perkins, J. *A Residence of Eight Years in Persia* (Andover, 1843).

Phillot, D.C. "Bibliomancy, divination, superstitions among the Persians," *Journal of the Asiatic Society of Bengal* 2 (1906), pp. 339-42.

Piemontese, Angelo Michele. "Gli Ufficiali Italini al servizio della Persia nel XIX secolo," in G. Borsa, P. Beonino Brocchieri, *Garibaldi, Mazzini et il Risorgimento nel resveglio dell'Asia et dell'Africa* (Milano: Franco Angeli, 1984), pp. 65-130.

Pirzadeh, *Safarnameh-ye Hajji Mohammad `Ali Pirzadeh*. 2 vols. Hafez Farmanfarmayan (Tehran: Daneshgah, 1343/1964).

Polak, J.E. *Persien, das Land und seine Bewohner*, 2 vols. (Leipzig, 1865 [Hildesheim-New York: Georg Olms, 1976]).

———. "Medicinische Briefe aus Persien," *Zeitschrift der k.k. Gesellschaft der Aerzte zu Wien* 9 (1859), pp. 138-40.

———. "Medicinische Briefe aus Persien," *Zeitschrift der k.k. Gesellschaft der Aerzte zu Wien* 11 (1859), pp. 173-75.

———. "Ueber den Gebrauch des Quecksilbers in Persien," *Wiener Medizinische Wochenschrift* 10 (1860), pp. 564-68.

———. "Lepra in Persien," *Virchows Archiv* 27 (1863), pp. 175-80.

Price, William. *Journal of the British Embassy to Persia*. 2 vols. in one (London: Thomas Thorpe, 1832).

Qasemi, Sayyed Farid ed. [Periodical] *Danesh* (Tehran: Markaz-e Gostaresh-e Amuzesh-e Resanehha, 1374/1995).

Qazvini, Mohammad Shafi`. *Qanun-e Qazvini – enteqad-e owza`-ye ejtema`i-ye Iran dowreh-ye Naseri*. ed. Iraj Afshar (Tehran: Talayeh, 1370/1991).

Rabino, H. L. "A Journey in Mazanderan (from Resht to Sari)", *Geographical Journal* 42 (1913), pp. 435-54.

Rasooli, Jay M. and Allen, Cady H. *The Life Story of Dr. Sa`eed of Iran* (Grand Rapids: Grand Rapids International Publications, 1958).

Rawlinson, Major H. C. "Notes on a March from Zohab ... to Khuzistan," *JGRS* 9 (1839), pp. 26-116.

Rees, J.D. *Notes of a Journey from Kasveen to Hamadan across the Karaghan Country* (Madras, 1885).

Reitlinger, Gerald. *A Tower of Skulls, a journey through Persian and Turkish Armenia* (London: Duckworth, 1932).

Rice, Clara. *Mary Bird in Persia* (London: CMS, 1916).

———. *Persian Women and Their Ways* (London: Seeley, Service & Co, 1923).

Rich, Claude James. *Narrative of a Residence in Koordistan ... and of a visit to Shirauz and Persepolis*. 2 vols. (London: James Duncan, 1836).

Richter-Bernburg, Lutz. "Avicenna gegen Pockenimpfung. Iranische Reaktion auf die Einführung westlicher Medizin im 19. Jahrhundert," in: Tilman Nagel ed., *Asien blickt auf Europa. Begegnungen und Irritationen* (Beirut, 1990), pp. 73-87.

Rivadeneyra, Adolfo. *Viaje al interior de Persia* 3 vols. (Madrid, 1880).

Roney Jr., James G. "The Occurrence of Trephining Among The Bakhtiari," *Bulletin of the History of Medicine* 28 (1954), pp. 489-91.

Rosen, Friedrich. *Persien in Wort und Bild* (Berlin: Schneider, 1926).

Ross, Elizabeth N. MacBean. *A Lady Doctor in Bakhtiyari Land* (London: Parsons, 1921).

Rubin, Micheal Allen. *The Formation of Modern Iran, 1858-1909: Communication, Telegraph and Society* (Yale University, unpublished thesis, 1999).

Sabar, Yona. *The Folk Literature Of The Kurdistani Jews: An Anthology* (New Haven: Yale UP, 1982).

Sadeq, `Isa. *Yadegar-e `Omr – Khaterati az Sargodhasht* 3 vols. (Tehran: Amir Kabir, 1345/1966).

Sadvandian, Cyrus. "The Inhabitants of Meydan-Gusfand", *The Journal of the Middle East Studies Society at Columbia University* 1 (1987), pp. 39-54.

Sa`dvandiyan, Sirus and Ettehadiyeh (Nezam-Mafi), Mansureh. *Amar-e Dar al-Khelafeh* (Tehran: Nashr-e Tarikh, 1368/1989).

Safari, Baba. *Ardabil dar Godhargah-e Tarikh* 3 vols. (Tehran, 1350-62/1971-83).

Sargis, Yacob Allahverdy. "Persia and Her Doctors," *Columbus Medical Journal* 25 (1901), pp. 583-88.

Sayyah, Hajj. *Khaterat-e Hajj Sayyah ya Dowreh-ye Khowf va Vahshat* ed. Hamid Sayyah (Tehran: Ebn Sina, 1347/1968).

Schindler, A.H. *Eastern Persian Irak* (London: Murray, 1898).

Schlimmer, Joh. L. *Terminologie Médico-Pharmaceutique: Française - Persane* (Tehran, 1874 [Tehran: Daneshgah, 1970]).

Schneider, D. *La médecine persane. Les médecins français en Perse. Leur influence* (Paris: Wellhof & Roche, 1911).

Schwartz, Benjamin ed. *Letters from Persia written by Charles and Edward Burgess 1828-1855* (New York: NY Public Library, 1942).

Sepehr, `Abdol-Hoseyn. *Mer'at al-Vaqaye`-ye Mozaffari va Yaddashtha-ye Malek al-Mo'arrekhin* ed. `Abdol-Hoseyn Nava'i (Tehran: Zarrin, 1368/1889).

Serena, C. *Hommes et Choses en Perse* (Paris: G. Charpentier, 1883).

Seyf, Ahmad. "Iran and Cholera in the Nineteenth century," *Middle Eastern Studies* 38 (2002), pp. 169-78.

Shabaz, Absalom D. *Land of the Lion and the Sun* (Madison, Wis., 1901).

Shahri, Ja`far. *Tarikh-e ejtema`i -Tehran dar qarn-e sizdahom*, 6 vols. (Tehran: Farhang-Rasa, 1368/1989).

Shakurzadeh, Ebrahim. *`Aqayed va Rosum-e `Ammeh-ye Mardom-e Khorasan* (Tehran: Bonyad-e Farhang-e Iran, 1346/1967).

Sheil, Lady. *Glimpses of Life and Manners in Persia* (London, 1856 [New York: Arno, 1973]).

Shekufeh beh enzemam-e Danesh. Nakhostin nashriyehha-ye zanan-e Iran (Tehran: Ketabkhaneh-ye Melli, 1377/1998).

Sheykh-Reza'i, Ensiyeh and Azari, Shahla ed. *Gozareshha-ye Nazmiyeh az Mahallat-e Tehran* (Tehran: Sazman-e Asnad-e Melli, 1377/1998).

Sirjani, Sa`idi. *Vaqaye`-ye Ettefaqiyeh. Gozareshha-ye khofyeh-nevisan-e englis* (Tehran: Now, 1361/1982).

Soane, Ely Bannister. *To Mesopotamia and Kurdistan in Disguise* (London: John Murray, 1912 [Amsterdam: Philo Press 1979]).

Soltani, Mohammad `Ali. *Joghrafiya-ye Tarikhi va Tarikh-e Mofassal-e Kermanshahan.* 3 vols. (Tehran: author, 1370/1991).

Southgate, H. *A Tour Through Armenia and Mesopotamia,* 2 vols. (New York: D. Appleton & Co, 1840).

Speer, Robert E. *Hakim Sahib, the foreign doctor; a biography of Joseph Plumb Cochran* (New York: Revell, 1911).

Stack, Edward. *Six Months in Persia.* 2 vols. (New York: G.P. Putnams, 1882).

Stark, Freya. *The Valley of the Assassins* (London, 1934 [New York, 2001).

Stileman, Rev. Charles Harvey. *The Subjects of the Shah* (London: CMS, 1902).

Stocqueler, J.H. *Fifteen Months' Pilgrimage through untrodden tracts of Khuzistan and Persia* (London: Saunders and Otley, 1832).

Stuart, Emmeline M. *Doctors in Persia* (London: CMS, n.d.).

Sykes, Ella. *Persia and its People* (London: MacMillan, 1910).

———. *Through Persia on a Side-Saddle* (Philadelphia: John MacQueen, 1898).

Sykes, Percy M. *Ten Thousand Miles in Persia or Eight Years in Iran* (New York: Charles Scribner's Sons, 1902).

Sykes, P.M. and Khan Bahadur Ahmad Din Khan. *The Glory of the Shia World. The Tale of a Pilgrimage* (London: MacMillan and Co., 1910).

Tahvildar, Mirza Hosein Khan. *Joghrafiya-ye Esfahan,* ed. M. Setudeh. (Tehran: Daneshgah, 1342/1963).

Taj al-Saltaneh. *Khaterat-e Taj al Saltaneh.* eds. Mansureh Ettehadiyeh and Sirus Sa`dvandiyan, and translated by Anna Vanzan and Amin Neshati as *Crowning Anguish. Memoirs of a Persian Princess from the Harem to Modernity.* (Washington, DC: Mage, 1993).

Tancoigne, J. M. *A Narrative of a Journey into Persia* (London: William Wright, 1820).

Tarbiyat [periodical] 3 vols. (Tehran, Ketabkhaneh-ye Melli, 1377/1998).

Tate, G. P. *The Frontiers of Baluchistan. Travels on the borders of Persia and Afghanistan* (London 1909 [Lahore: East & West Publishing Comp, 1976]).

Tholozan, J. D. *Note sur le développement de la peste bubonique dans le Kurdistan en 1871* (Paris, 1871).

———. *Histoire de la peste bubonique, 1er Mémoire- en Perse* 3 vols. (Paris: G. Masson, 1874).

———. *Sur deux petits épidémies de peste dans le Khorassan* (Paris: Gauthiers-Villars, n.d.)

———. *Prophylaxie du cholera en Orient. L'hygiène et la réforme sanitaire en Perse* (Paris: Masson, 1869).

———. *De la diphtérie en Orient et particulièrement en Perse* (Paris: Masson, 1878).

Ts., S. "Persidskie Doktora i Persidskie Patsienty," *Sovremennik* 47 (1854), pp. 155-71.

Ussher, John. *A Journey from London to Persepolis* (London: Hurst and Blackett, 1865).

Vahid. "Khaterat-e Vahid," *Vahid* 21-31 (1352-54/1973-75).

Vambéry, Arminius. *Voyages d'un Faux Derviche dans l'Asie Centrale* (Paris: Hachette, 1865).

-. *His Life and Adventures* (London: Fisher Unwin, 1884).

Varjavand, Parviz. *Sima-ye Tarikh va Farhang-e Qazvin*. 3 vols. (Tehran: Ney, 1377/1998).

Vaziri, Ahmad `Ali Khan, *Joghrafiya-ye Kerman* (Tehran, 1346/1967).

Waring, Edward Scott. *A Tour to Sheeraz* (London, 1807 [New York: Arno, 1973]).

Watelin, Louis-Charles. *La Perse Immobile* (Paris: Chapelot, 1921).

Waters, Lieut. Col. Geo. *Travel Reminiscences* (n.p., n.d.)

Weston, Harold F. "Persian Caravan Sketches," *National Geographic Magazine* 39/4 (1921), pp. 417-68.

Wigram, W.A. and Wigram, T.A. *The Cradle of Mankind. Life in Eastern Kurdistan* (London: A&C Black, 1936).

Williamson, J.W. *In A Persian Oil Field. A Study in Scientific and Industrial Development* (London: Ernest Benn, 1927).

Wills, C. J. *Persia As It Is* (London, 1886).

———. *In the Land of the Lion and the Sun* (London: Ward, Lock & Bowden, 1893).

Wilson, S.G. *Persian Life and Customs* (New York: Fleming. H. Revell, 1895).

Wishard, John G. *Twenty Years in Persia. A Narrative of Life under the Last Three Shahs* (New York: Fleming H. Revell, 1908).

Wolff, Joseph. *Researches and Missionary Labours* (London: James Nisbet & Co., 1835).

Wright, Denis. *The English Amongst the Persians* (London: I.B. Tauris, 2001).

———. *The Persians Amongst the English* (London: I.B. Tauris, 1985).

Ya Hoseyni, Sayyed Qasem, *Sad Sal-e Matbu`at-e Bushehr* [Bushire: Ershad-e Melli-ye Bushehr, 1374/1995]).

Yate, C .E. *Khurasan and Sistan* (London: William Blackwood & Sons, 1900).

Yonan, Isaac Malek. *Persian Women* (Nashville: Cumberland Presbyterian Publishing House, 1898).

Zarrabi, `Abdol-Rahim. *Tarikh-e Kashan*. ed. Iraj Afshar (Tehran: Ebn Sina, 1342/1963).

Zennaro, S. *Observations critiques au sujet du rapport de M. le Dr. Bartoletti sur les mesures à prendre contre la peste qui sévit en Perse par le Dr. S. Zennaro* (Constantinople: M. de Castro, 1872).

INDEX

'Abbas Mirza, 41, 43, 162, 163, 167, 168, 169
'Abbasak island, 211
'alaq, 145, 150
'Ali Akbar Khan, 192, 193
'Ali Qoli Mirza, 192, 206, 207
'Ali Ra'is al-Atebba, 175, 242
'arq-e madani, 32
'Ashqabad, 26
'attar, 78, 101, 130, 131, 134, 180, 220
'aynu'd-dik, 138
Abadan, 19, 23, 64, 202, 206
Abadeh, 196
abattoir, 227
ab-e do'a, 83
ab-e garm, 30
ab-e ma'dan, 30
ab-e qofl, 83
abeleh, 38, 43, 222
abji, 149
abortion, 50
abortus provocatus, 50
abshar-e bozorg, 27
Abu'l-Hasan Khan, 116, 175, 187
Adcock, 172
adviyeh-ye mosqateh-ye janin, 50
aegophonia, 177
aether, 165
Afghanistan, 18, 199, 212
Ahvaz, 14, 201
akaleh, 33
akeleh, 44
Al, 74, 96, 250
Albo, 173, 175, 187, 192, 207, 240, 242

alcoholism, 47
Aligi Salmakh, 98
Alphos, 36
amas-e zariyeh, 46
Amir Kabir, 41, 42, 173, 189, 190, 191, 204, 213, 225
amputation, 140, 164, 165
amraz-e jeldi, 31
amulets, 49, 56, 84, 85, 92, 93, 96, 125, 127
anatomy, 69, 82, 159, 162, 165, 174, 175, 176, 177, 182, 240
anemia, 38, 152
anesthesia, 140, 165
angina, 120
Anglo-Indian Telegraph Department, 126
Anglo-Persian Oil Company, 24, 173
anjoriyeh, 45
anthrax, 25
Antidotes, 120, 240
antipyrin, 143, 223
Anvar-e Naseriyeh, 176
APOC, 24, 173, 202
apoteyk, 218
Aqa Sayyed Ja'far Hakim-Bashi, 214
Ardabil, 14, 47, 80, 88, 90, 98, 104, 124, 159, 214, 215, 220, 230
areca, 35
Argus Persicus, 26, 27
Armenian, 31, 35, 38, 39, 45, 105, 106, 109, 142, 163, 187, 198, 199, 219, 220
army-surgeon, 163
asafetida, 50
asba, 24
Astaniyu, 189

Astarabad, 14, 30, 53, 102, 178, 203, 207, 230
Astarabadi, 53, 184
astrologer, 116, 117
asylum, 53, 54, 228
ateshak, 33
Azerbaijan, 14, 18, 30, 36, 43, 47, 81, 89, 104, 122, 131, 189, 207
bachchehbazi, 34
bad, 13, 14, 17, 38, 52, 57, 75, 161, 183
bad-e mobarak, 38
bad-e sorkh, 38
badkesh, 145, 151
Baghdad, 18, 25, 35, 36, 40, 41, 142
Bakhtiyari, 13, 29, 67, 143, 144, 173
Baluchis, 38, 39, 43, 144
Baluchistan, 14, 38, 56, 81, 144, 199, 212
Bam, 32
Bandar 'Abbas, 23, 29, 32, 133, 160, 209, 210, 212
Bander-e Gaz, 209
Barabar al-Sa'ah, 101
baraz, 36
barber, 29, 35, 43, 69, 77, 78, 127, 145, 146, 147, 148, 149, 150, 152, 153, 154, 156, 158, 159, 160, 161, 163, 192
Barfrush, 64
barhang, 128
barrenness, 48, 91, 168
Basil, 187, 247
Basra, 18, 40, 41

bathhouse, 30, 61, 63, 145, 151, 153, 160, 192, 228
bavasir, 47, 50, 135
beres, 36
Bertoni, 169
Bestam, 26, 47
Beyrout, 216, 219
beytal, 77, 78
bimarestan, 190
bimariha-ye jeldi, 33
bitumen, 160, 161
Board of Health, 206, 207
Bock, 178
Bojnord, 82
bonesetter, 78, 145, 159
boridan-e alat, 166
Borujerd, 64, 210
Bushire, 15, 19, 20, 22, 23, 26, 33, 38, 39, 44, 64, 140, 160, 165, 178, 188, 198, 199, 201, 204, 206, 207, 208, 209, 210, 211, 212, 216, 229, 230
Cabuzzi, 178
cairns, 85
calomel, 34, 114, 143, 167, 185, 223, 237
caries, 46, 144, 165
Caspian littoral, 14, 18, 22, 24, 29, 31, 47, 203, 212
Caspian Sea littoral, 152
Castaldi, 178, 206, 207
Cataract, 27
cauterization, 142
Cautery, 29
Cemeteries, 56, 61
chashm-e khorus, 50
chashm-i-khurus, 138
chemistry, 105, 175, 179, 187, 218, 220
chemists, 77, 180, 216, 218, 219, 220

chief army doctor, 191
China root, 119, 132
cholera, 13, 17, 18, 19, 20, 21, 51, 58, 64, 74, 88, 89, 130, 169, 174, 175, 178, 181, 194, 203, 204, 205, 206, 207, 208, 209, 210, 225, 229, 230, 232, 240, 241
chorea, 54, 71
Christian, 37, 41, 49, 54, 80, 84, 89, 105, 117, 126, 128, 129, 201, 213
chub-e chini, 132
Church Missionary Society, 102, 197, 198
Clay eating, 32
Cloquet, 17, 18, 169, 173, 206
CMS, 62, 102, 159, 197, 198, 199, 200, 201, 202, 204, 215, 222
colics, 120
conjunctivitis, 28
Cormick, 41, 162, 167, 168, 169, 189
couching, 136, 137, 139
cupping, 108, 120, 145, 150, 151, 153, 159, 161, 218
dagh, 29, 88
dagh-e ahan-e dagh, 29
daghineh, 29
Daleki, 114, 161
dallak, 43, 78, 145, 146
Damghan, 31, 43, 216, 220
Damsch, 172
Dana-i-daghi, 35
dandan-e kerm khordeh, 47

Dar al-Fonun, 26, 36, 42, 107, 173, 175, 177, 178, 179, 185, 187, 188, 192, 193, 199, 207, 214, 218, 234, 240, 242
dar al-shafa', 190
date palm, 50
dava va moshel-e senna, 21
dava-ye zananeh, 83
daya, 141
deafness, 121
Death certificates, 12
Deh Molla, 127
Deh Mulla, 27
demon, 53, 56, 57, 71, 75, 96
demonic possession, 56, 71
dentist, 154, 155, 214, 215
devil, 54, 56, 57, 162
Dezful, 14, 64, 161
dhu santariya, 45
diarrhea, 18, 21, 44, 45, 52, 83, 88, 109, 128, 240
diarrhea of surfeit, 18
diarrheic indigestion, 18
Dickson, 170, 171, 172
didan, 31, 115
diet, 13, 30, 46, 66, 76, 115, 121, 122, 123, 127, 128, 221
digestive, 121, 232, 239
diphtheria, 46, 206, 207
diploma, 102, 172, 195, 213, 217, 220
dissection, 177, 188
divanegi, 53
do`a-nevis, 90
doctor's fee, 124
Dolmage, 178
druggist, 21, 78, 115, 130, 131, 132, 161

dud ol-khall, 31
dum, 87
dust, 28, 30, 66, 83, 87, 166, 177
dysentery, 44, 45, 168, 191, 205
dyspepsia, 13
E'tezad al-Saltaneh, 43, 186, 192, 225
eczema, 13
Egypt, 18
ehtesab, 226
ejadat, 110
emaleh, 21, 121
enema, 21, 34, 63, 121, 238
epilepsy, 54, 56, 93
Erevan, 41, 109, 129, 133, 146, 204
Erysipele, 38
Erythema, 38
eshal, 45, 109
eshal-e damavi, 45
eshal-e khuni, 45
estekhareh, 117, 153
evil eye, 57, 72, 73, 92, 93, 96, 97
exorcist, 57
eye doctors, 77, 78, 136, 139
Fagergrin, 178
fairies, 70, 71, 80, 83, 84, 85, 92
Fakhr al-Atebba, 111, 171, 172, 183, 207
falbin, 92, 217
family doctor, 110
Fars, 26, 43, 81, 82, 143, 152, 161, 178, 207
fasad, 145
Fath 'Ali Shah, 13, 103, 146, 167
favus, 32
febris mucosa, 24
febris septica, 24

female healers, 78, 88, 141, 142
female physicians, 7, 113
Feuvrier, 7, 171
Fochetti, 173, 175
folus, 114, 122
France, 17, 18, 109, 170, 172, 179, 182, 187, 199, 216, 221, 222
fumigation, 166
fumigations, 35, 138
fungus, 32, 62
ganeh ganeh, 121
gangrene, 36, 160, 162, 166
gazonbor, 155
gel khordan, 32
gerd-e safid, 185
Germany, 18, 216, 221
Gilan, 8, 13, 14, 36, 42, 43, 72, 103, 189, 216
ginger, 53
glaucoma, 13, 28
goblins, 70
gondeh tavol, 25
gonorrhea, 33, 34, 48, 121
gowat, 57
granulation, 28, 164, 237
grape verjuice, 19
Great Britain, 18, 130, 168, 172, 203, 216, 221
growth rate, 11
Guinea worm, 32
gusht zadeh, 28
hafez al-sehheh, 206
hajjam, 151
Hajji Mirza Baba Shirazi, 183
hakem-e fowj, 189
hakim, 78, 100, 102, 104, 109, 112, 113,

114, 116, 149, 153, 160, 163, 169, 171, 180, 181, 185, 191, 223, 226
hakim-bashi, 169
hakim-bashi-ye hozur, 207
hakim-bashi-ye koll, 170
hakim-e hozur, 172
Hamadan, 13, 14, 18, 25, 41, 47, 64, 65, 105, 131, 166, 195, 196, 197, 198, 199, 200, 207, 208, 209, 210, 220
haqq al-qadam, 124, 236
harelip, 56
harem, 47, 106, 113, 117, 127, 162, 164, 167, 172
harqat al-bowl, 33
headache, 29, 52, 88, 94, 143, 238
hejamat-e ferangi, 145, 150
hemorrhoids, 50, 135
heyzeh, 18
hezal, 51
hobb al-qar', 31
homay-e hesbeh'i, 24
homay-e varami, 14
homreh, 38
hoqneh, 34
house calls, 91, 110, 124, 127, 174, 230
hozaz, 32
hydrophobia, 81
hysteria, 51, 162
IETD, 189, 196, 197
impotency, 50
India, 17, 18, 22, 23, 37, 129, 139, 160, 197, 210

Indo-European Telegraph Department, 7, 189, 196
Influenza, 26, 230
inhalation, 166
inoculation, 36, 38, 39, 43, 127, 138
Insanity, 53
International Sanitary Commission, 206
ir, 45, 103
Iraq, 16, 18, 41, 87, 105, 204, 207, 210, 213
Iritis, 28
Isfahan, 11, 13, 14, 18, 28, 31, 35, 41, 42, 45, 65, 74, 89, 92, 98, 104, 106, 109, 119, 133, 142, 146, 152, 155, 188, 190, 196, 197, 198, 199, 200, 207, 210, 222
Istanbul, 18, 178, 206, 214
jabbar, 159
jadugar, 92
jafr, 93
jarrah, 79, 109, 136, 139, 160, 161, 163, 181, 223
jarrah-bashi, 191
jarrah-e cheshm, 239
Jask, 210, 212
Jewish, 25, 84, 105, 106, 108, 115, 137, 141, 162, 163, 171, 173, 189, 200, 213, 216
Jews, 21, 25, 36, 49, 56, 70, 76, 77, 83, 92, 93, 97, 98, 105, 106, 162
jezam, 36
jinns, 54, 70, 71, 84, 86, 179, 235

jiveh, 129
joderi, 38
Jolfa, 41, 119, 142, 146, 159, 197, 204, 212
jonun, 53
Journal d'Hygiene, 208
kachali, 32
kadudaneh, 31
kahhal, 78, 136
kahir, 45
kalantar, 88, 225
kalbateyn, 155
Kalyan Shingrif, 34
Kampusan Pir, 207
kannas, 65
Karachi, 211
Karaj, 15
Karbala, 61, 93, 209, 210
karkon, 121
Kashan, 35, 41, 42, 105, 207
Kazulani, 189, 190
kefgirek, 25
keloruform, 165
Kengavar, 105
Keratitis, 27
kerm, 31, 46
kermak, 31
Kerman, 13, 14, 30, 32, 44, 46, 48, 62, 66, 85, 104, 129, 144, 188, 195, 197, 198, 199, 200, 201, 207, 208, 230
Kermanshah, 13, 14, 25, 26, 35, 36, 41, 103, 104, 145, 195, 198, 199, 200, 204, 207, 208, 210, 212, 217, 220, 229
Khalkhal, 36, 37
Khamseh, 36
Khaneqin, 209
Khar, 14
kholgh shodan, 18

khonaq, 45, 46
khoraj-e radi, 25
Khorasan, 13, 14, 18, 22, 26, 36, 38, 45, 92, 128, 193, 196, 207, 212, 244
Khoy, 81, 204, 207
khuni, 114
Khuzistan, 14, 38, 56, 204, 206, 209
komsuzak, 33
korsi, 63, 163
kuft, 33
kuft-e jeldi, 33
kufti, 33
Kurdish, 16, 76, 87, 88, 138, 168
Kurdistan, 11, 14, 22, 36, 54, 56, 57, 71, 83, 89, 105, 143, 207
Labat, 99, 169
lagheri, 51
Lar, 32
leeching, 149, 150, 152, 153, 154, 218
Leishmania tropica, 35
leprosy, 36, 37
license, 213, 214
life force, 73, 87, 96
Lingeh, 210
lithotomy, 48, 165, 176, 208
Loqman al-Mamalek, 219
love charms, 49
Luristan, 81, 207
Lurs, 54, 59, 81, 82, 154
Madraseh-ye Dar al-Shafa, 190
Mahallat, 30
mahkameh, 108
Majles, 205, 215, 216, 222, 224, 227
Majles-e Hefz al-Sehhat, 206

Majles-e Sehhat, 206
makhmalek, 44
Makhzan al-Adviyeh, 93, 101, 102
malaria, 13, 14, 15, 16, 17, 83, 89, 129, 194, 195, 205, 224, 232, 238, 240
mama, 141
manna, 21, 120, 121, 128, 142
Maragheh, 104, 110, 114, 207, 217
margamargi, 17
marg-e mowt, 17
margijeh, 45
mariz-khaneh, 190
marizkhaneh-ye dowlati, 190, 192, 194
marz-e mashur, 33
Mashad, 18, 19, 27, 34, 35, 37, 48, 50, 61, 66, 80, 128, 178, 188, 190, 193, 195, 196, 198, 199, 200, 201, 207, 210, 212, 226, 245
maw worm, 31
mayeh-ye panir-e shotor, 48
mazaj, 53, 184
Mazandaran, 13, 14, 19, 30, 42, 80, 109, 118, 121, 178, 207, 214
Measles, 44
Mecca, 18, 94, 126, 132, 209
mercury, 28, 34, 40, 114, 121, 129, 132, 166, 168, 181, 183, 186, 236
mesh mesh, 26
midwives, 50, 77, 141, 142, 179, 195
mineral springs, 30

Ministry of Public Instruction, 216, 220
Ministry of Science, 206
Ministry of the Interior, 210, 213
Mirza Ahmad Hakim-bashi-ye Tonakeboni, 214
Mirza Ahmad Tabib, 187, 214
Mirza Hasan Khan Moshir al-Dowleh, 193
Mirza Hesam al-Din Tabib, 208
Mirza Kazem Hakim-bashi, 21
Mirza Kazem Mahallati Shimi, 218
Mirza Mohammad Hakimbashi Kashani, 186
Mirza Mohammad Nazem al-Atebba, 193
Mirza Mohammad Vali Hakim-bashi, 190
Mirza Molla Hoseyn Hakim-Bashi, 193
Mirza Musa Khan Hakim-Bashi, 219
Mirza Nazar `Ali Hakim-Bashi-ye Qazvini, 103
Miyaneh, 26, 36, 59
Mohammad `Ali Mirza, 13, 41, 169, 172
Mohammad Shah, 30, 89, 90, 103, 105, 127, 168, 169, 190
Mohammad Taqi Shirazi, 181, 183, 184, 207, 225
Mohammarah, 23, 64, 195, 202, 210, 212

Mohammerah, 14, 173
mohreqeh, 24
monzej, 121, 239
Morbidity, 12
mordeh-shur, 65
Morel, 194
mortality rate, 11, 18, 22, 32, 42
moshel, 21, 52, 114, 121, 237
Mosul, 41
motbeqeh, 24, 224
Mozaffar al-Din Shah, 52, 84, 105, 170, 172, 219
mumiya, 160, 161
municipality, 12, 17, 227, 228, 229
Munis Effendi, 207
Musreh, 26
myrobalan, 237
nabat al-leyl, 45
nafas, 80, 87, 88, 159
namak-e ferengi, 185
Naser al-Din Shah, 43, 65, 83, 116, 153, 155, 164, 169, 170, 171, 173, 186, 187, 190, 192, 193, 205, 206, 214, 226, 236
Nasratabad, 88, 212
nazf al-dam, 102
Nazir-e Qanun va Shafa', 101
necrosis, 144, 165
nefat, 45
Nestorian, 54, 56, 57, 168, 193, 196, 199
Nestorians, 57
Nettle rash, 45
neurasthenia, 51
Nishapur, 31, 163
noma, 44
nowbeh, 14, 83, 224, 238

nozul-e ab-e marvarid, 27
nozul-e ab-e sabz, 28
ojaq, 88
omen, 52, 90, 111, 117, 118, 153, 155, 201
Ophthalmia, 13, 27, 28, 138, 208
Opium addiction, 47
Ottoman, 58, 178, 206, 207, 209
oxymel, 50, 52, 120, 121, 127, 184
panegyric, 116
Paratyphoid fever, 24
paris, 70, 83, 84, 235
passion play, 116
pearls, 119
pediculosis, 32
Pemphigus, 45
periostitis, 46
Persian Gulf, 14, 18, 23, 32, 196, 209, 210, 211
Persian teachers, 187, 242
pezeshk, 77, 100, 110, 136
pharmacology, 119, 175, 187, 218, 219, 220
pharmacopoeia, 102, 177, 178, 185
pharmacy, 130, 190, 195, 218, 220, 235
phlebotomy, 145, 150
Phthisis, 13, 25
physiology, 159, 175, 241
pis, 36
piyu, 32
plague, 13, 22, 23, 24, 51, 74, 176, 178, 181, 204, 205, 206, 207, 209, 210, 211, 232
pleurisy, 13

pneumonia, 13, 144
Polak, 7, 11, 18, 28, 31, 35, 36, 38, 41, 42, 44, 45, 46, 48, 67, 70, 79, 102, 103, 113, 121, 132, 151, 165, 169, 171, 173, 174, 175, 176, 177, 181, 183, 185, 186, 189, 190, 191, 205, 240, 241
potogav, 39
potoshotor, 39
poultice, 82, 160, 238
poyuk, 32
pregnancy, 48, 49, 85, 96, 134, 142
prescription, 37, 49, 52, 56, 91, 115, 117, 121, 124, 171, 186, 219, 236
public washers of the death, 12
pulse, 69, 112, 113, 115, 127, 128, 171, 172, 182
purgative, 21, 52, 114, 121, 143, 153, 237
Qa'en, 86
qabeleh, 141
Qaradagh, 36
Qashqa'i, 26
Qasr-e Shirin, 206, 212
qat`-e `ozv, 166
Qavanin-e `Alaj, 104
Qazvin, 45, 47, 59, 64, 109, 146, 161, 196, 198, 203, 207, 219, 235
qir, 161
Qom, 35, 47, 61, 83, 104, 146, 175, 207, 208, 210
qovveh-ye bah, 50
quacks, 78, 106, 107, 125, 213, 216

quarantine, 8, 19, 133, 196, 204, 206, 207, 208, 209, 210, 211, 212, 224
quick healing, 67
quinine, 14, 16, 17, 21, 69, 109, 121, 127, 129, 130, 131, 143, 152, 184, 185, 191, 221, 222, 223
rabies, 89, 208
rak zadan, 145
rammal, 92
rate of infant deaths, 11
rats bane, 21
recurrent fever, 26
rennet, 48, 51
reptiles, 82, 87
reshteh, 32, 90, 184
revand, 120, 121
rheumatism, 13, 29, 30, 31, 183
rickets, 46
ringworm, 32
rosary, 118
round worms, 31
rowzeh-khvan, 55
royal physician, 37, 40, 127, 169, 171, 181, 184
Russia, 17, 18, 19, 178, 203, 209, 212, 220, 221
sabal, 28
Sabzavar, 110, 163, 196, 207
sadliz, 52
sahaj-e jeld, 38
Sakhtsar, 30
salek, 35, 142
salmani, 145, 146
Salmonella, 24
salt, 19, 30, 52, 66, 121, 138, 185
salvarsan, 35
Salvatori, 188

samm al-far, 21
Sanitary Board, 205
Sanitary Council, 12, 22, 38, 104, 196, 206, 207, 208, 209, 211, 213, 224, 225, 244
Sanitation Council, 138, 209
Sarcocolla, 51
sarkeh, 52, 184
sarsaparilla, 119, 132
sartan-e juf-e dahan, 44
scabies, 14, 32, 33, 138, 220
scarification, 145, 151
Scarlet fever, 44
Schlimmer, 7, 18, 21, 25, 26, 31, 32, 38, 44, 47, 50, 51, 53, 101, 116, 142, 144, 152, 161, 166, 169, 173, 174, 175, 176, 177, 178, 186, 189, 191, 240, 241
Schneider, 169, 172, 187, 210, 219
Scrofula, 13
Seistan, 13, 14, 22, 35, 88, 195, 206, 212
sekanjebin, 52, 184
Semnan, 103, 207, 208
senekhchi, 159
Shah `Abdol-`Azim, 31, 237
Shahrud, 26, 27, 47, 207
Shanker, 33
Shariyar, 14
Sharpe, 189
shekasteh-band, 159
sherk, 38
Shiraz, 14, 18, 19, 21, 22, 26, 35, 37, 56, 70, 74, 87, 88, 130, 157, 165, 178, 189, 197, 198, 200, 204, 207, 208
shirkhesht, 21, 53, 120, 121
Shushtar, 14, 17, 18, 64, 161, 206, 209
siyah sorfeh, 37
Skinniness, 51
smallpox, 13, 38, 39, 40, 41, 42, 43, 64, 111, 167, 175, 206, 207, 213, 222
soap, 32, 45, 59, 138, 157, 158, 160
soothsayer, 86
sorkhcheh, 44
sowt-e bozi, 177
sphacelus, 36
spirits, 54, 56, 57, 71, 72, 80, 85, 179
Stagno, 178
sterility, 49
Stump, 215
suicide, 121
supernatural, 53, 71, 73, 74, 75, 76, 80, 90, 94, 97, 103, 167, 179, 181, 232
surgeon, 14, 41, 78, 79, 131, 145, 159, 160, 161, 163, 164, 165, 178, 181, 189, 191, 192, 193, 194, 202, 211, 229, 238
suzak, 33
suzanak, 33, 34, 48
syphilis, 33, 34, 44, 121, 132, 142, 166, 186
ta`vidh, 92
tab-e ghash, 21
tabi`at kardan, 18
tabib-bashi, 170
tabib-e jasmani, 79
tabib-e khasseh, 103
tabib-e rowhani, 79
Tabriz, 11, 18, 20, 26, 28, 36, 47, 65, 77, 81, 87, 90, 92, 107, 108, 110, 112, 121, 133, 136, 163, 170, 172, 174, 178, 181, 188, 189, 190, 195, 198, 199, 200, 204, 207, 219, 220, 225
tanqiyeh kardan, 114, 149
tanzif, 65, 226
tapeworm, 13, 31
taqereh-e solb-e kufti, 33
taranjabin, 50, 120
tarkeh-dava, 88
taryaqat, 120
tebb al-a'emmeh, 68
tebb al-nabi, 68
Tebb al-Reza, 101
Tebb al-Sadeq, 101
tebb-e larz, 14
tebb-e sonnati, 68
tebb-e yunani, 68
Tebb-e Yusefi, 102, 130
Tehran, 11, 12, 13, 14, 15, 17, 18, 25, 26, 31, 33, 35, 40, 41, 42, 44, 45, 46, 47, 49, 52, 55, 59, 61, 62, 65, 83, 90, 105, 106, 109, 110, 115, 116, 119, 121, 125, 128, 130, 134, 136, 141, 145, 146, 147, 152, 167, 170, 171, 174, 177, 183, 188, 189, 190, 192, 193, 194, 195, 196, 198, 199, 200, 202, 203, 205, 206, 207, 208, 210, 213, 214, 215, 216, 217, 218, 219, 220, 222, 224, 225, 226, 227, 228,

229, 234, 239, 244, 253
telesm, 92
teranjebin, 121
thavab, 203
theql-e sard, 18
Tholozan, 7, 22, 46, 164, 169, 170, 172, 173, 175, 176, 177, 205, 207, 209, 238, 240, 242
thread worm, 35
tigh, 149
tikeh-otoran, 88
Tohfeh-ye Hakim-e Mo'men, 101
tongue, 112, 115, 128, 149, 159, 182
tonsillitis, 33
trachoma, 14, 28, 62, 136, 137, 138
trephining, 55
Tuberculosis, 13, 25
tufan, 27
typhoid fever, 12, 13, 109, 201, 205
typhus, 12, 13, 24, 191
typhus fever, 12
Urumiyeh, 14, 21, 49, 55, 83, 139, 140, 152, 164, 168, 169, 178, 193, 196, 198, 199, 200, 207, 214
vaba, 17, 19, 26, 241, 256
vaba-ye pa'izi, 18
varam-e qarniyeh, 28
varam-e zariyeh, 46
Vata, 75
Vayu, 75
venereal disease, 13, 14, 33, 224, 243
venesection, 150, 228
vermifuge, 167
vitiligo, 36
washers of the dead, 65, 194, 207, 208
wind, 40, 74, 75, 181
witchcraft, 78, 92, 98
wounds, 67, 81, 109, 144, 161, 163, 164, 174, 180, 189
Yazd, 14, 42, 84, 197, 198, 199, 200, 201, 202, 207
Yezidi, 138
yobusat-e rotubat-e zojajiyeh, 28
yodurudupatas, 184, 207
zaft-e rumi, 161
zakhm-band, 163
zalu, 145, 150, 152
zanjabil, 53
zar, 57
Zenjan, 26, 36, 110, 125, 163, 207, 239
Zodiac, 98